Complex Cases in Structural Heart Intervention

Ofir Koren • Raj Makkar • Vivek Patel
Danon Kaewkes • Hasan Jilaihawi
Jubin Joseph
Editors

Complex Cases in Structural Heart Intervention

Springer

Editors
Ofir Koren
Smidt Heart Institute
Cedars-Sinai Medical Center
Los Angeles, CA, USA

Raj Makkar
Smidt Heart Institute
Cedars-Sinai Medical Center
Los Angeles, CA, USA

Vivek Patel
Smidt Heart Institute
Cedars-Sinai Medical Center
Los Angeles, CA, USA

Danon Kaewkes
Faculty of Medicine
Khon Kaen University
Khon Kaen, Thailand

Hasan Jilaihawi
Heart Valve Center
New York University Langone Health
New York, NY, USA

Jubin Joseph
Smidt Heart Institute
Cedars-Sinai Medical Center
Los Angeles, CA, USA

ISBN 978-3-031-05964-3 ISBN 978-3-031-05965-0 (eBook)
https://doi.org/10.1007/978-3-031-05965-0

This Springer imprint is published by the registered company Springer Nature Switzerland AG
The registered company address is: Gewerbestrasse 11, 6330 Cham, Switzerland

To my beloved wife, Regina, and our kids, Ilay and Emma,

Thank you for turning our life into a beautiful and pleasant adventure and supporting me with every new idea that pops into my head.

–Ofir–

About the Editors

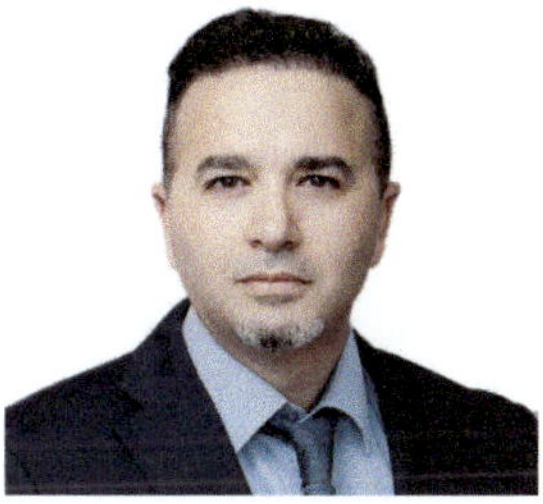

Koren Ofir, MD is a senior interventional cardiologist, researcher, and entrepreneur focusing on structural heart interventions. He has vast experience in coronary interventions, and, over the last few years, meticulously explored the field of structural heart intervention. Dr. Koren is a faculty lecturer at the Technion-Institute of Technology and a nominee for an associate clinical professor. He taught for many years and was repeatedly awarded as an outstanding lecturer by faculty, students, and colleagues. He conducted multiple national trials as a prime investigator and led as a subinvestigator for major international studies. Dr. Koren published numerous manuscripts and book chapters in leading peer-reviewed journals, presented them at major international conferences, and was awarded for his research achievements. Dr. Koren is the founder and CEO of D-flare, a company that aims to find a solution for heart failure patients.

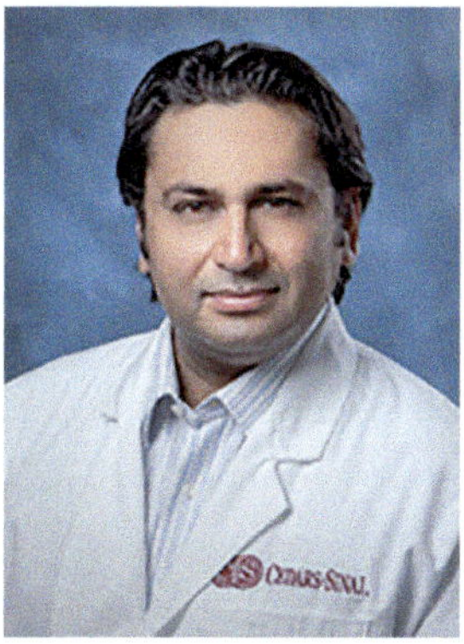

Raj Makkar, MD is a world-renowned leading expert in interventional cardiology and one of the most widely cited researchers on the management of valvular heart disease. He has performed the largest number of transcatheter valve implantation (TAVI) procedures worldwide and has led the field in the pursuit of the best patient outcomes. In 2020, he performed the most transcatheter mitral valve repair procedures with the MitraClip system in the United States. He has been the national principal investigator for numerous clinical trials in structural heart interventions. He has authored over 500 manuscripts, abstracts, and book chapters in peer-reviewed literature, including practice-changing contributions in *The New England Journal of Medicine* and *The Lancet*. Dr. Makkar is the director of the interventional cardiology division and the cardiology research program at Cedars-Sinai medical center and the vice president of the cardiovascular innovation center.

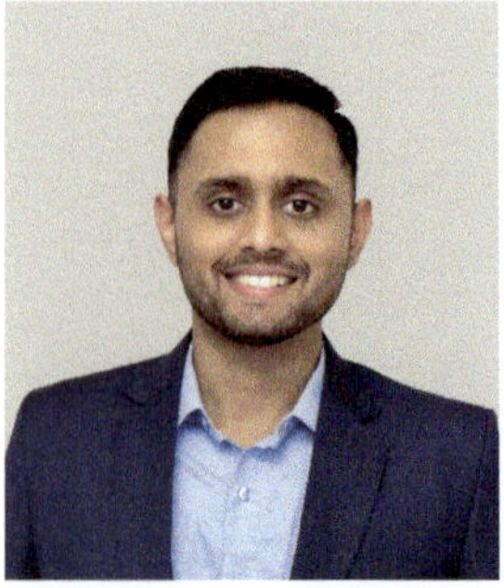

Vivek Patel, MS is a biomedical engineer who has a keen interest and expertise in transcatheter structural cardiovascular devices and imaging. Vivek has a strong level of knowledge, a diverse skill set, and solid research capabilities in structural heart disease intervention. Vivek Patel has contributed and reviewed multiple manuscripts for leading peer-reviewed journals. He has provided a key role in the national CT Imaging Core lab in numerous clinical transcatheter devices studies.

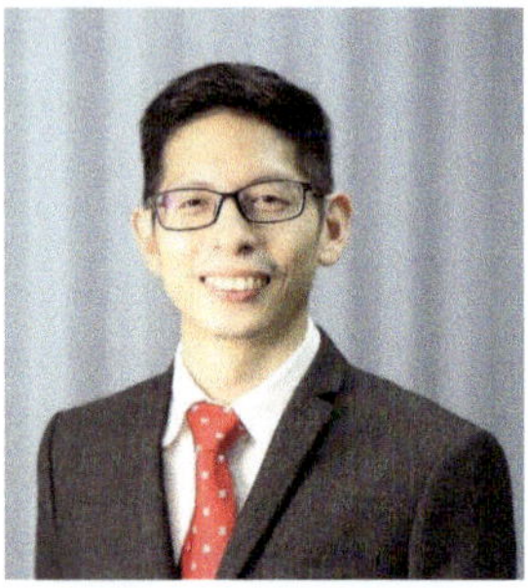

Danon Kaewkes, MD is a senior interventional cardiologist at the Department of Medicine of Khon Kaen in Thailand and a faculty member at Khon Kaen University. He has expertise in TAVR, edge-to-edge mitral repair procedure, and published multiple manuscripts in leading peer-reviewed journals. Dr. Kaewkes was a fellow in interventional cardiology at Cedars-Sinai Medical Center from 2019 to 2021.

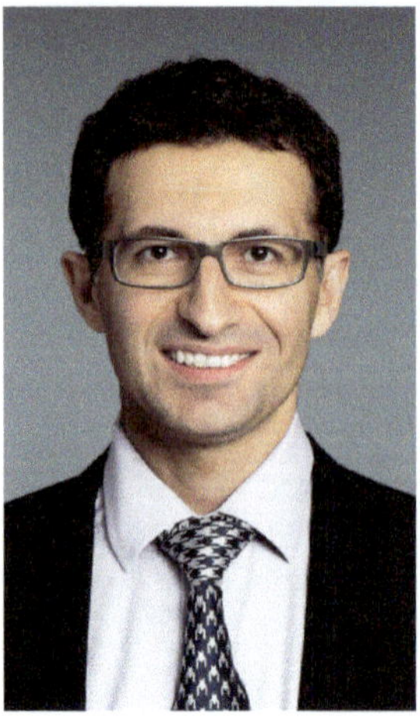

Hasan Jilaihawi, MD is a senior interventional cardiologist at Cedars-Sinai Medical Center. He was one of the first two cardiologists to perform TAVI in the UK and has been performing structural heart interventions for over 15 years. He is involved in all aspects of cardiology, with a particular interest in advanced imaging of structural heart disease, complex valvular and coronary intervention, and device and patient selection within the novel field of transcatheter valve therapies. His international reputation in the field has earned him the prestigious responsibility of running the CT Corelab for the pivotal US trial of the Portico device, the world's first fully repositionable and retrievable TAVR, as well as the CT Corelab for China's first TAVR trial. He is co-founder and Executive Director of China Structural

Week, the largest online educational meeting for structural heart intervention worldwide. He has authored more than 140 manuscripts in peer-reviewed journals, including *the New England Journal of Medicine*, *the Journal of the American College of Cardiology*, and *the European Heart Journal.*

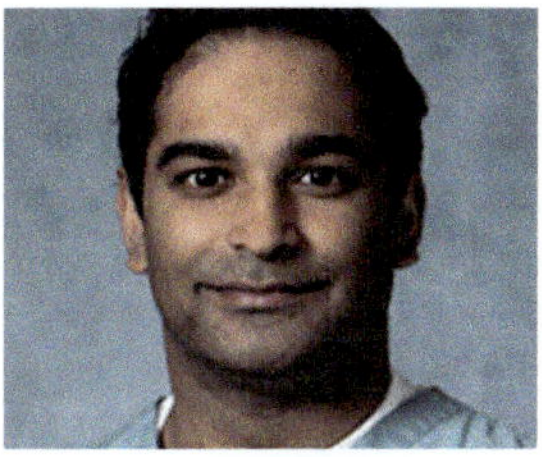

Jubin Joseph, MD is a senior interventional cardiologist with expertise in structural intervention. He completed undergraduate medical education at Cambridge and Oxford University before undertaking postgraduate clinical training in Oxford and London. Dr. Joseph has broad experience across the whole range of structural interventions. Since 2020, he has been working at Cedars-Sinai Medical Center with a particular focus on mitral and tricuspid intervention.

Our Team

The Interventional Cardiologists Team

Raj R. Makkar
Professor of Cardiology
Vice President of the Cardiovascular Innovation and Intervention
Executive Director of Cardiac Interventional Services
Co-Director of the Interventional Cardiology Research Program
Wen Cheng, MD
Professor of Cardiothoracic Surgery
Senior Cardiothoracic surgeon
Mamoo Nakamura, MD
Associate Professor of Medicine
Associate Director of the Cardiac Intervention Center
Tarun Chakravarty, MD
Associate Professor of Medicine
Senior Interventional Cardiologist
Hasan Jilaihawi
(Acting) Associate Professor of Medicine
Senior Interventional Cardiologist
Aakriti Gupta, MD
Interventional cardiologist

Our Nurse Practitioners

Jasminka Stegic, MSN, ACNP-BC, ANP-BC
Harutyunyan Izabela, MSN, AG-ACNP-BC
Friedman Michelle, ACNP-BC
Khaled Alsabaawi, MB BCh, CRC
Mitch Gheorghiu, MD, Director
Mondejar Pamela Grace S, MSN, FNP-C
Ok Linda, MSN, FNP-BC
Research Coordinators
Robinson Anna, MSN, FNP-BC
Salseth Tracy, MSN, CCRN, ACNP-BC

Our Research Coordinators

Mitch Gheorghiu, MD, Director
Khaled Alsabaawi, MB BCh, CRC
Artur Arakelyan, MD, CRA
Daniel Zumerkorn Hassan, MD, CRA
Dhairya Patel, BDS, MPH, CRA
Dzenana Slipac, BA, CRC
Elan Parada, CRA
Gabriella Mainea, MBA, CRA
Jason Yashar, BS, CRC
Kelly Salazar, BS, CRC
Keyur Golwala, MD, MPH, CRA
Navjot Sekhon, MD, CRC
Neecki Zand, BA, CRA
Quentin Wise, BA, CRA
Ripandeep S. Tiwana, MD, CRC
Rohan Sharma, BA, CRA

Our Cath Lab Staff

David Hildebrandt, BSN, MBA, Director
Aldrin Tolentino, BSN, Manager
Andrea Alarcon, Registered Nurse
Abdul Ahmed, Cardiovascular Tech
Alyssa Bueno, Radiologic Technologist
Billy Smith, Registered Nurse
Cat Tsai, Registered Nurse
Christina Brandt, Radiologic Technologist
Christopher Szafnicki, Registered Nurse
Cynthia Avalos, Cardiovascular Tech
Cynthia Dirkes, Registered Nurse
Debra Quarnberg, Registered Nurse
Genevieve Harlocker, Registered Nurse
Hannah McKay, Registered Nurse
Jansen Abarabar, Cardiovascular Tech, Lead
Jennifer Brown, Registered Nurse
Jennifer Timberlake, Registered Nurse
Jeremiah Sias, Registered Nurse
Jeremy Alexander, Registered Nurse
Jinho Kim, Registered Nurse
JoAnn Gironimi, Registered Nurse
Joel Bastillo, Radiologic Technologist
Keshal Patel, Registered Nurse
Kylene Baker, Radiologic Technologist
Lizza Migallos, Registered Nurse
Phillip Nevin, Registered Nurse

Our Past Fellows

Aaron Yung, MD
Abhijeet Dhoble, MD
Amin Manuchehry, MD
Atish Mathur, MD
Chirag Chauhan, MD
Danon Kaewkes, MD
David Lange, MD
Devanabanda Arvind Reddy, MD
Fangzhou Liu, MD
Grant Kim, MD
Gupta Aakriti, MD
Hasan Jilaihawi, MD
Hashim Gazi, MD
Heidi Reich, MD
Hirotsugu Mihara, MD
Hiroyuki Kawamori, MD

Huai Luo, MD
Hursh Naik, MD
Isic Kim, MD
James Yhip, MD
Jeff Tyler, MD
Joe Aragon, MD
Jorge Castellanos, MD
Jubin Joseph, MD
Justin Cox, MD
Kazuaki Okuyama, MD
Keita Koseki, MD
Larry Chan, MD
Luis Bowen, MD
Luke Oakley, MD
Luxhoj Andrew, MD
Mamoo Nakamura, MD
Manminder Bhullar, MD
Manminder Singh Bhullar, MD
Manu Uberoi, MD
Masaki Miyasaka, MD
Mike Shenoda, MD
Mohammad Kashif, MD
Nobuyuki Takahashi, MD
Ofir Koren, MD
Pranav Kansara, MD
Rahul Sharma, MD
Richard Cheng, MD
Sabah Skaf, MD
Sam Dawkins, MD
Sharon Shalom Natanzon, MD
Sunghan Yoon, MD
Takahiro Nomura, MD
Tarun Chakravarty, MD
Tomoki Ochai, MD
Vinny Ram, MD
Yigal Abramowitz, MD
Yoshio Kazano, MD
Yousif Ahmad, MD

Introduction

Structural heart interventions have grown exponentially over the past two decades as patients and physicians seek minimally invasive methods to treat a variety of cardiac pathologies. Due to an aging population and a decline in rheumatic heart disease, degenerative aortic stenosis and mitral regurgitation have emerged as the predominant valvular pathologies of the new era.

The transcatheter transfemoral technique for replacing stenotic and calcified aortic valves, and the transeptal edge-to-edge repair technique for treating regurgitant mitral valves have both demonstrated excellent procedural safety, clinical efficacy, and have been established as the gold standard therapies in certain patients.

These advances have helped to define the basic concepts for valvular heart interventions, and iterative improvements are constantly being pursued to improve patient outcomes and reduce procedural complications.

Our book provides a unique insight into the world of structural heart diseases using highly illustrated and detailed cases. We have included different clinical scenarios, discussed technical dilemmas, and shared our collective experiences as we continue to learn in this ever-evolving field.

We wish that these experiences may inform readers as they charter uncertain territory and ultimately benefit the patients we help.

Hope you enjoy the book and we wish you a pleasant reading.

Raj Makkar
Ofir Koren

Contents

Part II Mitral Valve

Part III Miscellaneous

Editors and Contributors

Editors

Ofir Koren, MD Smidt Heart Institute, Cedars-Sinai Medical Center, Los Angeles, CA, USA

Faculty of Medicine, Technion, Israel Institute of Technology, Haifa, Israel

Raj R. Makkar, MD Smidt Heart Institute, Cedars-Sinai Medical Center, Los Angeles, CA, USA

Vivek Patel, MS Smidt Heart Institute, Cedars-Sinai Medical Center, Los Angeles, CA, USA

Danon Kaewkes, MD Department of Medicine, Faculty of Medicine, Khon Kaen University, Khon Kaen, Thailand

Jubin Joseph, MD Smidt Heart Institute, Cedars-Sinai Medical Center, Los Angeles, CA, USA

Hasan Jilaihawi, MD Heart Valve Center, NYU Langone Health, New York, NY, USA

Contributors

Daniel Benhamou, BA Technion, Israel Institute of Technology, Haifa, Israel

Isabel Ben Guy Lithuania University of Health Sciences (LSMU), Kaunas, Lithuania

Daniel Eugene Cheng, MD Villanova School of Business, Villanova, PA, USA

Nathan Drillings, BS Psychobiology, University of California (UCLA), Los Angeles, CA, USA

Asaf Israeli, BSc Technion, Israel Institute of Technology, Haifa, Israel

Elli Izrailov, MD Bendigo Health, Bendigo, VIC, Australia

Siamak Kohan, MD Kaiser Permanente Los Angeles Medical Center, Los Angeles, CA, USA

Addee Lerner, BS David Geffen School of Medicine, University of California, Los Angeles, Los Angeles, CA, USA

Yonatan Moshkovits, MD, MPH Leviev Heart Center, Sheba Medical Center, Ramat-Gan, Israel

Edmund Naami, BS University of Illinois College of Medicine, Chicago, IL, USA

Robert Naami, MD University Hospitals Cleveland Medical Center, Cleveland, OH, USA

Bar Naiberg Santa Monica High School, CA, USA

Dhairya Patel Smidt Heart Institute, Cedars-Sinai Medical Center, Los Angeles, CA, USA

Alisa Leeds Rosenberg, BA, BS Biology Faculty, Pepperdine University, Malibu, CA, USA

Troy Sanders, BA David Geffen School of Medicine, University of California, Los Angeles, CA, USA

Rafael Skorka Smidt Heart Institute, Cedars-Sinai Medical Center, Los Angeles, CA, USA

Quentin Wise Interventional Cardiology, Cedars-Sinai Medical Center, Los Angeles, CA, USA

Daniel Zumerkorn Hassan Interventional Cardiology, Cedars-Sinai Medical Center, Los Angeles, CA, USA

Reviewers

Yigal Abramowitz, MD Cardiology Department, Soroka University Medical Center, Beer Sheva, Israel

Ahmed Al Badri, MD Cedars Sinai Medical Center, Los Angeles, CA, USA

Wen Cheng, MD Cedars Sinai Medical Center, Los Angeles, CA, USA

Arvind Reddy Devanabanda, MD Cedars Sinai Medical Center, Los Angeles, CA, USA

Mohamed Hassanein, MD Cedars Sinai Medical Center, Los Angeles, CA, USA

David Lange, MD, FACC, FSCAI Kaiser Santa Clara Medical Center, Santa Clara, CA, USA

Andrew Luxhoj, MD Cedars Sinai Medical Center, Los Angeles, CA, USA

Mamoo Nakamura, MD, FACC, FSCAI Cedars Sinai Medical Center, Los Angeles, California, USA

Sharon Shalom Natanzon, MD Cedars Sinai Medical Center, Los Angeles, CA, USA

Michael M. Shenoda, MD, FACC, FSCAI Interventional Cardiology and Structural Heart Disease, Santa Barbara Cottage Hospital, Santa Barbara, CA, USA

Hezzy Shmueli, MD Cardiology Department, Soroka University Medical Center, Beer Sheva, Israel

Siddharth Singh, MD, FASE Cedars Sinai Medical Center, Los Angeles, CA, USA

Sabah Skaf, MD, FASE Cedars Sinai Medical Center, Los Angeles, CA, USA

Abhimanyu Manu Uberoi, MD, MS, FACC, FSCAI Structural and Interventional Cardiology, Kaiser Northwest/Greater Portland Metro Region, Portland, OR, USA

Muhammad Zubair, MD Cedars Sinai Medical Center, Los Angeles, CA, USA

Part I
Aortic Valve

TAVR Procedure in a Patient with a Significant Large Aortic Valve Annulus

Danon Kaewkes, Robert Naami, and Andrew Luxhoj

1 Clinical Presentation

A 77-year-old male presented for a moderate aortic stenosis (AS) follow-up. The patient's medical history was notable for hypertension, hyperlipidemia, atrial fibrillation on a direct oral anticoagulant, and moderate AS regularly followed for 1.5 years. Three months prior to the follow-up, he underwent left-knee replacement surgery due to severe osteoarthritis at an outside hospital, which was complicated by cardiac arrest requiring cardiopulmonary resuscitation for 15 minutes and prolonged intubation for 15 days. He was told he did not have a myocardial infarction or stroke. Since discharge, he has continued to experience dyspnea with minimal exertion (5–10 steps).

2 Images and Supported Data

Transthoracic echocardiography (TTE) revealed normal left ventricular (LV) size and preserved LV systolic function with an LV ejection fraction of 55%. The aortic valve was trileaflet with moderate calcification. There was moderate to severe AS and mild aortic regurgitation. The aortic valve area (AVA) by the continuity equation was 0.81 cm^2, and the peak and mean gradient across the aortic valve were 45

D. Kaewkes (✉)
Department of Medicine, Faculty of Medicine, Khon Kaen University, Khon Kaen, Thailand

R. Naami
University Hospitals Cleveland Medical Center, Cleveland, OH, USA

A. Luxhoj
Cedars Sinai Medical Center, Los Angeles, CA, USA

O. Koren et al. (eds.), *Complex Cases in Structural Heart Intervention*,
https://doi.org/10.1007/978-3-031-05965-0_1

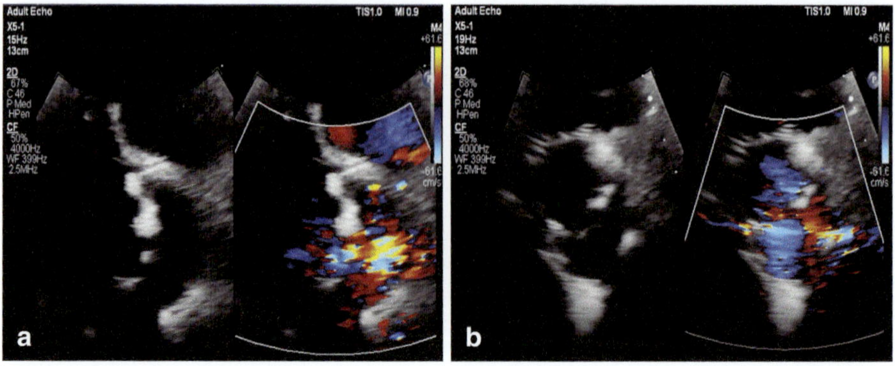

Fig. 1 Preprocedural transthoracic echocardiography. (**a**) Accelerated flow across the aortic valve consistent with severe AS in the parasternal long-axis, (**b**) short-axis view of aortic valve

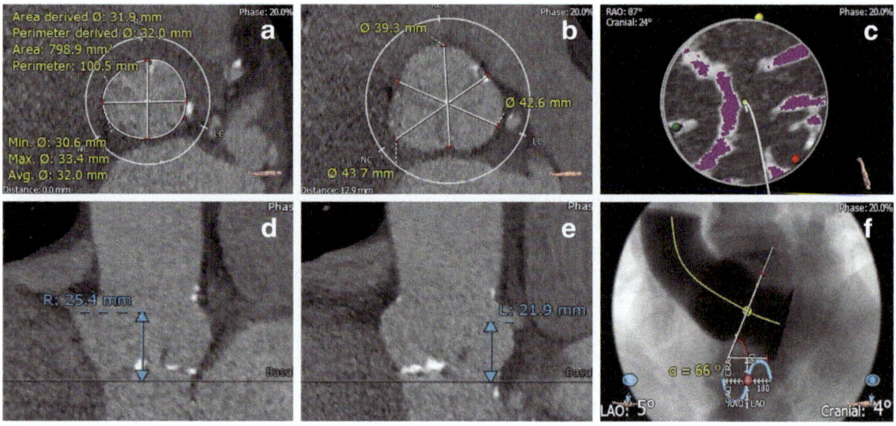

Fig. 2 Cardiac CT analysis. (**a**) Aortic annulus area and diameters; (**b**) sinus of Valsalva diameters; (**c**) aortic valve calcium; (**d**) right coronary height; (**e**) left coronary height; (**f**) aorto-ventricular angle

and 25 mmHg, respectively. Estimated pulmonary systolic pressure was 21 mmHg (Fig. 1). Cardiac computed tomography (CT) confirmed severe AS (AVA = 0.99 cm^2 by direct 3D planimetry). It showed a large aortic annulus with an area of 799 mm^2, a perimeter of 100 mm, and a mean diameter of 32 mm. The mean sinus of Valsalva, sinotubular junction, and LV outflow tract diameters were 42, 35, and 31 mm, respectively. The right and left coronary ostia were located 25 and 22 mm above the aortic annular plane, respectively. The calcium volume, measured over the annulus area using an 850 Hounsfield unit cut-off, indicated a moderate amount (187 mm^3) of calcium. A high aorto-ventricular angulation (66°) was also noted (Fig. 2). Iliofemoral arteries were adequate for transfemoral transcatheter aortic valve replacement (TAVR).

3 Preprocedural Consideration: Pitfalls, Dilemmas, and Challenges

"According to the heart team's assessment, the patient was 77 years old with moderate surgical risk as well as an oversized aortic annulus with respect to the available commercial transcatheter heart valves (THV). Based on our previous experiences, the balloon-expandable THV could be oversized to 32 mm. However, the patient strongly preferred TAVR to surgical aortic valve replacement. With this in mind, their aortic valve calcium seemed adequate for the THV anchoring, so we planned to perform TF TAVR with 29 mm Edward Sapien 3.

4 Technique

We successfully deployed the 29 mm Edward Sapien 3 using a standard TF TAVR technique along with 5 mL extra volume in the indeflator (Fig. 3). Postprocedural TEE revealed no central aortic regurgitation and no paravalvular leakage.

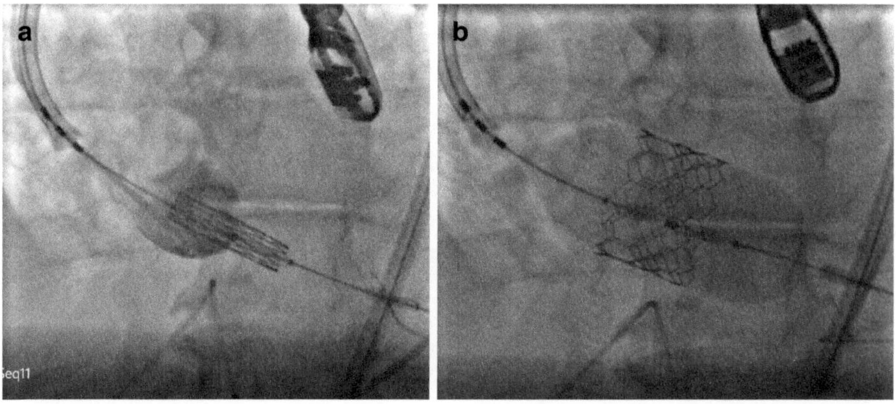

Fig. 3 Fluoroscopic images of TAVR procedure. (**a**) 29 mm Sapien-3 positioned at the aortic valve; (**b**) deployment of 29 mm Sapien-3 with 5 mL extra volume

5 Outcome and Follow-Up

Pre-discharge TTE presented normal LV systolic function. A good functioning bioprosthetic stented valve was detected in the aortic position. No paravalvular leakage was found (Fig. 4). The patient's symptoms improved and was discharged the next day.

6 Discussion

Currently, TAVR is an effective and less invasive treatment for patients with severe AS across all surgical risk categories [1]. Nonetheless, there is a paucity of choices for large aortic annuli. Using commercially available THVs beyond their limits for extra-large annuli (area ≥ 683 mm²; perimeter ≥ 94.2 mm) is considered off-label and may increase risks of THV embolization and PVL after implantation [2]. Several studies reported TAVR results in patients with extra-large annuli and found that TAVR using 29 mm Sapien 3 and 34 mm Evolut was safe and feasible. The device success rate was 94%, with acceptable rates of post-procedure paravalvular leakage and 30-day and 1-year mortality [2–5]. One study reported higher prevalences of significant paravalvular leakage, second valve implantation, and valve embolization in patients implanted with Evolut than those implanted with Sapien 3 [2]. However, using Evolut may prevent the valve from flipping upside down and obstructing blood flow. In addition, the strategy of using Sapien 3 instead of Evolut may be beneficial in cases with extensive annuli yet minimal leaflet calcification. In this patient, the valve calcification facilitated an anchoring of Sapien 3 and resulted in successful implantation without immediate complications. Our case demonstrated the feasibility of TAVR using a balloon-expandable valve in a patient with an extra-large aortic annulus. Preprocedural planning with cardiac CT is crucial for appropriately selecting patients, devices, and techniques.

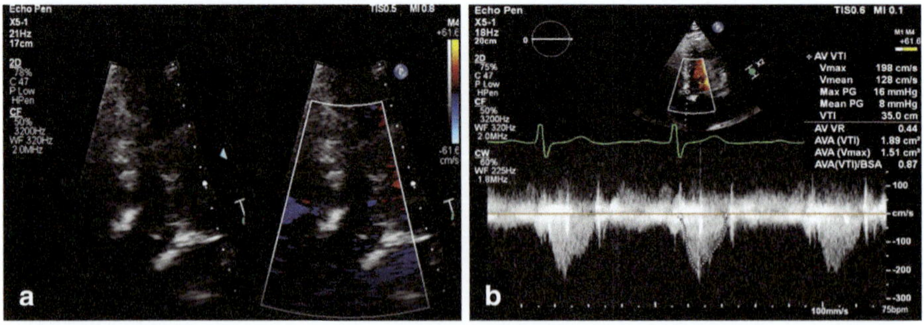

Fig. 4 Pre-discharge TTE. (**a**) A bioprosthetic stent valve can be seen in the aortic position without paravalvular leakage; (**b**) no significant gradient across the aortic valve

Key Points

- TAVR in patients with extra-large aortic annuli is feasible.
- In the real world, 29 mm Sapien 3 and 34 mm Evolut R are the commercially available THVs used off-label to treat patients with extra-large annuli.
- Preprocedural cardiac CT is crucial for selecting appropriate patients, devices, and techniques in patients with extra-large annuli.

References

1. Mack MJ, Leon MB, Thourani VH, Makkar R, Kodali SK, Russo M, Kapadia SR, Malaisrie SC, Cohen DJ, Pibarot P, Leipsic J, Hahn RT, Blanke P, Williams MR, McCabe JM, Brown DL, Babaliaros V, Goldman S, Szeto WY, Genereux P, Pershad A, Pocock SJ, Alu MC, Webb JG, Smith CR, Investigators P. Transcatheter aortic-valve replacement with a balloon-expandable valve in low-risk patients. N Engl J Med. 2019;380:1695–705.
2. Armijo G, Tang GHL, Kooistra N, Ferreira-Neto AN, Toggweiler S, Amat-Santos IJ, Keller LS, Urena M, Ahmad H, Tafur Soto J, Munoz-Garcia E, Regueiro A, Leenders GE, Tirado-Conte G, Sengupta A, McInerney A, Couture T, Cuevas Herreros O, Rodriguez-Gabella T, Kini A, Ahmed M, Zaid S, Gonzalo N, Nunez-Gil IJ, Munoz-Garcia AJ, Jimenez-Quevedo P, Fernandez-Ortiz A, Himbert D, Nietlispach F, Stella P, Dangas GD, Escaned J, Macaya C, Rodes-Cabau J, Nombela-Franco L. Third-generation balloon and self-expandable valves for aortic stenosis in large and extra-large aortic annuli from the TAVR-LARGE registry. Circ Cardiovasc Interv. 2020;13:e009047.
3. Miyasaka M, Yoon SH, Sharma RP, Maeno Y, Jaideep S, Taguri M, Kato S, Kawamori H, Nomura T, Ochiai T, Nemanpour S, Chakravarty T, Nakamura M, Wen C, Makkar R. Clinical outcomes of transcatheter aortic valve implantation in patients with extremely large annulus and SAPIEN 3 dimensions based on post-procedural computed tomography. Circ J. 2019;83:672–80.
4. Sengupta A, Zaid S, Kamioka N, Terre J, Miyasaka M, Hirji SA, Hensey M, Geloo N, Petrossian G, Robinson N, Sarin E, Ryan L, Yoon SH, Tan CW, Khalique OK, Kodali SK, Kaneko T, Shah PB, Wong SC, Salemi A, Sharma K, Kozina JA, Szerlip MA, Don CW, Gafoor S, Zhang M, Newhart Z, Kapadia SR, Mick SL, Krishnaswamy A, Kini A, Ahmad H, Lansman SL, Mack MJ, Webb JG, Babaliaros V, Thourani VH, Makkar RR, Leon MB, George I, Tang GHL. Mid-term outcomes of transcatheter aortic valve replacement in extremely large annuli with Edwards SAPIEN 3 valve. JACC Cardiovasc Interv. 2020;13:210–6.
5. Xiong TY, Liao YB, Li YJ, Chen F, Ou Y, Wang X, Wang ZJ, Li X, Zhao ZG, Meng W, Feng Y, Chen M. Treating patients with excessively large annuli with self-expanding transcatheter aortic valves: insights into supra-annular structures that anchor the prosthesis. Herz. 2020;46:166–72. https://doi.org/10.1007/s00059-020-04973-5.

TAVR in Patients with Bicuspid Aortic Valve

Ofir Koren, Edmund Naami, and Vivek Patel

1 Clinical Presentation

The patient is a 69-year-old male with a past medical history of aortic stenosis, chronic diastolic heart failure (NYHA Class III), paroxysmal atrial fibrillation (not anticoagulated), hypertension, hyperlipidemia, prostate cancer, and childhood tuberculosis. The patient was referred for an evaluation of aortic stenosis and to discuss treatment options. Recent left heart catheterization showed no significant obstructive artery disease. Given worsening shortness of breath, he was considered for aortic valve intervention.

1.1 Images and Supported Data

Pre-procedural TTE revealed an aortic valve area of 0.5 cm^2, mean gradient of 53 mmHg, a peak gradient of 80 mmHg, and preserved ejection fraction (Video 1, Fig. 3c). Cardiac reconstructed CT indicated an annular mean internal diameter of

Supplementary Information The online version contains supplementary material available at [https://doi.org/10.1007/978-3-031-05965-0_2].

O. Koren (✉)
Smidt Heart Institute, Cedars-Sinai Medical Center, Los Angeles, CA, USA

Faculty of Medicine, Technion, Israel Institute of Technology, Haifa, Israel
e-mail: Ofir.Koren@cshs.org

E. Naami
University of Illinois College of Medicine, Chicago, IL, USA

V. Patel
Smidt Heart Institute, Cedars-Sinai Medical Center, Los Angeles, CA, USA

O. Koren et al. (eds.), *Complex Cases in Structural Heart Intervention*,
https://doi.org/10.1007/978-3-031-05965-0_2

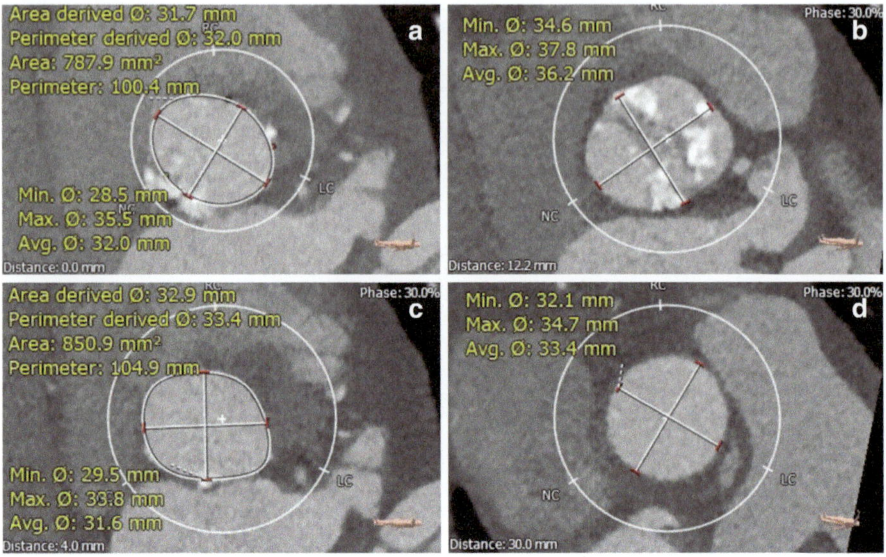

Fig. 1 Reconstructed CT images. (**a**) Bicuspid AV area of 787 mm^2 and a 100.4 mm perimeter. (**b**) The left and right coronary cusps are fused by calcified raphe. (**c**) The LVOT area is 850 mm^2. (**d**) Sinotubular junction area is 850 mm^2

32.0 mm, area of 787.9 mm^2, and perimeter of 100.4 mm. The following mean diameters were measured: 36.2 mm at the sinus of Valsalva, 31.6 mm at the left ventricular outflow tract, and 33.4 mm at the sinotubular junction dimension. The left ventricular outflow tract was measured with an area and perimeter of 850.9 mm^2 and 104.9 mm, respectively (Video 2, Fig. 1). The maximal diameter of the ascending aorta was measured to be 45.0 mm. The right and left coronary ostia originated 22.0 and 21.1 mm above the annular plane respectively. The aortic valve demonstrated severe calcification and measured 1961.8 Housefield units (Fig. 2).

1.2 Pre-Procedural Consideration

The patient was evaluated by CT surgery and deemed to be at low surgical risk; however, the patient adamantly refused cardiothoracic surgery. Thus, the patient was considered for transfemoral TAVR using FDA-approved Edwards Sapien S3 bioprosthesis. Transfemoral access was deemed feasible (Fig. 2f).

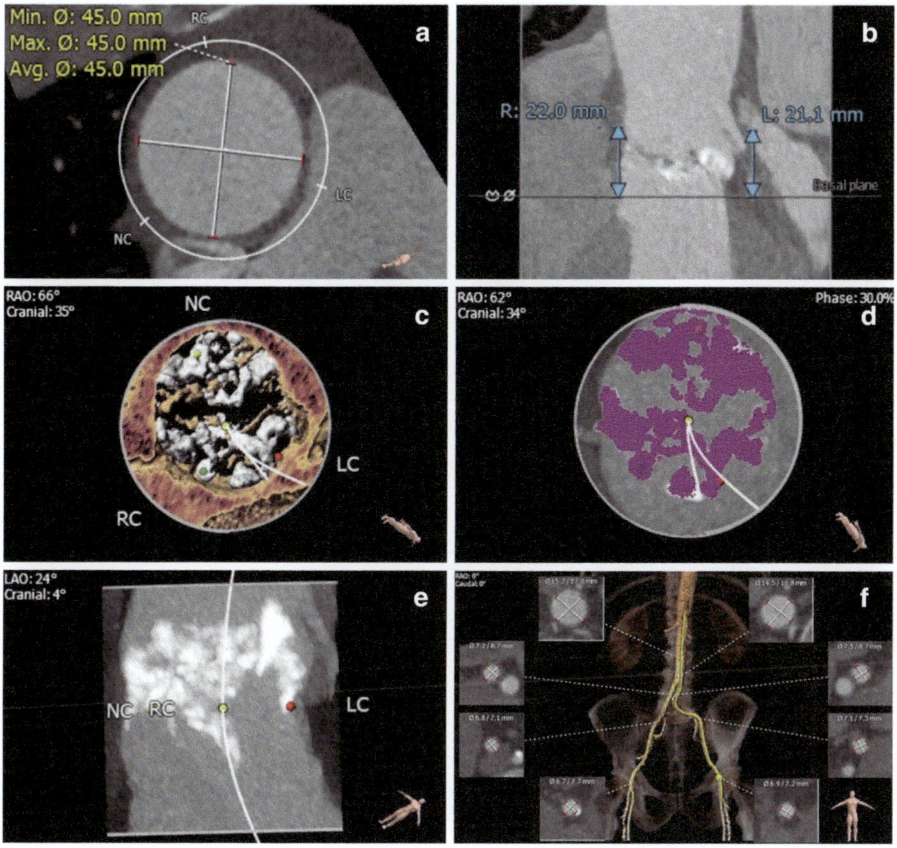

Fig. 2 Reconstructed CT images. (**a**) Maximal diameter of the ascending aorta, (**b**) the coronary artery height, (**c**) calcium distribution of the aortic valve, (**d**, **e**) the extent of valve calcification, (**f**) the dimension of the iliofemoral arteries

2 Outcome and Follow-Up

After initiating general anesthesia, a transesophageal echocardiographic probe was advanced into the mid-esophagus in order to obtain and record baseline images including aortic annulus measurements and aortic valve gradients (Fig. 3). Aortic annulus measurement was consistent with the previous CT angiographic study.

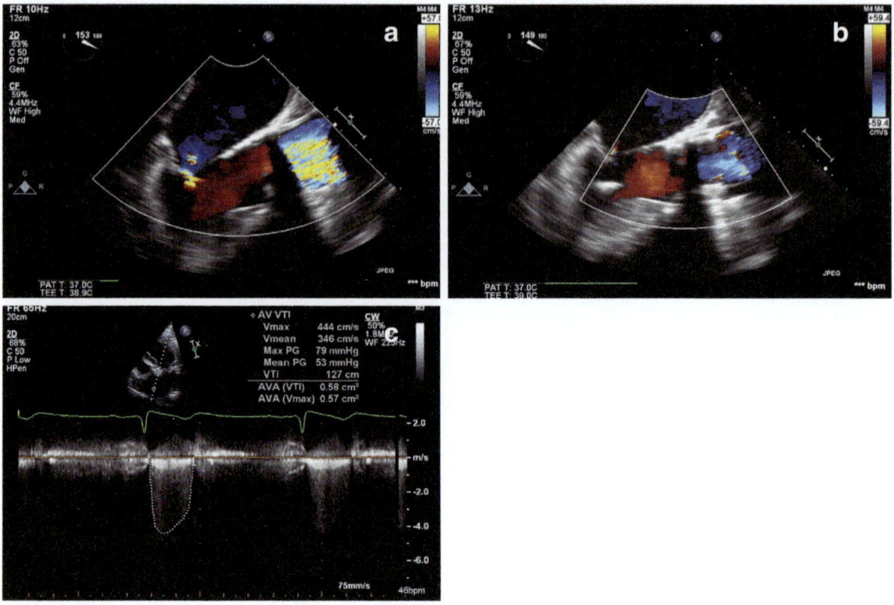

Fig. 3 TEE views before the TAVR procedure. (**a**, **b**) Aortic valve anatomy and color Doppler flow across aortic valve, (**c**) the pressure gradient over the AV

After obtaining femoral access, a 23 mm × 4.0 cm Z-Med II balloon was advanced across the stenotic aortic valve. With rapid pacing at 180 beats per minute, the balloon was inflated twice (Video 3, Fig. 4a, b). Next, a 29-mm Edwards Sapien S3 valve was positioned across the stenotic aortic valve, and was deployed using the standard technique (−5 mL in the inflation device) (Video 4, Fig. 4c). A post-procedure TEE revealed reduced aortic stenosis, no central aortic regurgitation, and no paravalvular regurgitation (Video 5).

TTE 30 days following the procedure measured a mean aortic valve gradient of 14 mmHg (Fig. 5). A cardiac reconstructed CT at 1-year follow-up demonstrated a well seated transcatheter heart valve (THV) within a calcified aortic annulus. The THV inner mean diameter and annulus area were 23.5 mm and 574.2 mm^2, respectively. The ascending aortic aneurysm showed no change in dimensions (Video 6, Fig. 6).

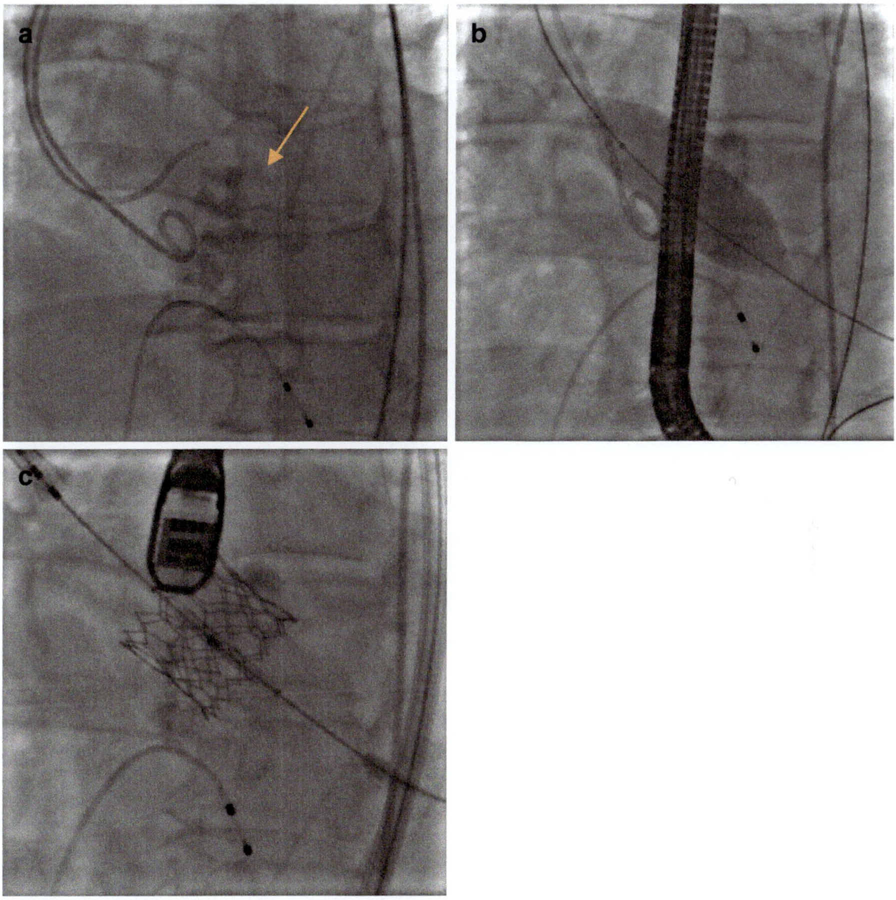

Fig. 4 Fluoroscopy views of the TAVR procedure. (**a**) The extent of calcification (yellow arrow), (**b**) pre-procedural AV dilatation, (**c**) a Sapien-3 THV seated in an aortic valve position

3 Discussion

Until recently, transcatheter aortic valve replacement in patients with bicuspid aortic valve stenosis had been the subject of controversy. The challenge of TAVR in bicuspid valves stems from the elliptical valve orifice that impedes device placement and asymmetric calcifications that serve as a potential embolic source during device deployment. Calcification is typically observed in the raphe and left cusp. Elevated left coronary cusp calcification has been associated with an increased risk for permanent pacemaker implantation following TAVR [1].

Previous studies have suggested that the first-generation TAVR valves had worse outcomes in patients with bicuspid aortic valves. However, newer-generation valves might have outcomes similar to those seen in patients with tricuspid valves [2].

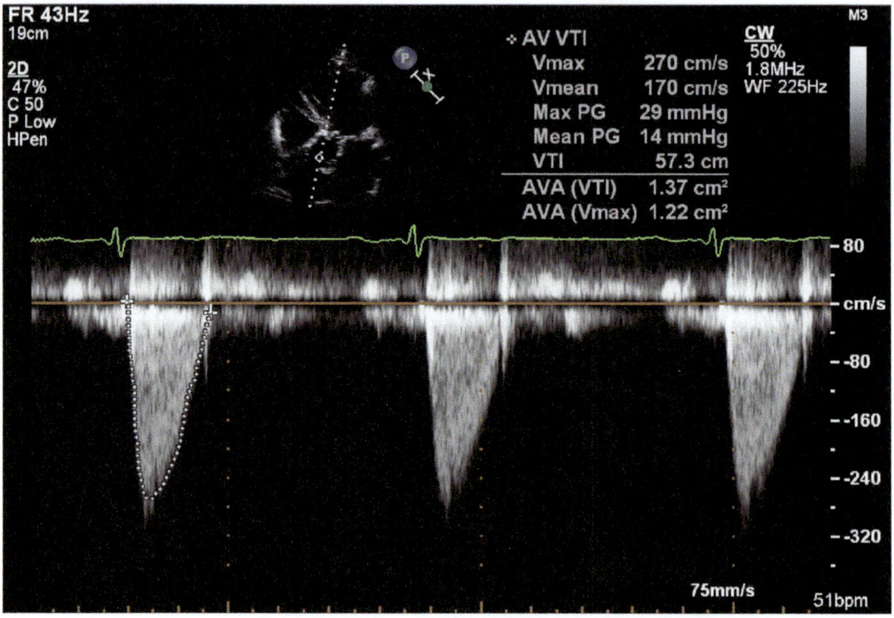

Fig. 5 TTE performed 30-day following the TAVR procedure shows a significant reduction in the mean velocity and pressure across the AV

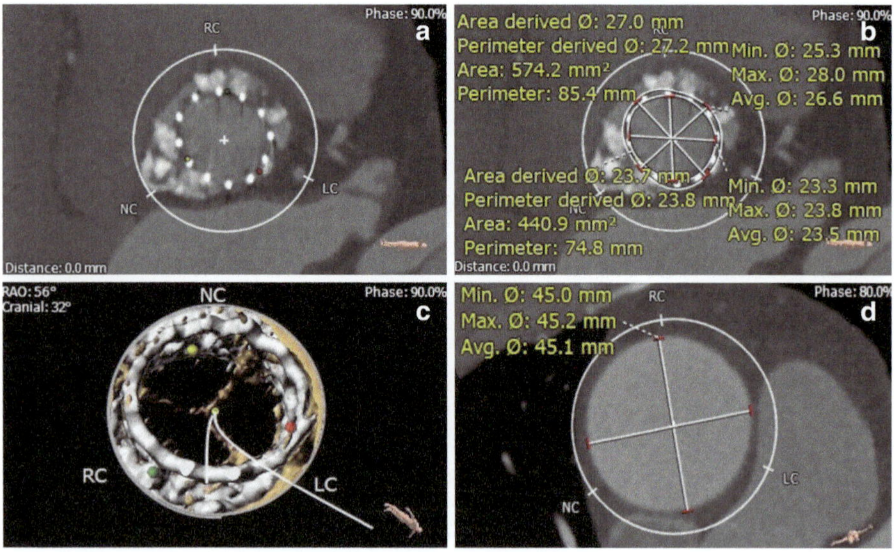

Fig. 6 Cardiac reconstructed CT at 1-year follow-up. (**a**, **c**) A well seated transcatheter heart valve (THV) within a calcified aortic annulus. (**b**) The THV inner mean diameter and annulus area was measured at 23.5 mm and 574.2 mm², respectively, (**d**) the ascending aortic aneurysm showed no change in dimensions

Preliminary studies have shown no significant difference in 30-day or 1-year mortality in patients who had undergone TAVR for bicuspid vs. tricuspid aortic stenosis, despite an increased 30-day risk for stroke in bicuspid patients [3]. Increased risk of stroke is attributed to emboli originating from the calcified bicuspid aortic valve.

An additional consideration in patients with bicuspid aortic valves undergoing TAVR is the potential for dilation of the ascending aortic root, leading to aortic aneurysm and dissection [4–6], which have been long- lasting arguments against TAVR [4–6]. In a subpopulation of bicuspid patients with a normal-sized ascending aorta, late adverse aortic events were considerably lower risk after isolated AVR, suggesting possible candidacy for TAVR [7]. It has been used to argue against TAVR in this subpopulation of patients. Current indications for surgical repair include (1) asymptomatic aneurysm >5 cm in diameter, (2) symptomatic aneurysm irrespective of size, (3) ascending aortic aneurysm >4.5 cm in patients undergoing aortic valve surgery, (4) a growth rate of >0.5 cm/year when the ascending aorta is <5.0 cm in diameter.

Nevertheless, the feasibility of TAVR in this subset of patients should be revisited. TAVR use has increased due to technological advances in valves while a clinical paradigm shift favoring less-invasive procedures has developed. In one study of patients with severe bicuspid aortic stenosis undergoing TAVR, there were minimal changes to the dimensions of their ascending aorta at follow-up, suggesting that progression of aortopathy in bicuspid aortic valve patients post-TAVR may not be clinically significant [8]. Importantly, this study excluded patients with an ascending aorta larger than 50 mm. There have also been cases of successful TAVR in severe bicuspid aortic stenosis with ascending aortic aneurysms [9]. Some argue that TAVR is a bridge to surgical valve replacement in patients with high surgical risk. Ultimately, larger studies with longer follow-up durations are needed to better understand the progression of ascending aortopathy in patients with bicuspid valves undergoing TAVR.

Key Points

- TAVR in bicuspid aortic stenosis patients (BAV) poses a significant challenge due to multiple anatomical complexities.
- Recent studies involving newer generation THV devices show a similar success rate and outcome as tricuspid AS patients.
- Meticulous pre-procedural planning using MDCT is essential to evaluate the anatomical changes in BAV patients and decide on the best therapeutic option.

References

1. Fujita B, Kütting M, Seiffert M, Scholtz S, Egron S, Prashovikj E, et al. Calcium distribution patterns of the aortic valve as a risk factor for the need of permanent pacemaker implantation after transcatheter aortic valve implantation. Eur Heart J Cardiovasc Imaging. 2016;17(12):1385–93. https://academic.oup.com/ehjcimaging/article/17/12/1385/2680067.

2. Yoon S-H, Bleiziffer S, De Backer O, Delgado V, Arai T, Ziegelmueller J, et al. Outcomes in transcatheter aortic valve replacement for bicuspid versus tricuspid aortic valve stenosis. J Am Coll Cardiol. 2017;69(21):2579–89. https://www.sciencedirect.com/science/article/pii/S0735109717360412.
3. Makkar RR, Yoon S-H, Leon MB, Chakravarty T, Rinaldi M, Shah PB, et al. Association between transcatheter aortic valve replacement for bicuspid vs tricuspid aortic stenosis and mortality or stroke. JAMA. 2019;321(22):2193–202. https://jamanetwork.com/journals/jama/fullarticle/2735503.
4. Fernandes S, Khairy P, Graham DA, Colan SD, Galvin TC, Sanders SP, et al. Bicuspid aortic valve and associated aortic dilation in the young. Heart. 2012;98(13):1014–9. https://heart.bmj.com/content/98/13/1014.
5. Fedak PWM, Verma S, David TE, Leask RL, Weisel RD, Butany J. Clinical and pathophysiological implications of a bicuspid aortic valve. Circulation. 2002;106(8):900–4. https://doi.org/10.1161/01.cir.0000027905.26586.e8.
6. Roberts CS, Roberts WC. Dissection of the aorta associated with congenital malformation of the aortic valve. J Am Coll Cardiol. 1991;17(3):712–6. https://www.sciencedirect.com/science/article/pii/S0735109710801883.
7. Disha K, Rouman M, Secknus M-A, Kuntze T, Girdauskas E. Are normal-sized ascending aortas at risk of late aortic events after aortic valve replacement for bicuspid aortic valve disease? Interact Cardiovasc Thorac Surg. 2016;22(4):465–71. https://academic.oup.com/icvts/article/22/4/465/2363426.
8. Jung J-H, Kim H-K, Park J-B, Lee S-P, Koo B-K, Kim Y-J, et al. Progression of ascending aortopathy may not occur after transcatheter aortic valve replacement in severe bicuspid aortic stenosis. Korean J Intern Med. 2021;36(2):332–41. https://doi.org/10.3904/kjim.2019.089.
9. Maeda K, Kuratani T, Shimamura K, Yamada Y, Toda K, Sawa Y. Transcatheter aortic valve replacement as a bridge to surgical aortic valve replacement in a younger patient with extremely high surgical risk. J Card Surg. 2021;36(1):386–9. https://doi.org/10.1111/jocs.15138.

Acute Aortic Dissection Due to Access Site Tortuosity

Ofir Koren, Alisa Leeds Rosenberg, and Abhimanyu Manu Uberoi

1 Clinical Presentation

The patient is an 89-year-old male with a history of hypertension, hyperlipidemia, mitral regurgitation, renal insufficiency, intermittent heart block status-post pacemaker placement, and severe symptomatic bicuspid aortic stenosis with severely dilated ascending aorta.

2 Images and Supported Data

Reconstructed computed tomography (CT) pre-TAVR demonstrated a bicuspid aortic valve with an annular mean diameter of 30.9 mm, area of 722.4 mm^2, and perimeter of 97.5 mm (Fig. 1a, b). The sinus of Valsalva was measured to have a mean diameter of 43.8 mm, an area of 1568.3 mm^2, and a perimeter of 141.6 mm (Fig. 1c, d). Additionally, the CT scan demonstrated dilated morphology of the ascending

Supplementary Information The online version contains supplementary material available at [https://doi.org/10.1007/978-3-031-05965-0_3].

O. Koren (✉)
Smidt Heart Institute, Cedars-Sinai Medical Center, Los Angeles, CA, USA

Faculty of Medicine, Technion, Israel Institute of Technology, Haifa, Israel
e-mail: Ofir.Koren@cshs.org

A. L. Rosenberg
Biology Faculty, Pepperdine University, Malibu, CA, USA

A. M. Uberoi
Structural and Interventional Cardiology, Kaiser Northwest/Greater Portland Metro Region, Portland, OR, USA

O. Koren et al. (eds.), *Complex Cases in Structural Heart Intervention*,
https://doi.org/10.1007/978-3-031-05965-0_3

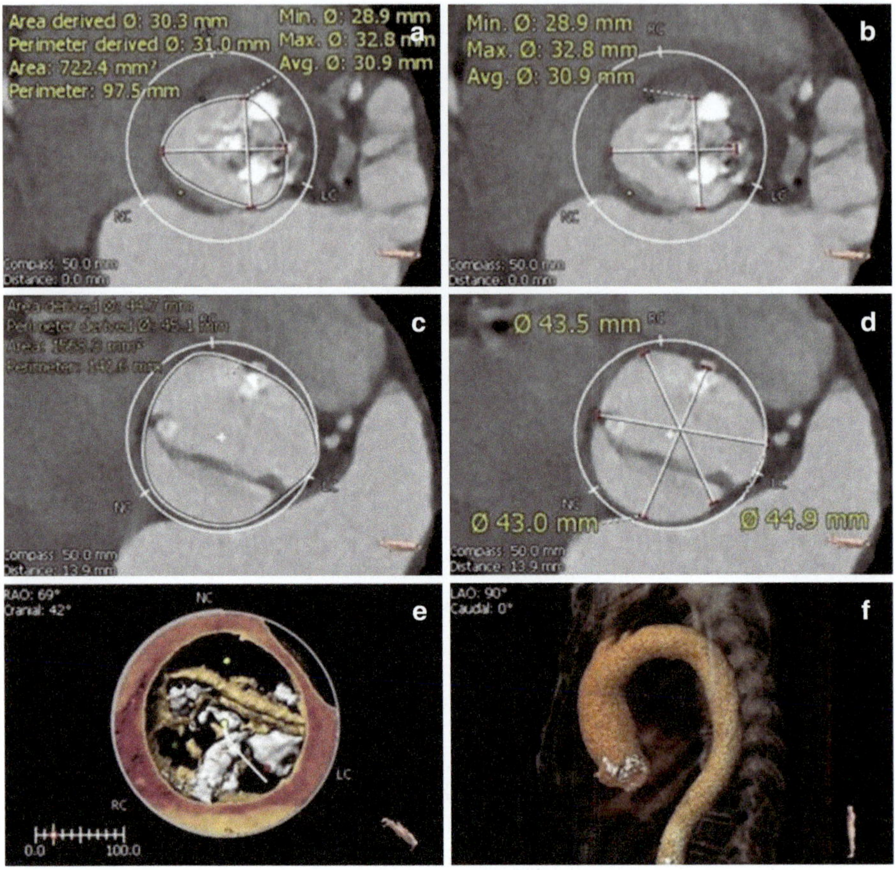

Fig. 1 Reconstructive CT analysis pre-TAVR. (**a**) Bicuspid annulus valve size. (**b**) Annulus diameter. (**c**, **d**) SOV size and diameter. (**e**) Annulus morphology in hockey puck view. (**f**) Anatomy of the ascending aorta with dilating ascending aorta

aorta (Fig. 1e, f), high tortuosity of the common iliac arteries (CIA), particularly the left CIA, and vascular calcification (Fig. 2). The tangent curve of the left CIA was 91° compared to 53° for the right CIA. The left and right CIA dimensions were 8.3 mm × 9.7 mm and 7.3 mm × 9.8 mm, respectively. The dimensions of the left and right common femoral arteries were 7.4 mm × 7.7 mm and 7.8 and 8.0 mm, respectively (Fig. 3).

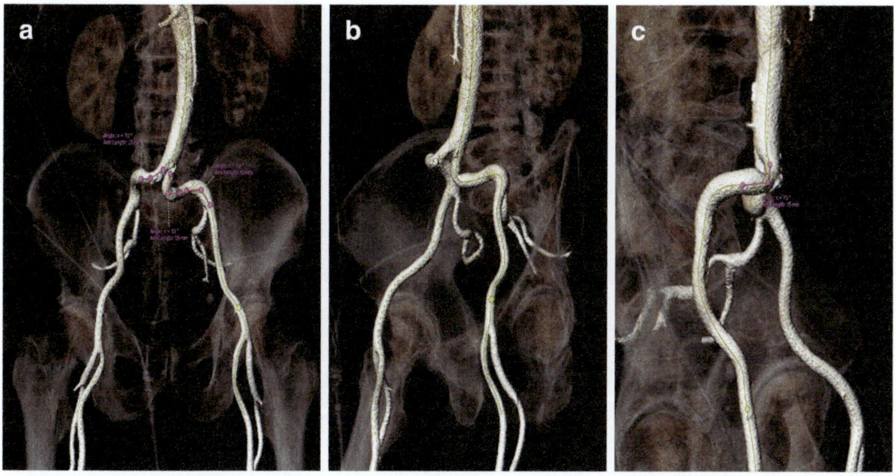

Fig. 2 Reconstructed CT analysis of the iliofemoral arteries indicating high tortuosity of the common iliac arteries. (**a**) Anterior-posterior view. (**b**) Left anterior oblique view. (**c**) Right anterior oblique view

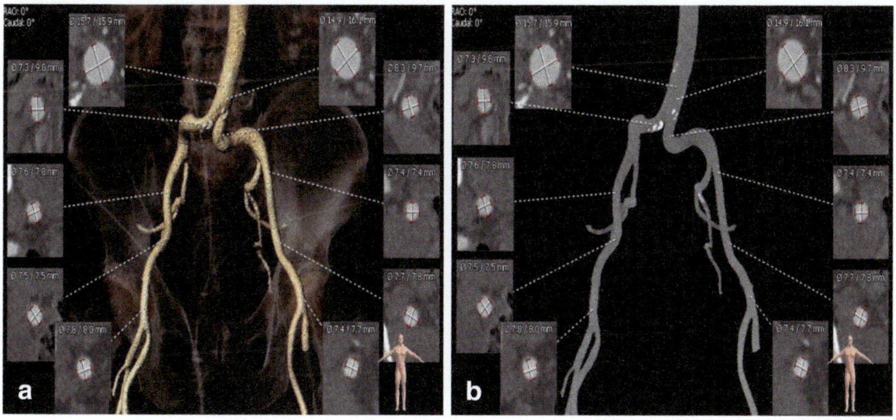

Fig. 3 Assessment of the minimal lumen diameter and calcification of the iliofemoral artery using reconstructed CT. (**a**) Volume rendering view. (**b**) Calcification mode

3 Procedure and Outcome

We used the right femoral access to deliver a 29-mm Sapien 3 Commander valve system and positioned it across the stenotic aortic valve. Due to technical difficulties in crossing the AV, balloon dilatation was performed (Video 1). The valve was deployed in the standard technique with rapid pacing at 180 beats per minute (Video 2). A post-procedure TEE revealed no central aortic regurgitation and moderate paravalvular leak (PVL) (Fig. 4a). The valve delivery system was then taken out.

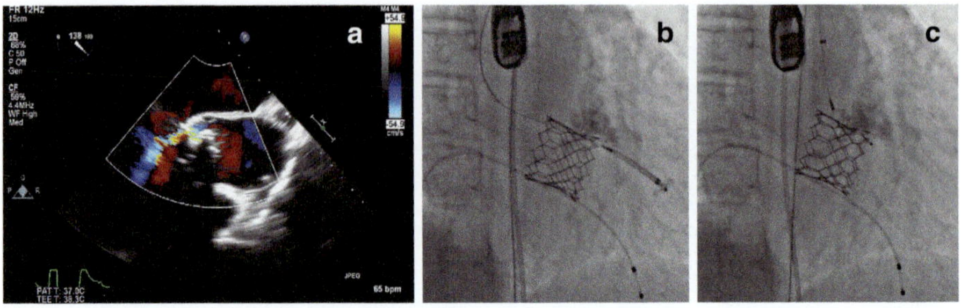

Fig. 4 TAVR procedural images. (**a**) Posterior paravalvular leak (PVL) following a TAVR procedure treated with a 12 mm closure Amplatzer Vascular Plug (AVP) II device. (**b**) The procedure involved a wire crossing of the PVL (yellow arrow). (**c**) Retraction of the device to full deployment over the PVL

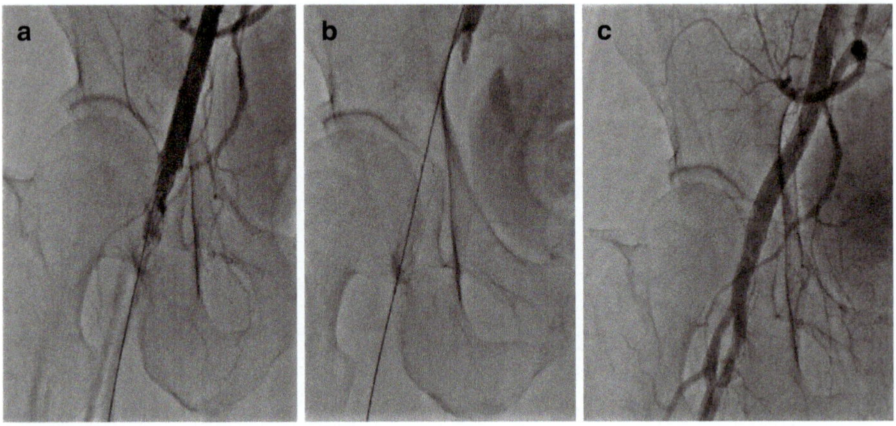

Fig. 5 Angiography of the right iliac artery. (**a**) An up-and-over technique was used, indicating no antegrade blood flow at the femoral bifurcation level. (**b**) Following balloon dilatation and multiple stenting of the external iliac and femoral arteries. (**c**) We achieved restoration of the blood flow to the lower extremity and controlled the anterograde dissection to the upper extremity

The PVL was closed with a 12-mm Amplatzer Vascular Plug II device (Fig. 4b, c, Videos 3, 4 and 5). Following device removal, no blood flow was noted in the right femoral artery (Fig. 5a, Video 6) due to plaque detachment. By stenting the right iliofemoral vessels with 9.0 × 60 mm and 9.0 × 40 mm Absolute Pro self-expanding stents and stenting the right profunda femoral artery using a 4.0 mm × 12 mm Xience Alpine drug-eluting stent (Video 7), normal blood flow was restored. The final result showed normal blood flow restoration (Fig. 5b, c, Video 8). Procedural TEE demonstrated a Type B dissection involving the descending aorta and extending to the left subclavian artery. We could not determine the distal extension of the dissection in the descending aorta, and after considering open vascular surgical repair versus percutaneous approaches we decided to pursue the latter, given the high risk for an open procedure with prohibitive comorbidities.

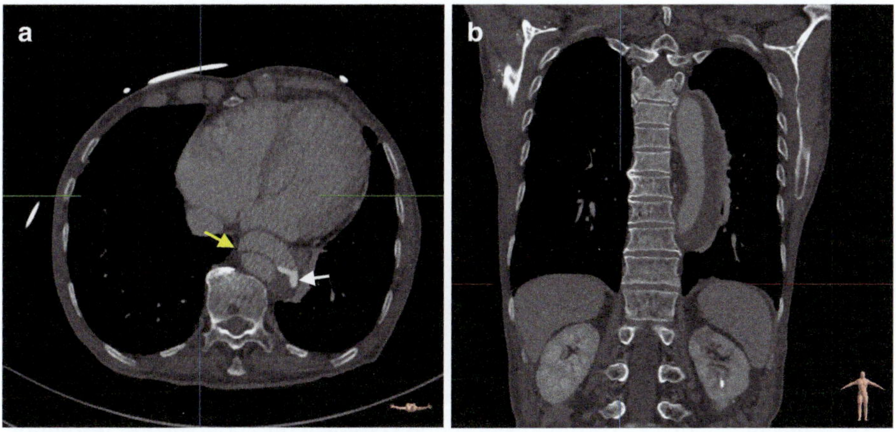

Fig. 6 Computed tomography angiography images. (**a**) Type B acute aortic dissection (yellow arrow). (**b**) Extended toward the descending aorta to its origin at the right iliac artery. The false lumen at the left pulmonary artery level is mostly thrombosed (white arrow on Figure **a**) with a small focus of true lumen

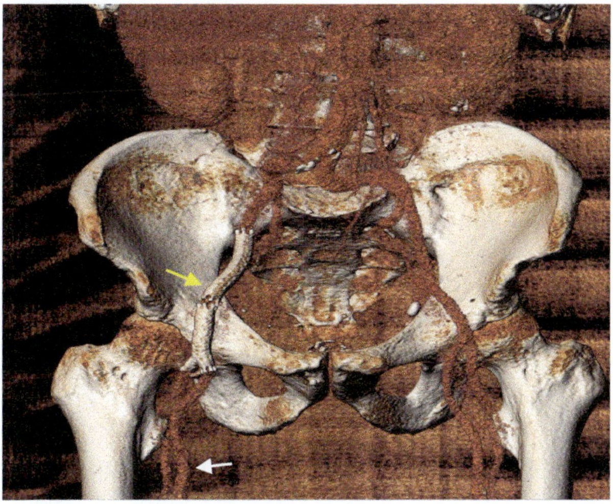

Fig. 7 Reconstructed CT angiography of the pelvic region post iliac. The blood flow to the femoral arteries below the inguinal region was restored (white arrow) following the placement of two stents at the right iliac artery (yellow arrow)

Post-procedural CT angiogram demonstrated a Type B aortic dissection extending into the abdominal aorta to the right common iliac artery level. Largely, the false lumen was thrombosed at the level of the thorax with minimal patency distally (Fig. 6a, b). Also appreciated was a stable, previously known 45 mm ascending aortic aneurysm and patency of the stented peripheral vessels (Fig. 7).

During the 1-year follow-up, the patient stated that he did not have symptoms such as chest pain, paroxysmal nocturnal dyspnea, orthopnea, dizziness, nor palpitations. He stated that he can ride a stationary bike and remains active around the house. TTE showed an ejection fraction of 64%, a mean and peak transaortic gradient of 10 and 20 mmHg, respectively, and severe mitral regurgitation with mean and peak gradients of 6 and 12 mmHg, respectively. The ascending aorta was stable at 4.82 cm^2.

4 Discussion

Vascular complications are commonly grouped into major and minor complications [1]. The incidence of combined vascular complication during TAVR is grossly estimated to be slightly above 4% of the total procedures. Over the last years, the incidence has declined with increased operator experience.

Minor complications usually result in localized and temporary events such as access site bleeding (3–5%) or distal embolization with spontaneous resolution. Major complications such as flow-limiting dissection (0.6–1.9%), stenosis, rupture (<1%), A-V fistula, and pseudoaneurysm often require multiple blood transfusions and surgery [2].

Major vascular complications increased both short and long-term morbidity, directly affecting the patients quality of life, and are an independent risk factor for in hospital mortality and increased mortality 1-year from discharge [2].

Several factors are known to increase the likelihood of vascular complications: the site of arterial access, the size of the sheath (especially sheath >19F), calcification of the artery, minimal vessel luminal diameter, vessel tortuosity, female gender, and the inexperience of the medical center. Among all risk factors, tortuosity is the only factor that cannot be objectively measured, requiring operators to use visual judgment and choose alternative access when feasible [3, 4].

Patients who experience vascular complications during TAVR are likely to develop worse outcomes, especially when it comes to 30-day and 1-year mortality rates [2]. Patients with vascular complications are also predisposed to many other conditions such as renal failure, infection, and neuropathies [1, 2].

Key Points

- Ultrasound-guided arteriotomy should be used for all cases to help optimize the puncture site to ensure Perclose sutures have the highest likelihood of success (i.e., avoidance of anterior plaques or large hanging atheromatous disease for the perclose to grab).
- In heavily calcified arteries, slow and deliberate serial dilation could be used to facilitate adequate acceptance of large-bore sheaths, theoretically minimizing the risk of dissection of endothelial disruption.
- When managing tortuous arteries, pre-procedure planning is imperative. Concentric calcification may be challenging to traverse and may require lesion or Concentric vessel preparation before insertion of a large-bore catheter (i.e., PTA ± concomitant stenting, Shockwave, etc.). Sequential upgrading of wire stiffness is another option (Meier wire, Amplatz super stiff, safari, confide,

Lunderquist, etc.). Stiffer wires increase the risk of penetrating calcified plaque (dependent on how the artery will foreshorten), and increasing dissection risk.
- In highly calcified arteries, a single Perclose technique can be employed. After deploying this suture, limited femoral angiography can be performed with the wire in place. If the remaining degree of extravasation is excessive, the operator can choose to deploy a second perclose or prolong manual pressure.

References

1. Depboylu BC, Yazman S, Harmandar B. Complications of transcatheter aortic valve replacement and rescue attempts. Vessel Plus. 2018;2(9):26.
2. Mangla A, Gupta S. Vascular complications post-transcatheter aortic valve procedures. Indian Heart J. 2016;68(5):724–31.
3. Raptis DA, Beal MA, Kraft DC, Maniar HS, Bierhals AJ. Transcatheter aortic valve replacement: alternative access beyond the femoral arterial approach. Radiographics. 2019;39(1):30–43.
4. Pascual I, Carro A, Avanzas P, Hernández-Vaquero D, Díaz R, Rozado J, Lorca R, Martín M, Silva J, Morís C. Vascular approaches for transcatheter aortic valve implantation. J Thorac Dis. 2017;9(Suppl 6):S478.

TAVR in Highly Horizontal Aorta of a Bicuspid AS Patient

Ofir Koren, Daniel Eugene Cheng and Andrew Luxhoj

1 Clinical Presentation

The patient is an 80-year-old male with a history of chronic diastolic heart failure NYHA class III–IV, hypertension, hyperlipidemia, coronary artery disease status-post several percutaneous coronary interventions, atrial fibrillation/flutter status-post ablation, obesity, diabetes mellitus, and aortic stenosis that endorsed fatigue, dyspnea on exertion, and increasingly frequent episodes of lightheadedness over the past few years. He denied chest pressure, paroxysmal nocturnal dyspnea, orthopnea, dizziness, palpitations, fevers, chills, and recent infections. The patient was referred to our center for further evaluation of candidacy for transcatheter aortic valve replacement.

Supplementary Information The online version contains supplementary material available at [https://doi.org/10.1007/978-3-031-05965-0_4].

O. Koren (✉)
Smidt Heart Institute, Cedars-Sinai Medical Center, Los Angeles, CA, USA

Faculty of Medicine, Technion, Israel Institute of Technology, Haifa, Israel
e-mail: Ofir.Koren@cshs.org

D. E. Cheng
Villanova School of Business, Villanova, PA, USA

A. Luxhoj
Structural Interventional Cardiology Fellow, Cedars Sinai Medical Center, Los Angeles, CA, USA

O. Koren et al. (eds.), *Complex Cases in Structural Heart Intervention*, https://doi.org/10.1007/978-3-031-05965-0_4

2 Images and Supported Data

Pre-procedural TTE revealed an aortic valve area of 0.8 cm^2 (Video 1), a mean gradient of 40 mmHg, a peak gradient of 63 mmHg, and preserved ejection fraction. Cardiac reconstructed CT indicated an annular mean internal diameter of 26.2 mm, area of 545.9 mm^2, and perimeter of 85.3 mm. The following mean diameters were measured: 40.45 mm at the sinus of Valsalva, 39.1 mm at the STJ, and 26.5 mm at the LVOT (Fig. 1). The maximal diameter of the ascending aorta was 45.6 mm. The aortic valve was found to have type 1 bicuspid morphology with annular and LVOT calcification (Video 4). Quantitation of the calcium using 850 Hounsfield units as a threshold indicated a volume of 287.3 mm^3 over the AV annulus. The coronary ostia originated at 22.1 and 9.1 mm (for the RCA and LCA, respectively) above the annular plane (Fig. 2). A coplanar CT view illustrated a high aorto-ventricular angulation

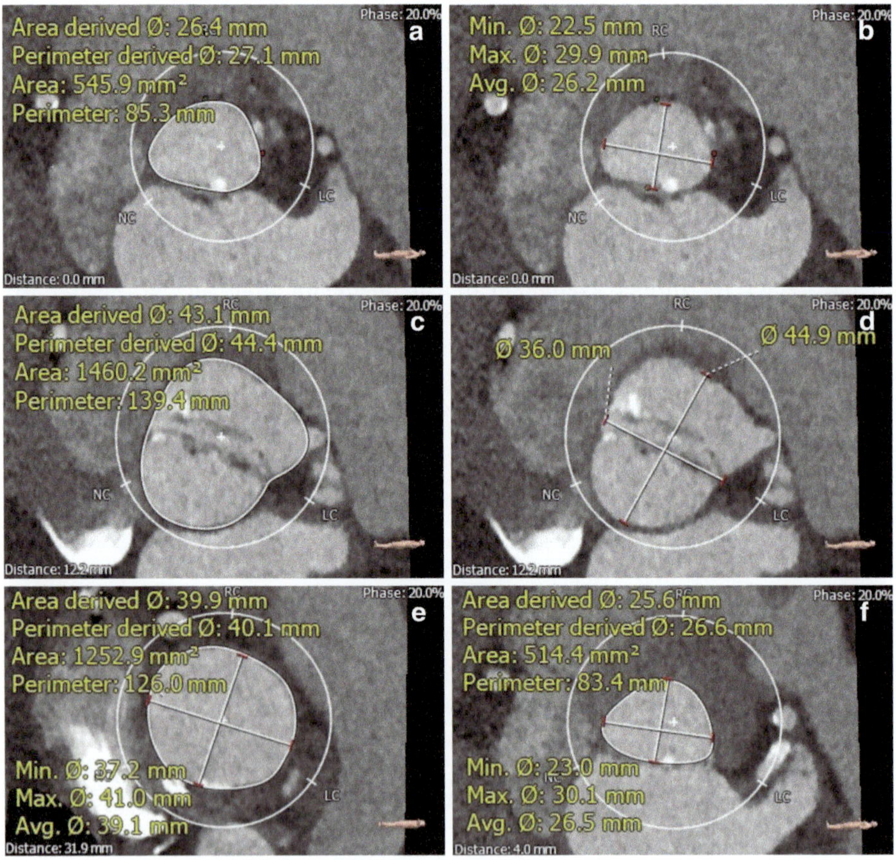

Fig. 1 Pre-TAVR CT reconstruction. (**a**, **b**) Area, perimeter, and diameter measurement of the AV annulus. (**c**, **d**) The SOV, (**e**) the sinotubular junction, (**f**) the LVOT

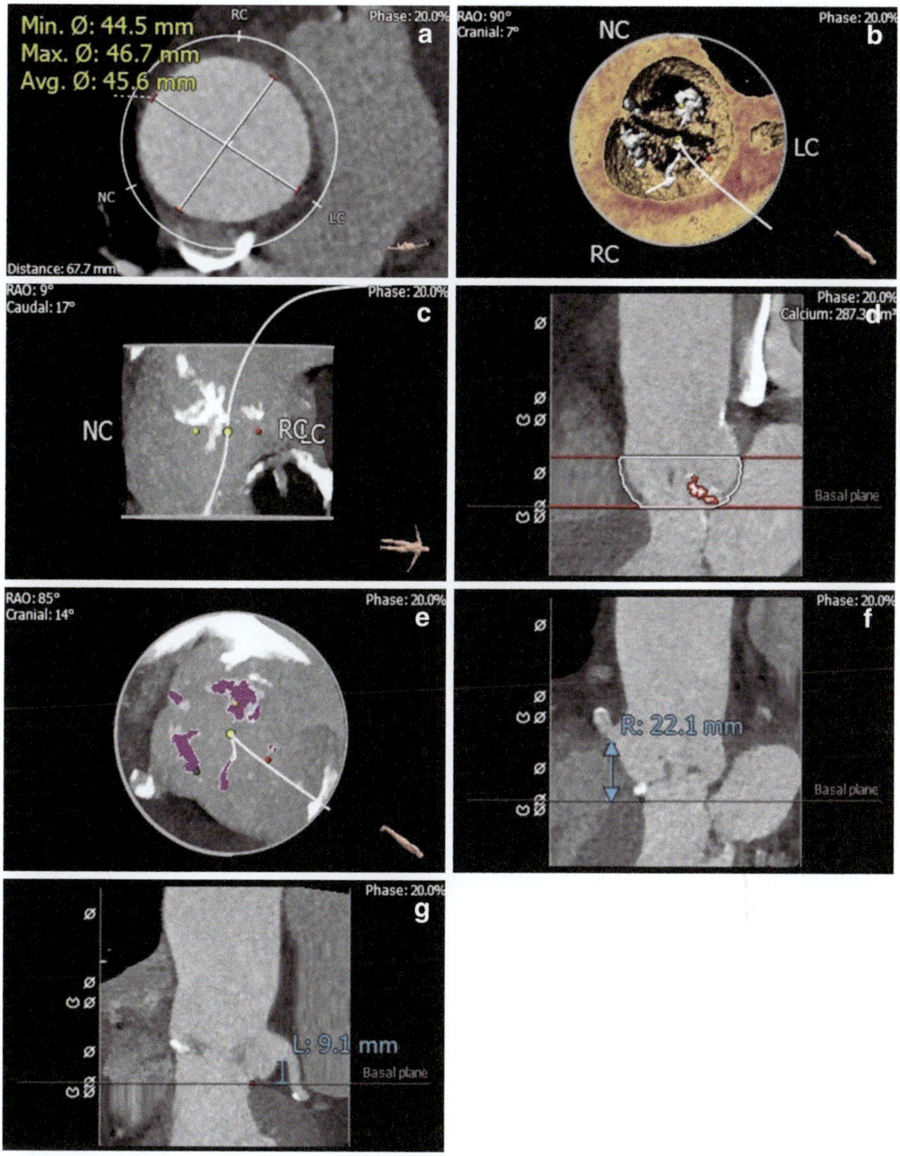

Fig. 2 Reconstructed CT analysis pre-TAVR. (**a**) Maximal diameter of the ascending aorta. (**b**) Hockey puck VR view of a type 1 bicuspid aortic valve with a calcified fusion of the left and right cusps (white arrow). (**c–e**) Annular and LVOT calcification assessment using a HU850 threshold. (**f**, **g**) Coronary artery height above the annular plane. Note the low left coronary height (9.1 mm)

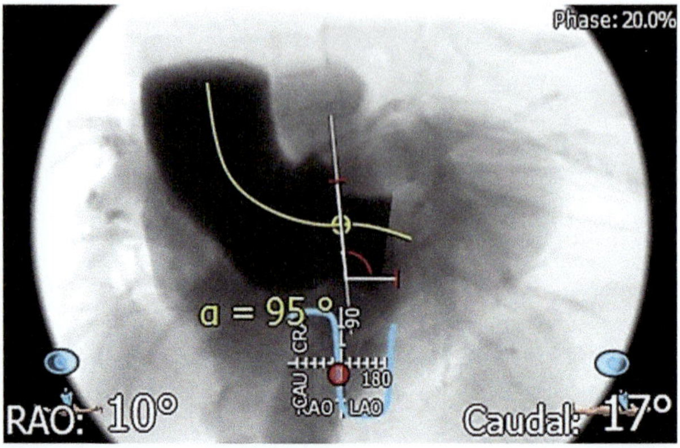

Fig. 3 Coplanar CT view of aortic root. Measurements of aorto-ventricular angulation indicating a 95° angle

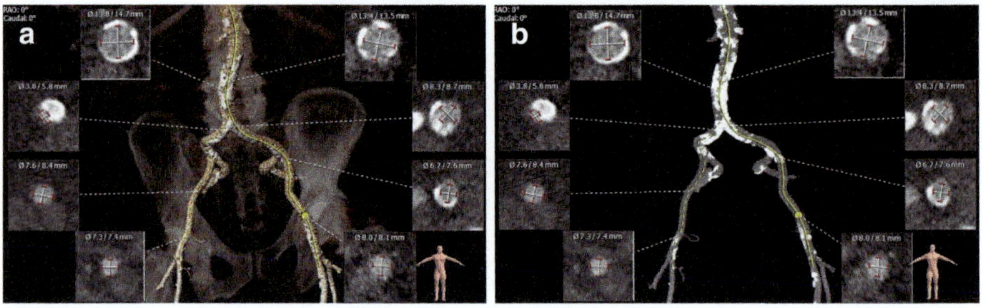

Fig. 4 CT analysis of the abdominal aorta and the iliofemoral arteries. (**a**) CTA indicated significant tortuosity. (**b**) Calcification at the abdominal aorta and common iliac branches

of 95° (Fig. 3). The iliofemoral and abdominal aortic arteries demonstrated severe calcification. The right and left common iliac arteries were measured as 3.8 × 5.8 mm and 6.7 × 7.6 mm, respectively (Fig. 4). Left heart catheterization demonstrated non-obstructive coronary artery disease (Videos 2 and 3).

3 Procedure and Outcome

The patient was evaluated by cardiothoracic surgery and deemed to have moderate surgical risk and was therefore appropriate for transcatheter aortic valve replacement using a 29-mm Edwards Sapien S3 valve. Pre-procedural transesophageal echocardiography demonstrated a severely stenotic, bicuspid aortic valve as well as a large and aneurysmal sinus of Valsalva (Fig. 5). We decided not to use cardioembolic protection due to unfavorable anatomy. After gaining femoral access, a 23 mm × 4 cm Edwards balloon was advanced across the stenotic aortic valve, and valvuloplasty was performed before valve deployment (Fig. 6, Video 4). The valve

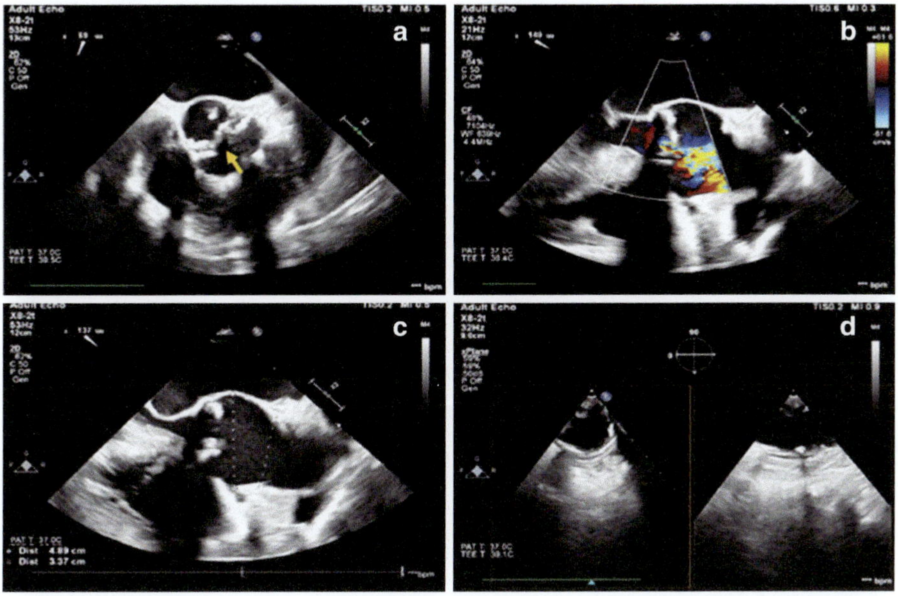

Fig. 5 Pre-procedure TEE. (**a**) Severe stenotic and calcified bicuspid aortic valve with a calcified raphe between the right and left coronary arteries (yellow arrow). (**b**) Color Doppler over the aortic valve indicates severe stenosis. (**c**) Large and aneurysmal sinus of Valsalva (white dashed lines). (**d**) Atheromatous plaques over ascending aorta

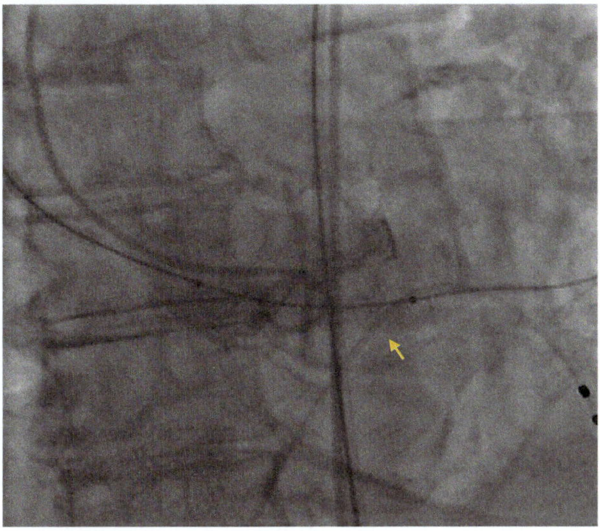

Fig. 6 Cardiac fluoroscopy during valvulotomy. Note the Edwards 23 × 40 mm balloon used for the pre-TAVR valvulotomy (yellow arrow)

was then deployed in the standard technique with 3 mL in the inflation device (Fig. 7, Video 5). A post-procedure TEE revealed mild paravalvular regurgitation (Fig. 8, Video 6). Therefore, we decided to dilate the valve above the nominal volume. The delivery system was re-prepped and used to post-dilate the valve with an extra 3 mL volume (Video 7). At the end of the procedure, the patient exhibited ventricular escape rhythm with a narrow complex escape at 60 beats per minute. The patient displayed focal neurological deficits following the procedure, suggesting a minor cardioembolic cerebrovascular accident. However, the patient improved upon discharge.

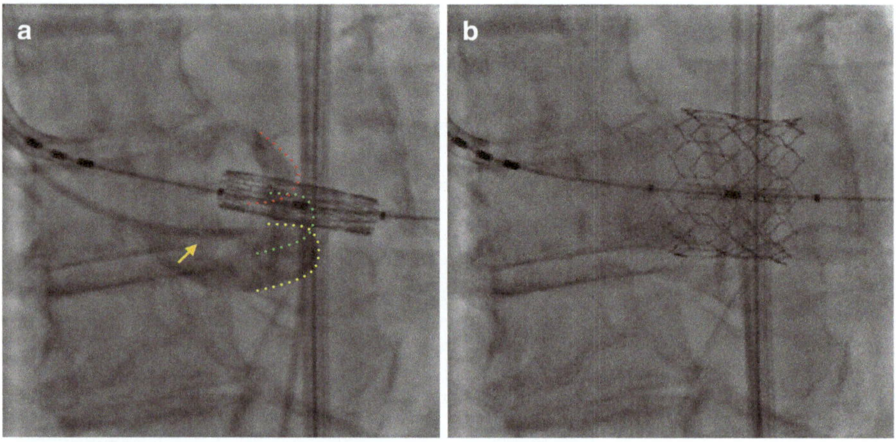

Fig. 7 Cardiac fluoroscopy during TAVR. (**a**) The positioning of the balloon-expandable THV in aortic position. (**b**) Final deployment. The pigtailed catheter (yellow arrow Figure **a**) in the RCC and the alignment of THV in respect to the three cups (dashed yellow line represents NCC, green line represents the RCC, and red line represents LCC)

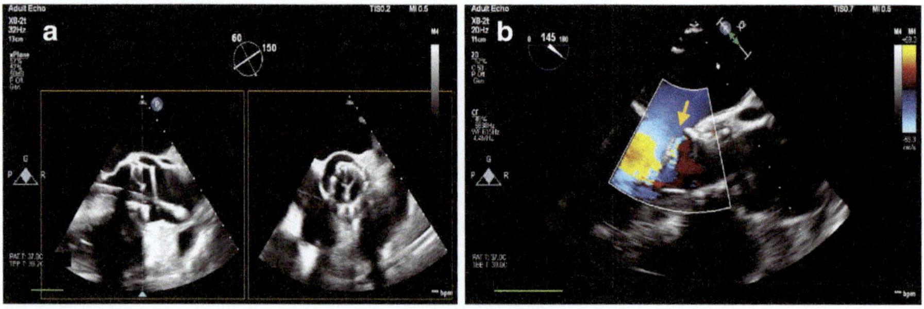

Fig. 8 Post-procedure TEE. (**a**) Well seated bioprosthetic balloon-expandable THV in the aortic position. (**b**) Trivial to mild posterior valvular regurgitation (yellow arrow)

4 Discussion

The normal aortic valve has three leaflets that open and close, allowing blood flow from the heart to the aorta. The bicuspid valve has only two functioning leaflets. With this anomaly, the valve does not function perfectly. However, it may work adequately for years, even to late adulthood, with no obvious signs of a problem. The actual cause of BAVD is not completely clear. The two-leaflet valve develops in the early stages of pregnancy. Roughly 2% of the population has BAVD, which is more than twice as common in males as in females [1, 2]. The latest studies suggest that a connective tissue disorder causes BAVD. Ascending aortic aneurysms and abnormal thoracic aortas are associated with BAVD. Aortic dimensions are enlarged in BAVD, and the ascending aortic morphology differs between bicuspid aortic valves and tricuspid aortic valves. The degree of aortic angulation (AA) is greater in BAVD [3].

The AA degree poses significant anatomic and technical challenges to successfully positioning and deploying the transcatheter aortic valve (TAVR). The balloon-expandable Edwards Sapien Valve has the advantage of active-flexion catheter steerability and a shorter stent frame, thereby facilitating the positioning and deployment of the TAVR valve in horizontal aortas (AA >70°) [4]. Patients with AA >70° are usually excluded from clinical trials of self-expanding TAVR valves, such as the Medtronic CoreValve. A transaortic TAVR approach through a mini-thoracotomy is also recommended for extremely horizontal aorta [5].

Key Points

- Bicuspid aortic valves are frequently associated with greater AA degrees than tricuspid aortic valves.
- Aortic angulation >70°, and horizontal ascending aorta, usually exclude the use of self-expanding transcatheter valves due to the difficulty of positioning and deploying these valves.
- Balloon-expandable valves using a steerable delivery system can facilitate successful valve deployment in extremely horizontal aortas, AA = 95°.

References

1. Masri A, Svensson LG, Griffin BP, Desai MY. Contemporary natural history of bicuspid aortic valve disease: a systematic review. Heart. 2017;103(17):1323–30.
2. Kong WK, Bax JJ, Michelena HI, Delgado V. Sex differences in bicuspid aortic valve disease. Prog Cardiovasc Dis. 2020;63(4):452–6.

3. D'ostrevy NI, Ngo H, Magnin B, Azarnoush K, Cassagnes L, Camilleri L. Bicuspid and tricuspid aortic valve do not have the same ascending aorta morphology. Clin Anat. 2018;31(5):693–7.
4. Abramowitz Y, Maeno Y, Chakravarty T, Kazuno Y, Takahashi N, Kawamori H, Mangat G, Cheng W, Jilaihawi H, Makkar RR. Aortic angulation attenuates procedural success following self-expandable but not balloon-expandable TAVR. JACC Cardiovasc Imaging. 2016;9(8):964–72.
5. Okuyama K, Jilaihawi H, Mirocha J, Nakamura M, Ramzy D, Makkar R, Cheng W. Alternative access for balloon-expandable transcatheter aortic valve replacement: comparison of the transaortic approach using right anterior thoracotomy to partial J-sternotomy. J Thorac Cardiovasc Surg. 2015;149(3):789–97.

Retrograde Approach for AV Wire Crossing

Ofir Koren, Robert Naami, and Jubin Joseph

1 Clinical Presentation

The patient is a 70-year-old male with a history of coronary artery disease, end-stage renal disease on dialysis, essential hypertension, hyperlipidemia, paroxysmal atrial fibrillation (without anticoagulation due to gastrointestinal bleed), heart failure with preserved ejection fraction NYHA Class III–IV, severe mitral regurgitation status post MitraClip procedure, and severe aortic stenosis status post-transcatheter aortic valve replacement using 34-mm Evolut Pro prosthetic heart valve in 2018 (Videos 1 and 2). He is currently admitted for acute, chronic decompensated heart failure. He presents to the hospital with severe and worsening shortness of breath. He reports experiencing exertional distress with only a few steps.

Supplementary Information The online version contains supplementary material available at [https://doi.org/10.1007/978-3-031-05965-0_5].

O. Koren (✉)
Smidt Heart Institute, Cedars-Sinai Medical Center, Los Angeles, CA, USA

Faculty of Medicine, Technion, Israel Institute of Technology, Haifa, Israel
e-mail: Ofir.Koren@cshs.org

R. Naami
University Hospitals Cleveland Medical Center, Cleveland, OH, USA

J. Joseph
Smidt Heart Institute, Cedars-Sinai Medical Center, Los Angeles, CA, USA

O. Koren et al. (eds.), *Complex Cases in Structural Heart Intervention*,
https://doi.org/10.1007/978-3-031-05965-0_5

2 Images and Supported Data

Cardiac reconstructed CT estimated the aortic annulus inflow to have a mean internal diameter of 31.1 mm, area of 776.9 mm^2, and perimeter of 99.7 mm (Fig. 1a, b). The estimated SOV area and ascending maximal aorta diameter were estimated to be 403.2 mm^2 and 43.3 mm, respectively (Fig. 1c, d). We used the Hockey puck mode to assess THV sizing (Fig. 1e, f).

The right and left coronary ostia originated at 27.4 and 30.9 mm above the THV inflow, respectively (Fig. 2a, b). The distance of a virtual 29-mm Sapien-3 valve THV to the LCA and RCA ostium was 7.1 and 9.0 mm, respectively (Fig. 2c, d).

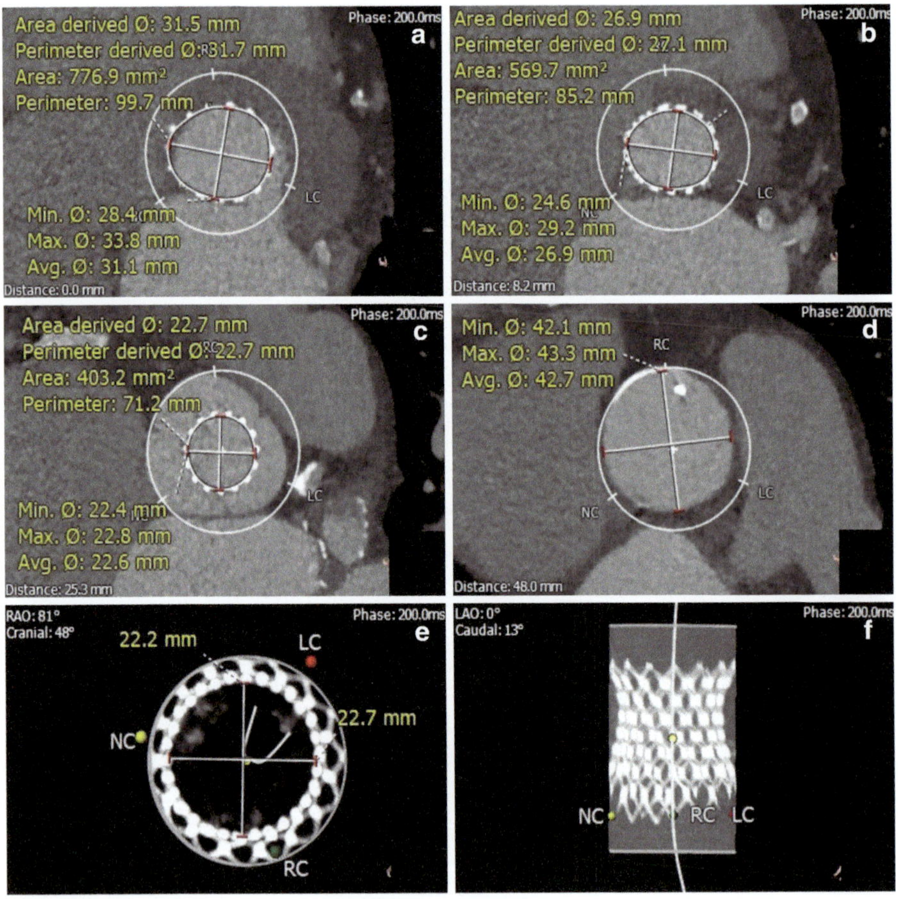

Fig. 1 Reconstructed CT analysis before the procedure. (**a**) The annulus inflow dimensions. (**b**) The estimated native annulus size. (**c**) The SOV area. (**d**) Maximal diameter of ascending aorta. (**e**) The true internal diameter in Hockey puck mode for THV sizing. (**f**) STJ and LVOT calcification in MIP

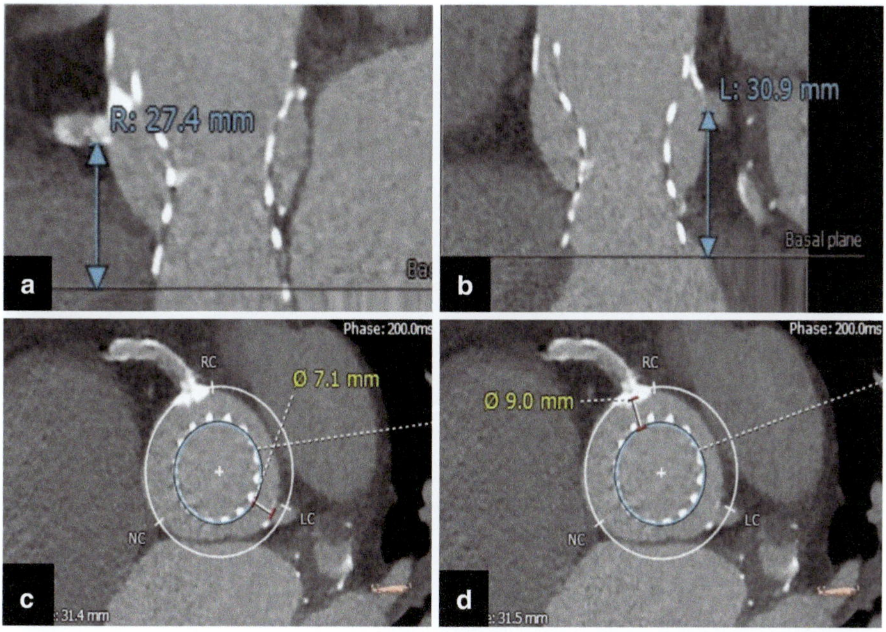

Fig. 2 RCA height from inflow of THV. (**a**) and the LCA (**b**) LCA height from inflow of THV. The distance of the LCA (**c**) and the RCA (**d**) ostium from a 29 mm S3 virtual valve

Before the procedure, TTE revealed severely depressed left ventricular systolic function with EF 25% (compared to 55% in the previous study) as well as severe aortic valve bioprosthetic stenosis (peak transaortic gradient 69 mmHg, mean transaortic gradient is 43 mmHg) and trivial paravalvular regurgitation (Video 3, Fig. 3a) without evidence of hypoattenuated leaflet thickening (HALT). Additionally, one MitraClip was seen on the anterior and posterior leaflets of the mitral valve associated with severe mitral regurgitation (Fig. 3b, c). Pre-procedural coronary angiography illustrated no obstructive lesion (Fig. 4, Videos 4–6).

3 Pre-Procedural Consideration: Pitfalls, Dilemmas, and Challenges

The patient was evaluated by cardiothoracic surgery and deemed to have moderate surgical risk and appropriate for transcatheter aortic valve replacement (TAVR). Therefore, the patient underwent transfemoral TAVR using FDA-approved 29-mm Edward Sapien S3 bioprosthesis.

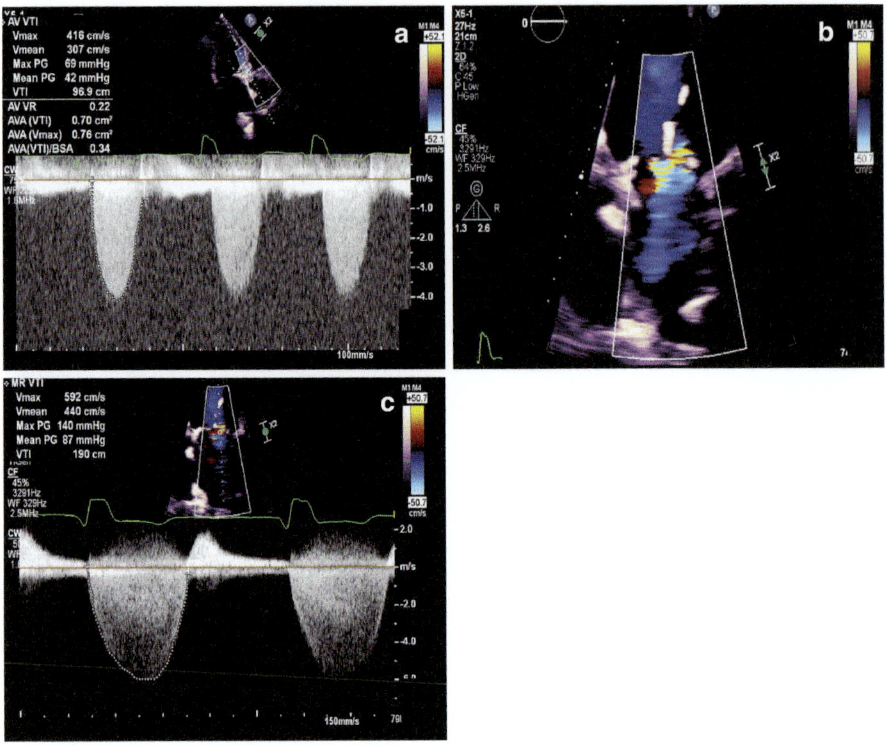

Fig. 3 Transthoracic echocardiography before the procedure. (**a**) Severe bioprosthetic stenosis with high pressure gradient and small AV area. (**b**, **c**) The volume and pressure overload shift to the mitral valve creating severe regurgitation flow

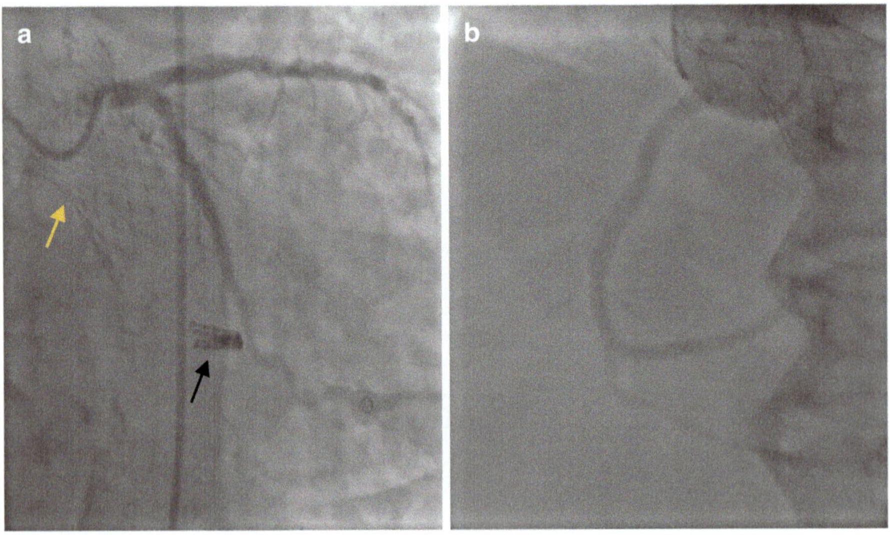

Fig. 4 Coronary angiogram before the procedure. (**a**) No significant obstructing lesions in LCA. (**b**) No significant obstructing lesions in RCA. Note the prior self-expandable THV located at the aortic valve (orange arrow) and single clip at the MV area (black arrow)

4 Procedure and Outcome

The patient was brought to the cardiac catheterization laboratory and placed under moderate sedation by the anesthesiologist. Shortly after this, there was profound hypotension requiring chest compression. Resuscitation was performed, including chest compressions.

We proceeded with the valve replacement procedure using the transfemoral approach alongside ongoing cardiopulmonary resuscitation and pressure recovery. However, we could not cross the stenotic aortic valve despite using a variety of wires as the orifice area was too small (Video 7). Therefore, we opted to perform antegrade crossing using the transseptal approach. We made a transseptal puncture using the Bayliss Versacross system and passed a wire across the medial orifice of the mitral valve (Video 8, Figs. 5a and 6a, b). Through this, a Berman end-hole catheter was advanced into the LV and placed in the LVOT. Then, we used a balance wire to cross the aortic valve antegrade and placed it in the ascending aorta.

We used a snare wire via the femoral sheath to capture the balance wire and externalize it (Fig. 5b). An MPA catheter was introduced over the balance wire and into the left ventricle (Videos 9 and 10). We then used an Amplatz extra-stiff wire and advanced it into the LV cavity via the MPA catheter. A 29-mm Edwards Sapien S3 valve delivery system was positioned across the stenotic aortic valve. With rapid pacing, the valve was deployed in the standard technique with nominal inflation (Video 11, Figs. 5c and 6c). Post-procedure transesophageal echocardiogram revealed no central aortic regurgitation and no paravalvular regurgitation. The patient returned to the coronary intensive care unit.

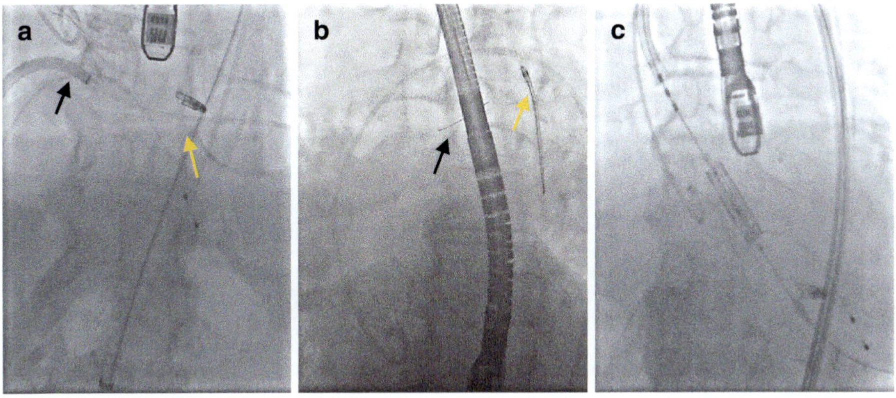

Fig. 5 Fluoroscopy of the procedure. Crossing the AV in the standard retrograde approach failed, thereby necessitating a change to an anterograde approach. (**a**) Transeptal puncture (black arrow) was used to cross into the left-sided chamber and approach the bioprosthetic valve from the ventricle side (orange arrow). (**b**) Following the successful crossing of the AV from the ventricle side to ascending aorta, a snare wire (orange arrow) was used to hook the wire (black arrow) at AA and pass it to the ventricle. (**c**) A balloon-expanding THV was delivered over the new wire positioned in the left ventricle and the THV was successfully deployed over the prior self-expandable valve

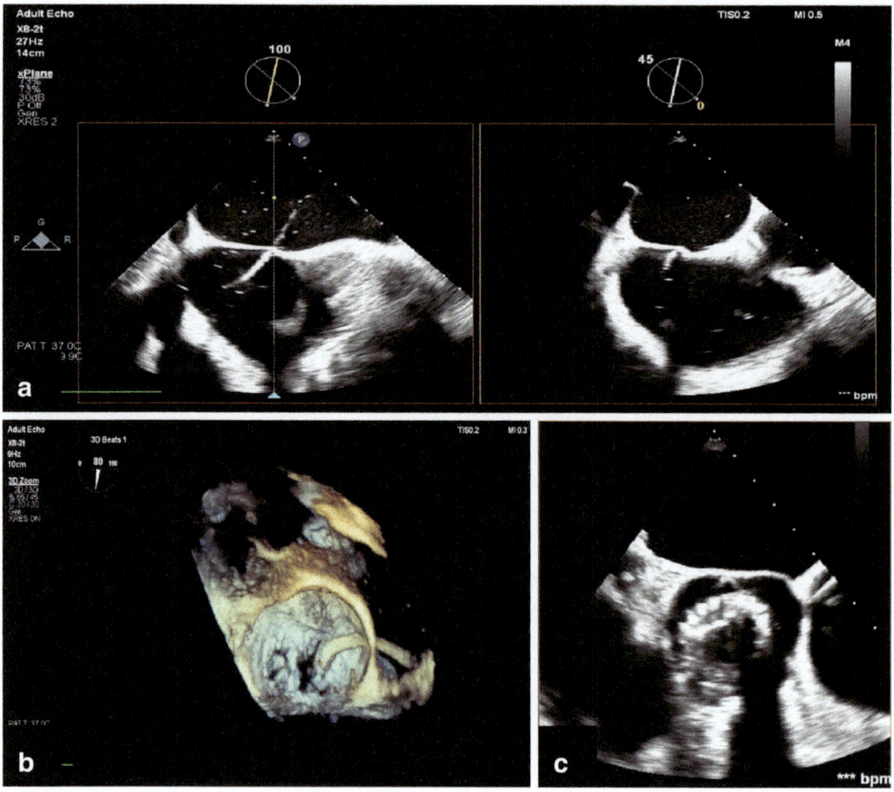

Fig. 6 Procedural TEE imaging. (**a–c**) Transseptal puncture using TEE guided for proper positioning of the new balloon-expanding valve

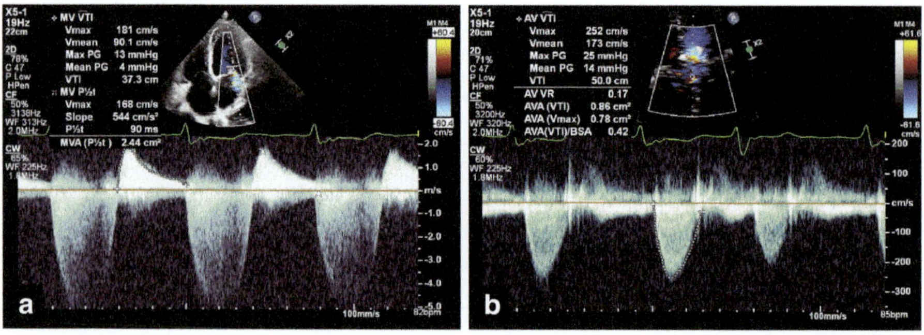

Fig. 7 Transthoracic echocardiography at follow-up. (**a**) A well seated balloon-expanding THV with a significant reduction in the gradient over the AV. (**b**) Early signs of volume and pressure overload improvement over the mitral valve

Follow-up TTE demonstrated a well-seated bioprosthetic aortic valve with a substantial reduction in transaortic gradients (peak 25 mmHg, mean 43 mmHg) and improvement in mitral regurgitant flow (Video 12, Fig. 7). Several days following his procedure, the patient demonstrated no neurological deficits or signs of decompensated heart failure. He was discharged home in stable condition.

5 Discussion

The retrograde crossing of a severely stenotic aortic valve (AV) is crucial in the transfemoral transcatheter aortic valve replacement (TAVR) procedure. Crossing the native valve can be time-consuming and technically challenging [1–4]. Risk factors associated with difficulty crossing include significant small AV area, extreme aortic arch angulation, severe valvular calcification, and bicuspid morphology. Physiologically, the critically stenosed leaflets are immobile, producing a high-velocity systolic jet that impedes the wire crossing into the AV valve [5]. Additionally, valve crossing, especially in a forceful fashion, increases the risk of cerebral embolisms. In one study assessing patients undergoing retrograde catheterization of the aortic valve, 22% of individuals demonstrated focal abnormalities on magnetic resonance imaging. Moreover, 3% of these patients presented with clinically apparent neurological deficits [6].

There are various techniques to cross the aortic valve in a retrograde fashion. The telescopic catheter technique, widely used in tortuous and calcified coronary vessels, has been useful [7]. Here, the straight-tipped wire, with the wire tip placed in LV, is loaded with a guiding catheter. The proximal portion of this catheter is connected to a Y-connector with a diagnostic pigtail catheter placed across the guiding catheter. With the increased backup force provided by the guiding catheter, the inner pigtail catheter can cross the aortic valve. An alternative technique is using a pigtail catheter and J-wire combination. The catheter is placed 3–4 cm above the aortic valve (AV) and turned anteriorly in the 30° RAO view. The J-wire is subsequently pushed out of the pigtail catheter to form a u-shaped curve above the AV. With rotation, the vertex of the curved J-wire will easily find an orientation to pass the AV [8].

Key Points

- The traditional and the widely used retrograde approach to cross stenotic AV may be challenging in a case of highly calcified or critical AS.
- The operator should be familiar with the anterograde technique when attempts to cross the AV using the retrograde approach fail or in urgent situations.

References

1. Otto CM. Valvular aortic stenosis: disease severity and timing of intervention. J Am Coll Cardiol. 2006;47(11):2141–51.
2. Chin CW, Pawade TA, Newby DE, Dweck MR. Risk stratification in patients with aortic stenosis using novel imaging approaches. Circ Cardiovasc Imaging. 2015;8(8):e003421.
3. Kalusche D, Betz P, Roskamm H. Disorders of intraventricular conduction in patients with calcified aortic valve diseases: pre-and postoperative incidence and effect on prognosis following aortic valve replacement. Z Kardiol. 1986;75(3):147–50.
4. Omran H, Schmidt H, Hackenbroch M, Illien S, Bernhardt P, von der Recke G, Fimmers R, Flacke S, Layer G, Pohl C, Lüderitz B. Silent and apparent cerebral embolism after retrograde catheterisation of the aortic valve in valvular stenosis: a prospective, randomised study. Lancet. 2003;361(9365):1241–6.

5. Kasel AM, Shivaraju A, von Scheidt W, Kastrati A, Thilo C. Anatomic guided crossing of a stenotic aortic valve under fluoroscopy: "right cusp rule, part III". JACC Cardiovasc Interv. 2015;8(1 Part A):119–20.
6. Lesh MD, Van Hare GF, Scheinman MM, Ports TA, Epstein LA. Comparison of the retrograde and transseptal methods for ablation of left free wall accessory pathways. J Am Coll Cardiol. 1993;22(2):542–9.
7. Ruparelia N, Prendergast BD. Transcatheter aortic valve implantation - what the general physician needs to know. Clin Med (Lond). 2015;15(5):420–25. https://doi.org/10.7861/clinmedicine.15-5-420.
8. Chambers J, Bach D, Dumesnil J, Otto C, Shah P, Thomas J. Crossing the aortic valve in severe aortic stenosis: no longer acceptable? J Heart Valve Dis. 2004;13(3):344–6.

Balloon Burst During a Sapien-3 THV Inflation

Ofir Koren, Ran Eliaz, and Hasan Jilaihawi

1 Clinical Presentation

The patient is an 82-year-old male with a past medical history of coronary artery disease (treated with coronary bypass grafting), interstitial lung disease, hypertension atrial fibrillation (on Eliquis), chronic diastolic heart failure (NYHA Class IV), and chronic kidney disease. The patient denies any chest pain, orthopnea, and paroxysmal nocturnal dyspnea. Over several months, the patient developed a significant worsening of his shortness of breath, experiencing dyspnea with minimal exertion and no relief with adjustment of diuretic therapy.

2 Images and Supported Data

TTE revealed an aortic valve area of 0.7 cm^2, mean gradient of 36 mmHg, peak gradient of 62 mmHg, and preserved ejection fraction. There were no regional wall motion abnormalities at rest or with dobutamine-stress. The estimated pulmonary artery

Supplementary Information The online version contains supplementary material available at [https://doi.org/10.1007/978-3-031-05965-0_6].

O. Koren (✉)
Smidt Heart Institute, Cedars-Sinai Medical Center, Los Angeles, CA, USA

Faculty of Medicine, Technion, Israel Institute of Technology, Haifa, Israel
e-mail: Ofir.Koren@cshs.org

R. Eliaz
Schulich Heart Program, Sunnybrook Health Sciences Centre, Toronto, ON, Canada

H. Jilaihawi
Heart Valve Center, NYU Langone Health, New York, NY, USA

O. Koren et al. (eds.), *Complex Cases in Structural Heart Intervention*,
https://doi.org/10.1007/978-3-031-05965-0_6

pressure was 43 mmHg. A subsequent coronary angiogram showed severe aortic calcification, proximal LCX stenosis (~80%), proximal LAD stenosis (20%), mid-LAD bifurcation stenosis with the first diagonal artery (60–70%), and patent SVG-RCA bypass graft. TEE before the procedure showed moderate mitral regurgitation and mild aortic insufficiency, respectively (Fig. 1, Videos 1 and 2). Cardiac reconstructed CT indicated an annular mean internal diameter of 27.5 mm, area of 550.8 mm^2, and perimeter of 84.4 mm. The following mean diameters were measured: 35.2 mm at the Sinus of Valsalva, 28.1 mm at the STJ, and 27.1 mm at the LVOT (Fig. 2). The coronary ostia originated at 21.3 and 16.3 mm (for the RCA and LCA) above the annular plane (Fig. 3). Significant calcium deposition was noticed mainly on aortic valve leaflets and aortic arch (Figs. 3 and 4). The STJ was found to have protuberant calcification with a height of 26.5 mm. Quantifying of the calcium using 850 Hounsfield units as a threshold indicated a 311.8 mm^3 volume of calcium over the AV annulus (Fig. 3). We noticed a focal dissection in the right external iliac artery.

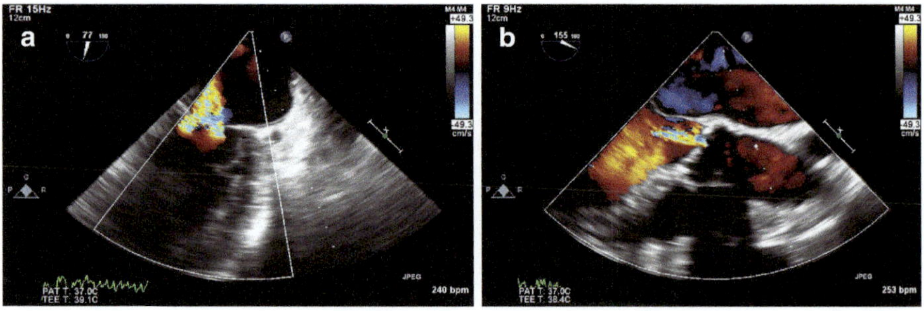

Fig. 1 TEE pre-procedure. (**a**) Moderate mitral regurgitation seen on ME Mitral commissural view. (**b**) Mild aortic insufficiency seen on ME AV LAX view

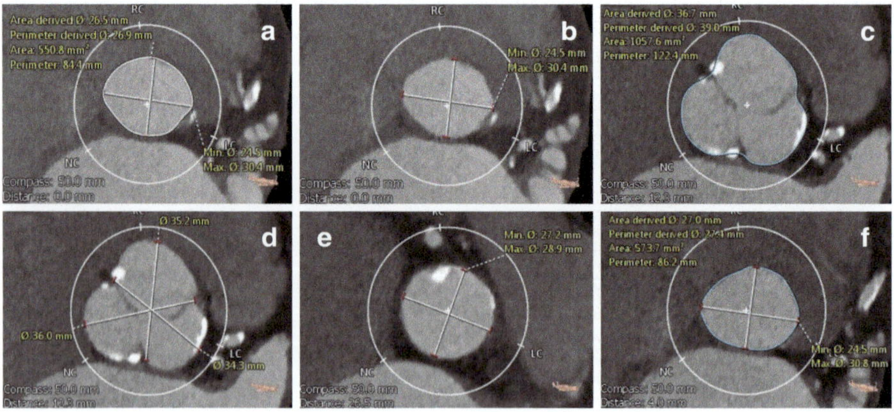

Fig. 2 Reconstructed CT analysis pre-TAVR. (**a**) AV annular area and perimeter. (**b**) AV annular diameter. (**c**) SOV area and perimeter. (**d**) SOV diameters. (**e**) Sinotubular junction diameter. (**f**) LVOT diameter

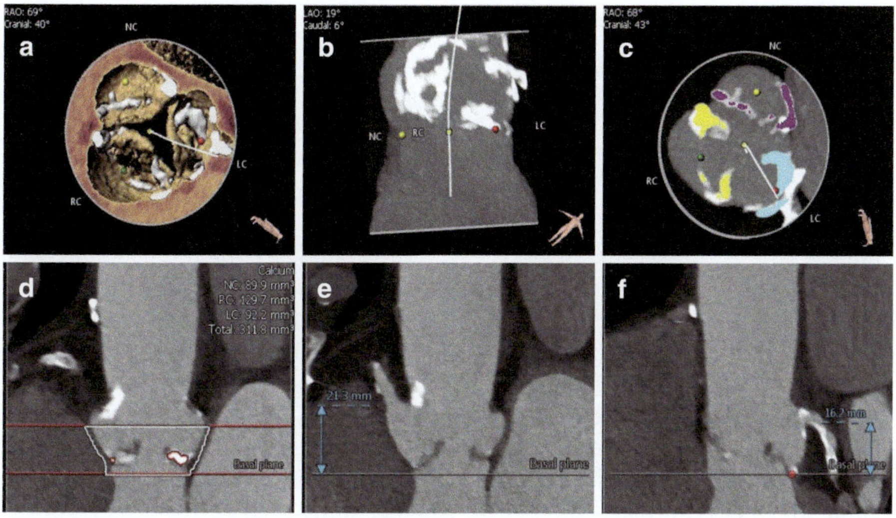

Fig. 3 Calcium quantification and distribution over the annulus and the aortic root measured by reconstructed CT analysis before the TAVR procedure. (**a**) AV annulus calcification seen on Hockey puck VR view. (**b**) Aortic root calcification seen on Hockey puck MIP view. (**c**, **d**) Cross-section and long axis views of the AV annulus cross-section at HU850 threshold. (**e**, **f**) Coronary heights and calcium distribution at the coronary level

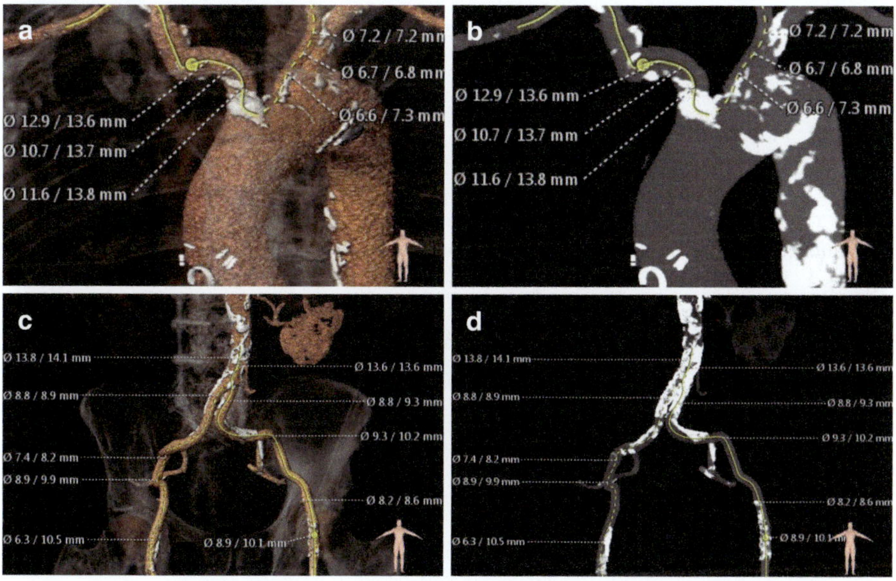

Fig. 4 Calcium distribution in aortic arch, abdominal aorta, and iliac system on reconstructed CT. (**a**) Aortic arch (dimmed view). (**b**) Aortic arch (calcification view). (**c**) Abdominal aorta and iliac system (dimmed view). (**d**) Abdominal aorta and iliac system (calcification view)

3 Procedure and Outcome

Following evaluation by the heart team, patient was deemed high risk for surgery due to severe interstitial lung disease. Instead, patient was referred for transfemoral TAVR using a 29-mm Edward Sapien S3 bioprosthetic valve. The THV was advanced and deployed in standard technique with rapid pacing at 180 beats per minute. During deployment, the delivery balloon for the valve ruptured at maximal inflation (Fig. 5, Video 3). Evaluation of the valve showed normal functioning with minimal perivalvular leak (Figs. 6 and 7, Video 4). There was no evidence of pericardial effusion or root injury. However, the sheath and valve system could not be completely removed from the arterial access site due to balloon rupture. Due to this, vascular surgery was consulted, and they successfully performed an emergent exploration of the left common femoral artery with the extraction of the Sapien balloon and device (Fig. 8). Selective left femoral arteriography was then performed, demonstrating excellent vessel patency with no distal dissection or thrombus propagation which was further suported by Doppler ultrasound (Figs. 8 and 9). The

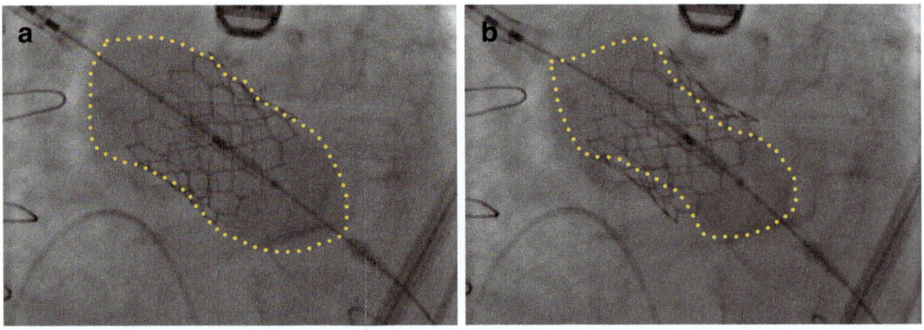

Fig. 5 The deployment of a 29 mm Sapien-3 balloon-expandable THV over the AV annulus. (**a**) THV inflated over an intact balloon (dashed yellow line). (**b**) Balloon burst during THV deployment

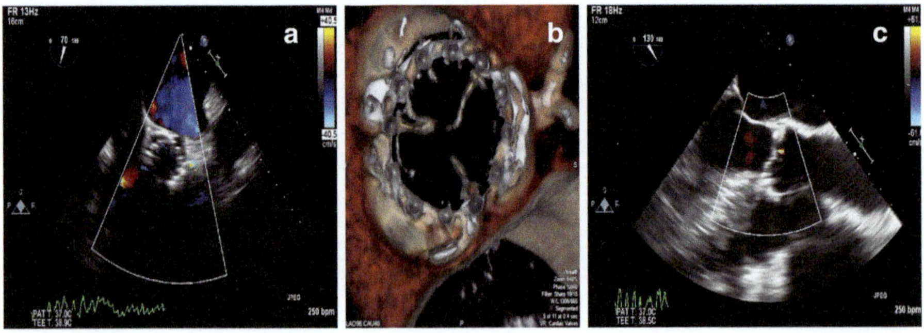

Fig. 6 Well seated Sapien-3 balloon-expandable THV over the AV annulus with no evidence of significant PVL. (**a**) ME AV SAX TEE view following the THD deployment. (**b**) Reconstructed TEE at follow-up. (**c**) ME LAX doppler TEE view

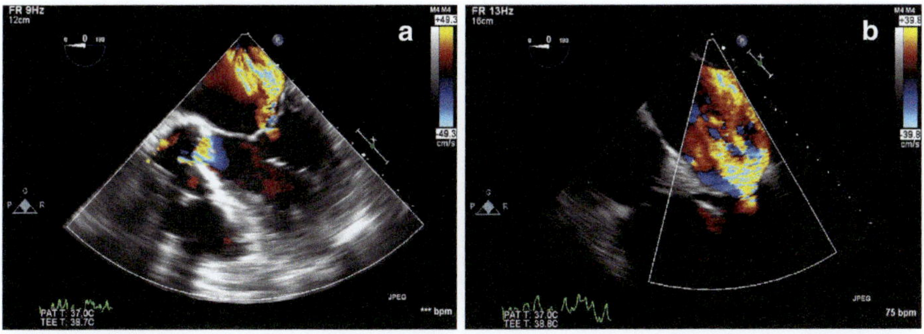

Fig. 7 ME 4C TEE view. (**a**) Mitral regurgitation before TAVR procedure. (**b**) Mitral regurgitation after TAVR procedure

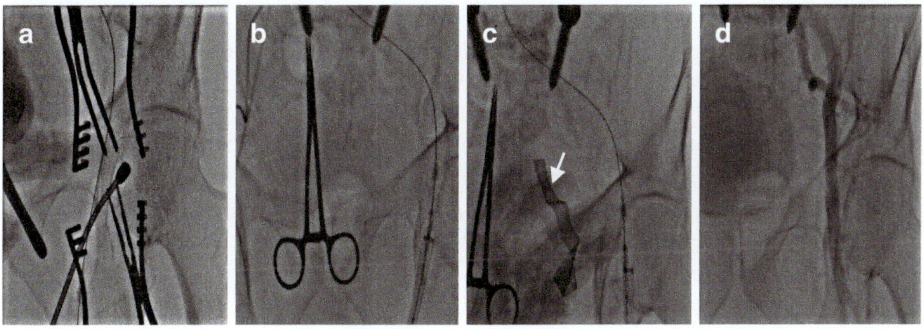

Fig. 8 Procedural images. (**a**) Open left common femoral arteriotomy to remove the burst THV balloon. (**b**) Atraumatic vascular clamp over the proximal part of the common femoral artery in the inguinal region. (**c**) Pericardial patch (white arrow) trimmed as an ellipse and sutured to the arteriotomy. (**d**) Angiography revealing patern left external iliac artery

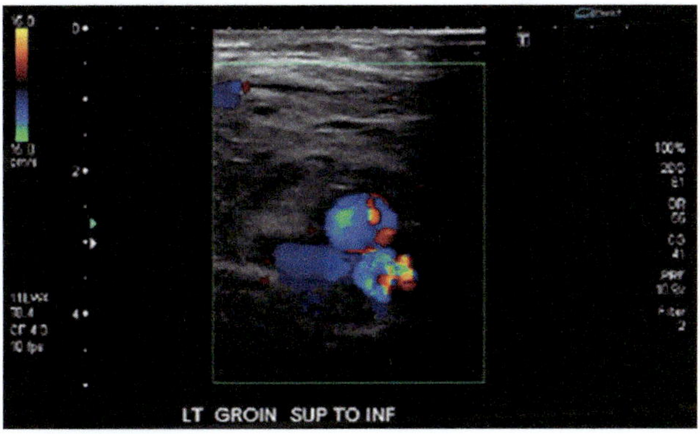

Fig. 9 Left femoral Doppler ultrasound indicating intact flow and no evidence of vascular dissection or pseudoaneurysm

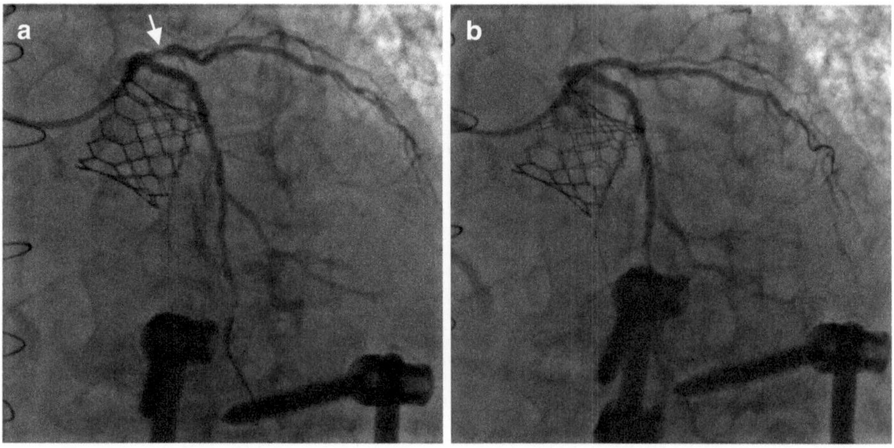

Fig. 10 Coronary angiography at follow-up. (**a**) A significant lesion along proximal segment of the LAD artery (white arrow). (**b**) After treated with drug eluting stent

remainder of the patient's hospitalization was uneventful as the patient remained hemodynamically stable. The patient developed ischemic chest pain during 1-year follow, requiring percutaneous coronary intervention and drug-eluting stent placement (Fig. 10).

4 Discussion

Balloon rupture of a transcatheter heart valve is a rare but serious complication during transcatheter aortic valve replacement (TAVR). In part, such an event makes the procedure substantially more complex with worse outcomes. Balloon rupture may lead to procedure failure due to difficulty retrieving the patient's delivery system and can be associated with other complications such as vascular injury, bleeding, surgical intervention, and death.

The mechanisms of intraoperative balloon rupture during TAVR can be an equipment malfunction, as seen with the Edwards SAPIEN 3 Ultra delivery system [1]. Still, other factors such as rapid or overinflation of the balloon, sharp calcific disease at the level of the aortic arch or valve, misalignment between the stent frame and delivery shaft, presence of a bicuspid aortic valve, aortic tortuosity, and protruding stents from the proximal right or left main coronary arteries are much more common [2–4]. Calcific disease at the valve, STJ, or LVOT is the most commonly encountered scenario and should be considered during pre-procedural planning.

Avoiding balloon rupture requires diligence both before and during the operation. Preoperative preparation includes accurate annular sizing to avoid balloon overinflation, assessing degrees of calcific disease, and accounting for above mentioned risk factors for balloon rupture.

Intraoperatively, operators should be familiar with feasible solutions at their disposal when balloon rupture does occur. It depends on whether the valve has remained attached to the delivery system, the degree of success of valve deployment, and how the remaining device should be removed [5, 6]. These considerations can determine if the balloon and delivery system can be removed as a single unit, the plausibility of exit through the point of access, and whether to consult surgical colleagues to provide alternative strategies. Alternative exit strategies include transapical removal and iliofemoral arteriotomy [7, 8].

Key Points

- Balloon rupture during TAVR is a rare but potentially serious complication.
- Recognizing high-risk patients and preoperative planning is essential.
- Risk factors include severe calcific disease and rapid/excessive balloon inflation.
- Device extraction strategies are specific to each procedure and patient.

References

1. Edwards lifesciences SAPIEN 3 ultra delivery system. Biomedical safety & standards. 2019;49:137–9.
2. Percutaneous balloon aortic valvuloplasty. Acute and 30-day follow-up results in 674 patients from the NHLBI Balloon Valvuloplasty Registry. Circulation. 1991;84(6):2383–97.
3. Blanke P, Reinöhl J, Schlensak C, Siepe M, Pache G, Euringer W, Geibel-Zehender A, Bode C, Langer M, Beyersdorf F, Zehender M. Prosthesis oversizing in balloon-expandable transcatheter aortic valve implantation is associated with contained rupture of the aortic root. Circ Cardiovasc Interv. 2012;5(4):540–8.
4. Kadoya Y, Zen K, Kuwabara K, Ito N, Yamano T, Nakamura T, Matoba S. Pinhole balloon rupture during valve alignment in TAVR using SAPIEN 3. JACC Cardiovasc Interv. 2019;12(12):1188–9.
5. Kubo S, Fuku Y, Shimamoto T, Kuwayama A, Ohya M, Amano H, Maruo T, Goto T, Komiya T, Kadota K. Vascular injury caused by retrieval of ruptured and detached balloon valvuloplasty catheter during transcatheter aortic valve replacement. JACC Cardiovasc Interv. 2017;10(15):1593–5.
6. Mustafa A, Farooq V, Manoly I, Hassan R, Fraser DG. Recurrent balloon rupture during Transcatheter Aortic Valve Replacement (TAVR)—implication for access site choice. Heart Lung Circ. 2015;24(11):e193–4.
7. Sawaya FJ, Roy A, Neylon A, Spaziano M, Hovasse T. An unusual complication after rupture of the SAPIEN 3 valve balloon during transcatheter aortic valve replacement. JACC Cardiovasc Interv. 2016;9(8):e79–81.
8. Pasala TK, Elmann EM, Ng AF, Song D, Ruiz CE. Transapical retrieval of a ruptured and immobilized TAVR balloon. In: Seminars in thoracic and cardiovascular surgery, September 1, vol 31, no 3. Amsterdam: Elsevier; 2019. p. 470–2.

Sapien-3 THV Dislodgment During Balloon Inflation

Ofir Koren, Edmund Naami, and Vivek Patel

1 Clinical Presentation

The patient was an 88-year-old male referred by his cardiologist to evaluate of worsening aortic stenosis and aortic regurgitation. Past medical history was remarkable for ascending aortic aneurysm (4.8 cm), diastolic heart failure (NYHA Class III–IV), atrial fibrillation (on Xarelto), hyperlipidemia, prostate cancer, GERD, and PAH. The patient complained of fatigue, dyspnea on exertion, intermittent edema of lower extremities, 2–3 pillow orthopnea, and intermittent dizziness. He denied chest pain, presyncope/syncope, palpitations, fevers, chills, recent infections or recent CHF-related hospitalizations.

Supplementary Information The online version contains supplementary material available at [https://doi.org/10.1007/978-3-031-05965-0_7].

O. Koren (✉)
Smidt Heart Institute, Cedars-Sinai Medical Center, Los Angeles, CA, USA

Faculty of Medicine, Technion, Israel Institute of Technology, Haifa, Israel
e-mail: Ofir.Koren@cshs.org

E. Naami
University of Illinois College of Medicine, Chicago, IL, USA

V. Patel
Smidt Heart Institute, Cedars-Sinai Medical Center, Los Angeles, CA, USA

O. Koren et al. (eds.), *Complex Cases in Structural Heart Intervention*,
https://doi.org/10.1007/978-3-031-05965-0_7

2 Images and Supported Data

TTE showed normal LV systolic function (67% EF), severe AS (AV peak velocity is 427 cm/s, mean transaortic gradient 47 mmHg, aortic valve area by continuity equation using VTI and Vmax 1.1 cm^2), and moderate-to-severe AR. TEE before the procedure showed severe aortic insufficiency with reconstructed CT measuring the ascending aortic aneurysm at 4.86 cm (Figs. 1 and 2, Videos 1 and 2). Cardiac reconstructed CT indicated an annular mean internal diameter of 27.5 mm, an area of 601.4 mm^2, and a perimeter of 87.3 mm. The following mean diameters were measured: 38.4 mm at the sinus of Valsalva, 35.3 mm at the STJ, and 26.6 mm at the LVOT. Quantitation of the calcium using 850 Hounsfield units as a threshold

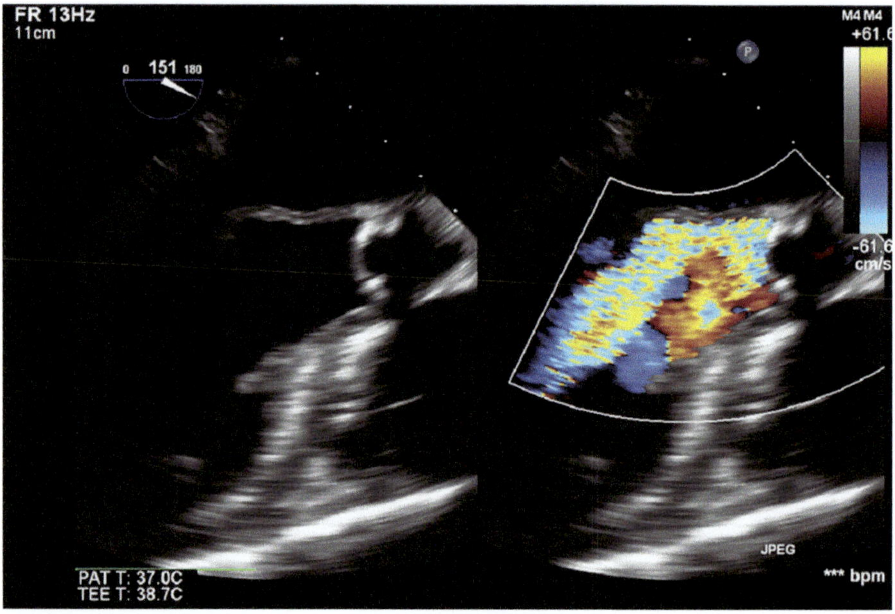

Fig. 1 Severe aortic insufficiency seen on mid-esophagus AV long axis TEE view

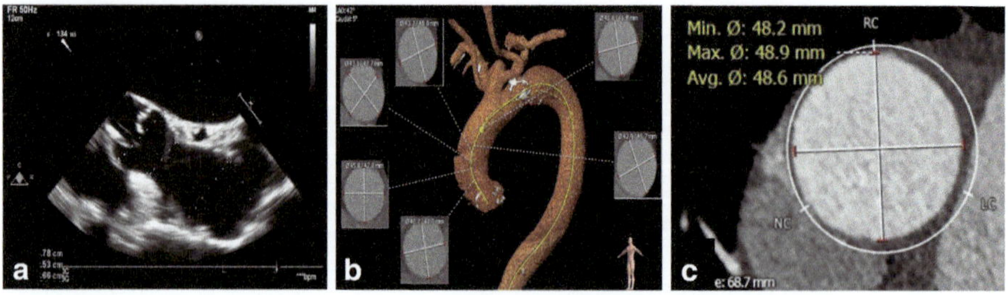

Fig. 2 Assessment of the ascending aortic aneurysm in different imaging modalities. (**a**) Mid-esophagus AV long axis TEE view. (**b**) CT reconstruction of the aortic arch with cross-sectional diameter measurements at various heights. (**c**) Cross-sectional diameter measurement at maximal distance

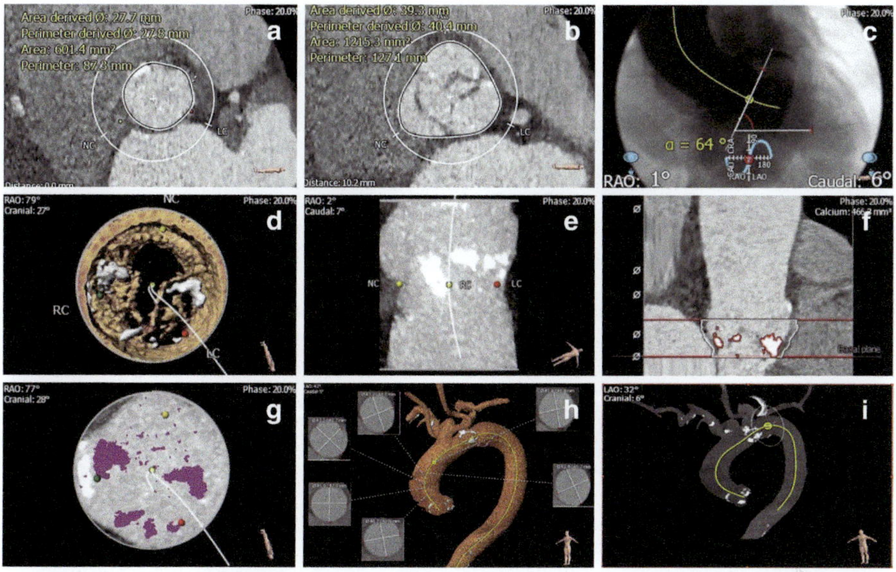

Fig. 3 Reconstruction CT measurements of the aortic valve and root. (**a**) AV annulus area and perimeter. (**b**) SOV area and perimeter. (**c**) Aortic root angulation. (**d**) Hockey puck en face VR indicating distribution of calcium plaques over the RCC and the LCC. (**e**) Hockey puck MIP side view. (**f**) Calcification assessment using HU850 threshold indicating 466.3 mm^3 volume of calcium. (**g**) Hockey puck en face MIP view. (**h**) Arch dimensions. (**i**) Arch calcification

indicated 466.3 mm^3 volume over the AV annulus. The aortic root angulation was 60° (Fig. 3). Reconstructed CT of the abdominal aorta and branches showed significant tortuosity of the common iliac arteries and significant calcification at abdominal aorta bifurcation.

3 Procedure and Outcome

The patient was evaluated by CT surgery and deemed to have intermediate surgical risk and therefore underwent transfemoral TAVR using a 29-mm Edwards Sapien 3 (S3) bioprosthesis. The valve was positioned across the stenotic aortic valve. At that point, we did not notice any ectopy or loss of capture. During balloon dilation (less than 20%), the THV embolized to the ascending aorta (Fig. 4, Video 3). Given the dilated ascending aorta (>40 mm diameter), the bioprosthetic valve was pulled back and deployed in the infrarenal abdominal aorta (Fig. 5, Video 4). Aortogram was performed below the deployed valve, which showed no dissection or leak (Video 5). Another valve, 29-mm Sapien S3, was then passed across the aortic annulus and successfully deployed with rapid ventricular pacing (Fig. 6, Videos 6 and 7). Post-deployment, there were excellent hemodynamics and trivial regurgitation. In the early postoperative period, the patient complained of worsening shortness of breath and substernal CP, cough, and groin pain. While initially stable, the patient

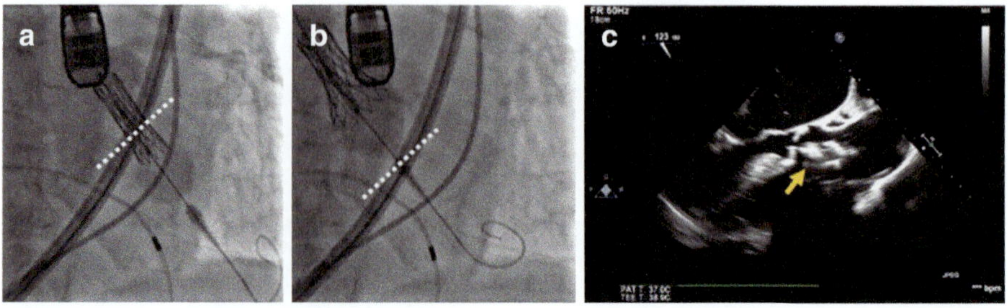

Fig. 4 THV displacement during deployment. (**a**) THV positioning at the AV annular plane (dashed lines) pre-balloon inflation. (**b**) THV displacement toward ascending aorta. (**c**) THV displacement (yellow arrow) seen on ME AV LAX TEE

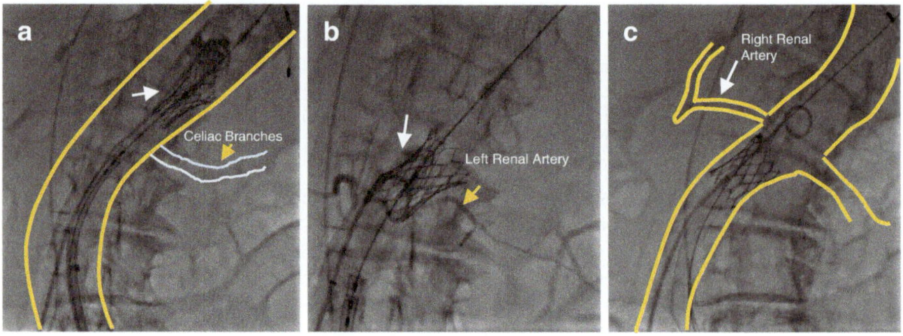

Fig. 5 Deployment of partially inflated THV. (**a**) Re-positioning of the undetached and partially inflated THV (white arrow) in the abdominal aorta (yellow lines) on its way below the celiac arteries (yellow arrow), (**b**) below the renal arteries (yellow arrow), (**c**) inflated at its final position (yellow arrow). The THV was further deflated to allow pulling back across descending aorta and reinflated below the renal arteries ostia

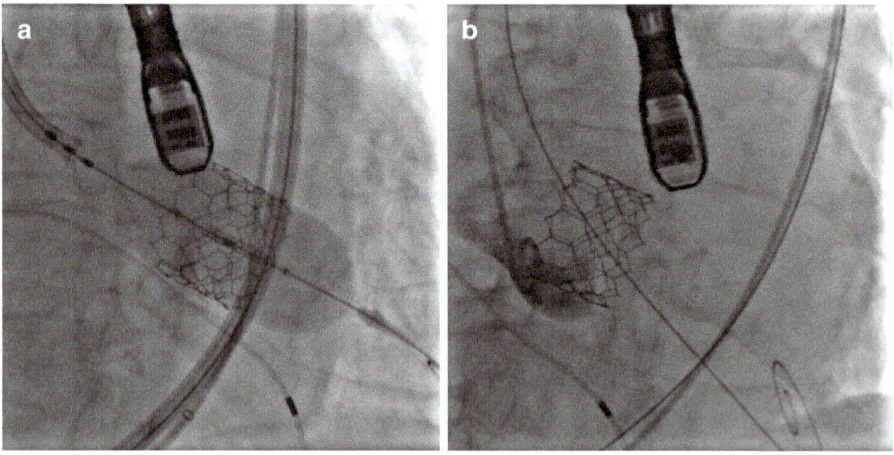

Fig. 6 Successful inflation of a second Sapien-3 THV over a native AV. (**a**) THV during balloon inflation. (**b**) Firmly attached THV over the AV annulus. The THV deployed slightly deeper into the LVOT with rapid inflation. No extra volume was needed

developed hypotension in the CCU and was sent for an urgent CT angiogram, which revealed type B aortic dissection, extending from the distal left subclavian to aortic bifurcation with contained rupture and left hemothorax (Fig. 7). He was taken urgently to the OR and underwent successful chest tube placement and thoracic endovascular aortic repair (TEVAR) using Medtronic Navion (Fig. 8). During the

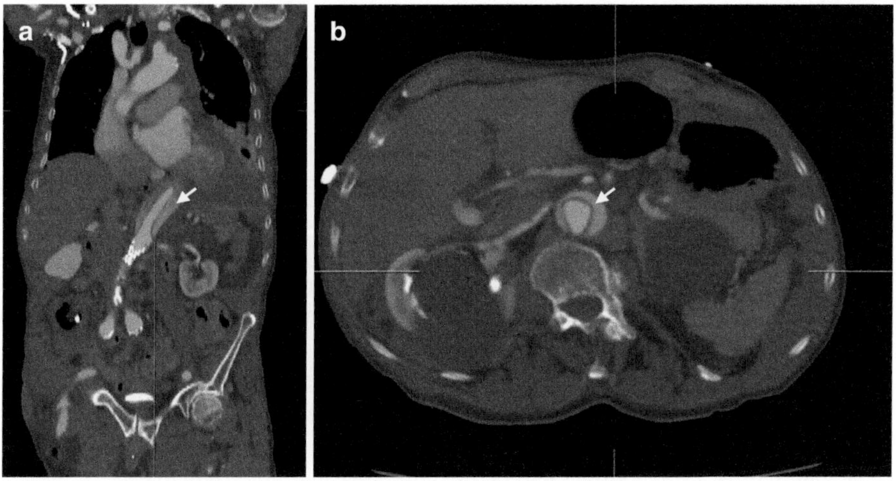

Fig. 7 Type B aortic dissection extending from the distal left subclavian to aortic bifurcation above the renal arteries. Note, the false lumen (white arrow). (**a**) Sagittal CT view. (**b**) Cross-section CT view

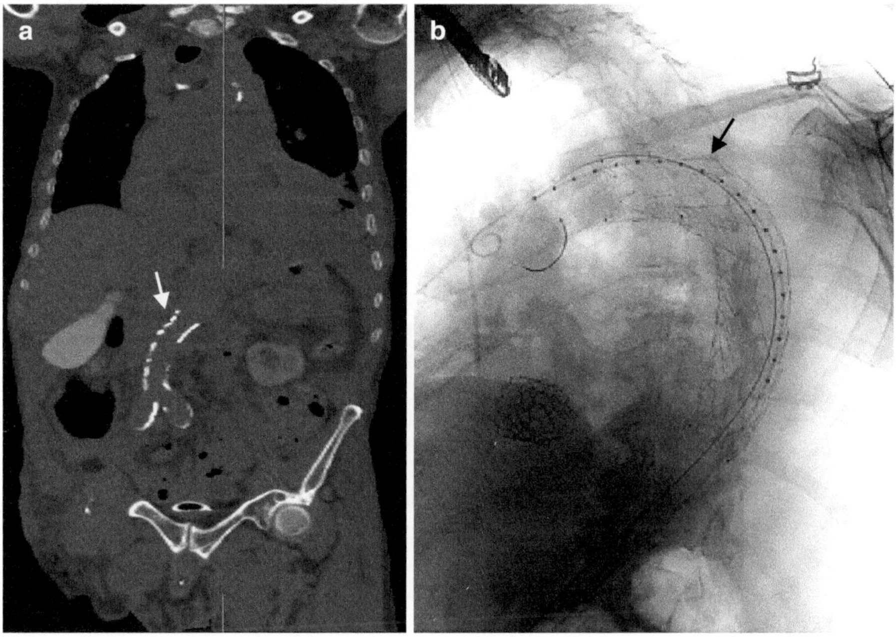

Fig. 8 Thoracic endovascular aortic repair (TEVAR) of the descending aorta. (**a**) Longitudinal CT view (white arrow). (**b**) X-ray (black arrow)

same hospitalization, the patient dropped to a heart rate of 30 bpm with frequent symptomatic pauses. He was transferred back to the CCU and taken for urgent pacemaker placement. A consecutive CT angiogram confirmed no retroperitoneal bleed or new fluid collections. The patient was discharged home 12 days after the TAVR procedure. The patient passed away 16 months after discharge while in hospice hospital.

4 Discussion

Valve migration and embolization are relatively rare but potentially devastating complications of transcatheter aortic valve implantation, with studies estimating an incidence rate of approximately 1% [1]. Potential causes of valve dislodgment include sizing errors, large annuli, limited or asymmetric valve, pacing failures, post-dilation, and device malpositioning (e.g., failure to disengage the prosthesis and delivery system) [2, 3]. The co-existence of moderate to severe aortic regurgitation creates a dynamic jet across the AV, interfering with valve deployment. To overcome these anatomical and hemodynamic situations, we recommend placing the THV firmly into the LVOT and ensuring that the deployment (either balloon-expandable or self-expanding) will carry on rapidly and not gradually.

Furthermore, operators must select an appropriately sized prosthetic valve, ensure precise positioning, and observe technical aspects of each device. Balloon-expandable valves for example require effective rapid pacing while self-expanding valves rely on high device placement. While most dislodgement events occur intraoperatively or shortly after completion of the procedure, delayed embolization has been described to occur up to 43 days postoperatively [4–7]. Treatment strategies can depend on the location of the prosthesis. Percutaneous management has shown to be sufficient for prostheses located in the aorta, whereas embolization into the left ventricle often requires conversion to open-heart surgery. Ultimately, implantation of a second transcatheter heart valve during the same procedure has been effective and is considered first-line treatment [8, 9].

Key Points

- Valve migration is a rare phenomenon that occurs mostly during the procedure. It poses a catastrophic consequence and is challenging to address.
- Meticulous pre-procedural planning should be focused on the entire aortic root dimension, particularly the annulus and the LVOT.
- Asymmetrical valve calcification, pacing failure, and device malpositioning are known risk factors.
- Operators should be familiar with all percutaneous and surgical solutions for dislodged THV.

References

1. Kim WK, Schäfer U, Tchetche D, Nef H, Arnold M, Avanzas P, Rudolph T, Scholtz S, Barbanti M, Kempfert J, Mangieri A, Lauten A, Frerker C, Yoon SH, Holzamer A, Praz F, De Backer O, Toggweiler S, Blumenstein J, Purita P, Tarantini G, Thilo C, Wolf A, Husser O, Pellegrini C, Burgdorf C, Antolin RAH, Díaz VAJ, Liebetrau C, Schofer N, Möllmann H, Eggebrecht H, Sondergaard L, Walther T, Pilgrim T, Hilker M, Makkar R, Unbehaun A, Börgermann J, Moris C, Achenbach S, Dörr O, Brochado B, Conradi L, Hamm CW. Incidence and outcome of peri-procedural transcatheter heart valve embolization and migration: the TRAVEL registry (TranscatheteR HeArt Valve EmboLization and Migration). Eur Heart J. 2019;40(38):3156–65. PMID: 31230081. https://doi.org/10.1093/eurheartj/ehz429.
2. Masson JB, Kovac J, Schuler G, Ye J, Cheung A, Kapadia S, Tuzcu ME, Kodali S, Leon MB, Webb JG. Transcatheter aortic valve implantation: review of the nature, management, and avoidance of procedural complications. JACC Cardiovasc Interv. 2009;2(9):811–20. PMID: 19778768. https://doi.org/10.1016/j.jcin.2009.07.005.
3. Binder RK, Webb JG. Transcatheter heart valve migration and embolization: rare and preventable? Eur Heart J. 2019;40(38):3166–8. PMID: 31377802. https://doi.org/10.1093/eurheartj/ehz562.
4. Nkomo VT, Suri RM, Pislaru SV, Greason KL, Sinak LJ, Holmes DR, Mathew V, Rihal CS. Delayed transcatheter heart valve migration and failure. JACC Cardiovasc Imaging. 2014;7(9):960–2. PMID: 25212804. https://doi.org/10.1016/j.jcmg.2014.02.010.
5. Clavel MA, Dumont E, Pibarot P, Doyle D, De Larochellière R, Villeneuve J, Bergeron S, Couture C, Rodés-Cabau J. Severe valvular regurgitation and late prosthesis embolization after percutaneous aortic valve implantation. Ann Thorac Surg. 2009;87(2):618–21. PMID: 19161796. https://doi.org/10.1016/j.athoracsur.2008.06.059.
6. Pang PY, Chiam PT, Chua YL, Sin YK. A survivor of late prosthesis migration and rotation following percutaneous transcatheter aortic valve implantation. Eur J Cardiothorac Surg. 2012;41(5):1195–6. Epub 2012 Jan 6. PMID: 22228843. https://doi.org/10.1093/ejcts/ezr195.
7. Radu C, Raffoul R, Brochet E, Himbert D. Delayed migration of a transfemorally implanted aortic bioprosthesis. J Thorac Cardiovasc Surg. 2012;143(1):e1–3. Epub 2011 Oct 11. PMID: 21996299. https://doi.org/10.1016/j.jtcvs.2011.09.014.
8. Makkar RR, Jilaihawi H, Chakravarty T, Fontana GP, Kapadia S, Babaliaros V, Cheng W, Thourani VH, Bavaria J, Svensson L, Kodali S, Shiota T, Siegel R, Tuzcu EM, Xu K, Hahn RT, Herrmann HC, Reisman M, Whisenant B, Lim S, Beohar N, Mack M, Teirstein P, Rihal C, Douglas PS, Blackstone E, Pichard A, Webb JG, Leon MB. Determinants and outcomes of acute transcatheter valve-in-valve therapy or embolization: a study of multiple valve implants in the U.S. PARTNER trial (Placement of AoRTic TraNscathetER Valve Trial Edwards SAPIEN Transcatheter Heart Valve). J Am Coll Cardiol. 2013;62(5):418–30. Epub 2013 May 15. PMID: 23684680. https://doi.org/10.1016/j.jacc.2013.04.037.
9. Ussia GP, Barbanti M, Ramondo A, Petronio AS, Ettori F, Santoro G, Klugmann S, Bedogni F, Maisano F, Marzocchi A, Poli A, Napodano M, Tamburino C. The valve-in-valve technique for treatment of aortic bioprosthesis malposition an analysis of incidence and 1-year clinical outcomes from the Italian CoreValve registry. J Am Coll Cardiol. 2011;57(9):1062–8. PMID: 21349397. https://doi.org/10.1016/j.jacc.2010.11.019.

Valve Emboli Due to Non-Captured Pacing

Ofir Koren, Edmund Naami, and Jubin Joseph

1 Clinical Presentation

The patient is a 75-year-old male evaluated for worsening shortness of breath. The patient's past medical history is remarkable for hypertension, coronary artery disease, aortic valve stenosis, glaucoma, and a 20-year smoking history. The patient has been experiencing worsening fatigue and dyspnea on exertion for the past 6 months.

2 Images and Supported Data

TTE revealed a severe calcific aortic valve, a mean gradient of 40 mmHg, a peak gradient of 64 mmHg, and preserved ejection fraction (Fig. 1). Coronary angiogram showed nonobstructive coronary disease (Fig. 2). Cardiac reconstructed CT indicated an annular mean internal diameter of 24.2 mm, area of 452.9 mm^2, and perimeter of 76.3 mm. The following means diameters were measured: 32.4 mm at the

Supplementary Information The online version contains supplementary material available at [https://doi.org/10.1007/978-3-031-05965-0_8].

O. Koren (✉)
Smidt Heart Institute, Cedars-Sinai Medical Center, Los Angeles, CA, USA

Faculty of Medicine, Technion, Israel Institute of Technology, Haifa, Israel
e-mail: Ofir.Koren@cshs.org

E. Naami
University of Illinois College of Medicine, Chicago, IL, USA

J. Joseph
Senior Interventional cardiologist, Assistant Professor, Cedars Sinai Medical Center, Los Angeles, California, USA

O. Koren et al. (eds.), *Complex Cases in Structural Heart Intervention*,
https://doi.org/10.1007/978-3-031-05965-0_8

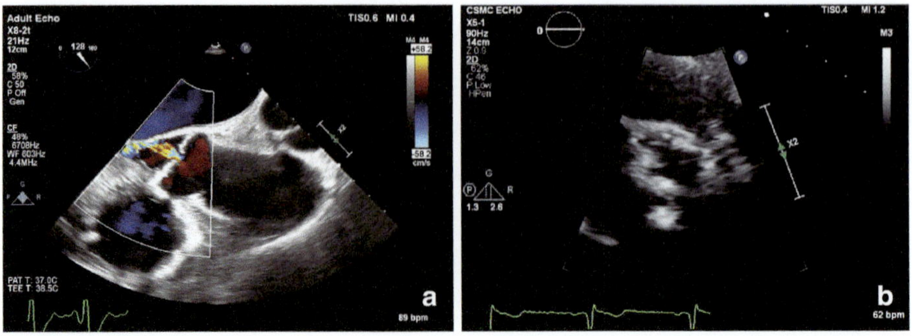

Fig. 1 TEE imaging before TAVR procedure. (**a**) Severe stenotic and calcified AV seen on ME LAX TEE view. (**b**) SAX TTE view

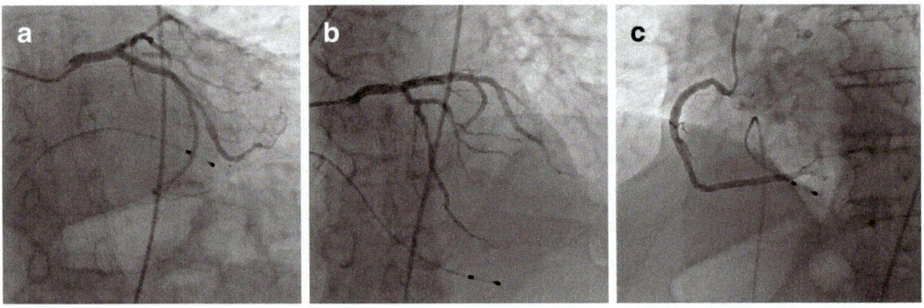

Fig. 2 Coronary angiography indicating nonobstructive coronary artery disease. (**a**, **b**) Left coronary artery, (**c**) the right coronary artery

sinus of Valsalva, 30.1 mm at the STJ, and 23.4 mm at the LVOT. The aortic diameter was 40 mm above the annulus with maximal aortic diameter of 33.3 and 36.3 mm, respectively (Fig. 3). Quantifying the calcium using 850 Hounsfield units as a threshold indicated a 240.1 mm^3 volume of calcium over the AV annulus (Fig. 4).

3 Procedure and Outcome

The heart team evaluated the patient and found him suitable for transfemoral TAVR using a 26-mm Edwards Sapien S3 bioprosthesis. The delivery system and THV were positioned across the stenotic aortic valve using standard technique. With rapid pacing at 180 beats per minute, the valve was deployed. However, at 50% deployment, the pacemaker lost capture, and the patient experienced a PVC leading to THV embolization before full deployment (Fig. 5, Video 1). At this point, the patient was stable. The valve was then maneuvered into the descending aorta (Video 2). The size of the descending aorta was assessed using TEE and found to be 25–26 mm,

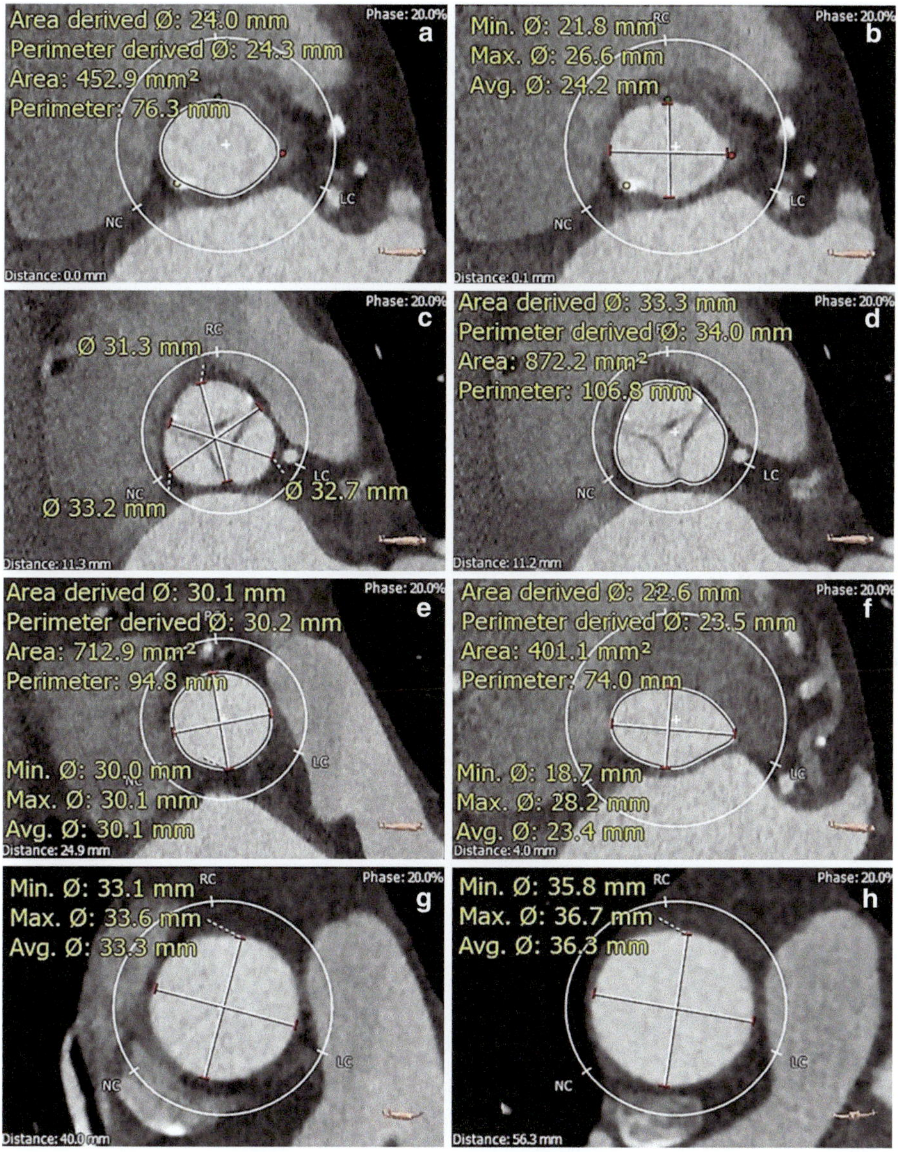

Fig. 3 Reconstructed CT analysis pre-TAVR. (**a**) AV annular area and perimeter. (**b**) AV annular diameter. (**c**) SOV area and perimeter. (**d**) SOV diameters. (**e**) Sinotubular junction diameter. (**f**) LVOT diameter. (**g**) Aortic diameter at 40 mm above annulus. (**h**) Maximal aortic diameter

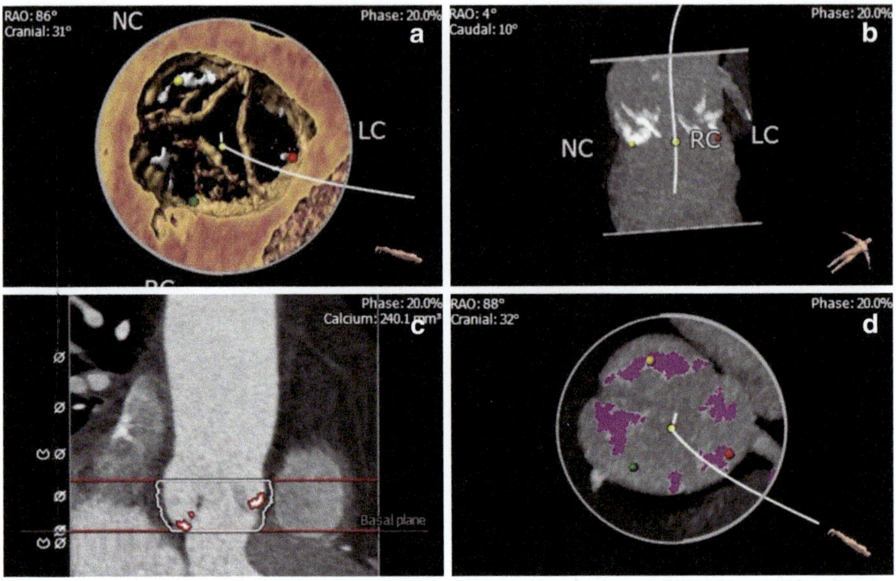

Fig. 4 Calcium quantification and distribution over the annulus and the aortic root in various modes. (**a**) AV annulus in sagittal cross-section view (Hockey Puck VR mode). (**b**) Longitudinal calcification mode (Hockey Puck MIP mode). (**c**) Longitudinal view and (**d**) sagittal view using an 850 Hounsfield unit as a threshold

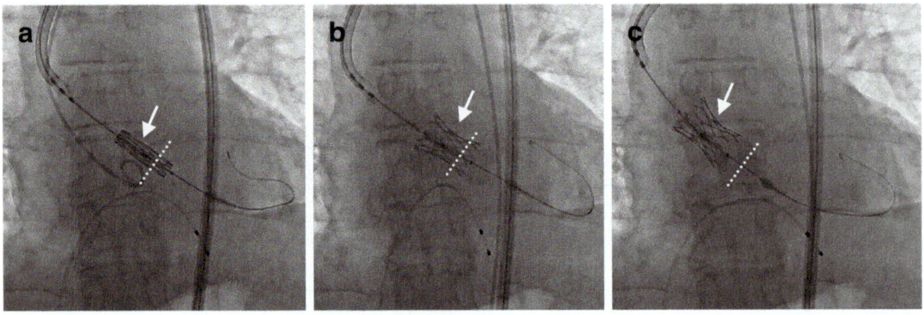

Fig. 5 TAVR procedure. (**a**) Balloon-expandable THV (white arrow) positioned over the AV annulus (dashed white line) before balloon inflation. (**b**) During balloon inflation. (**c**) The displacement of the inflated THH toward the ascending aorta

appropriate for a 26 mm Sapien Ultra transcatheter valve. The valve was successfully deployed in the descending aorta guided by TEE and an aortogram (Figs. 6 and 7, Video 3). Following deployment, the valve was well-positioned without paravalvular leak and no extravasation outside of the aorta. A second 26 Ultra transcatheter valve was then prepared, passed across the aortic annulus, and deployed under rapid ventricular pacing (Fig. 6, Video 4). There were excellent hemodynamics, trivial regurgitation, and minimal gradient (Fig. 7, Video 5). The patient was stable and tolerated the procedure at discharge and 30-day follow-up (Fig. 8).

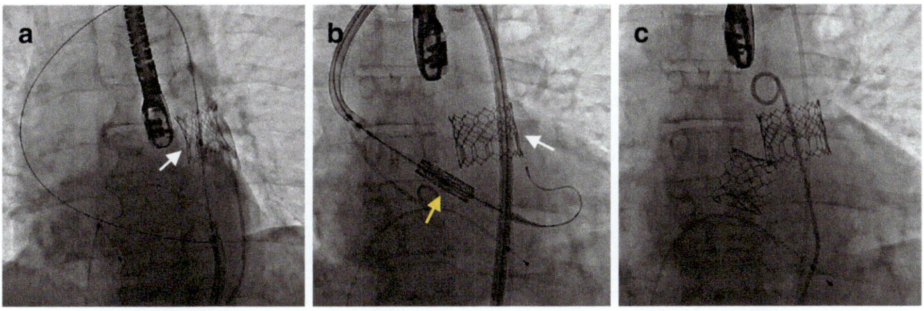

Fig. 6 TAVR procedure. (**a**) Repositioning the partially inflated balloon-expandable THV (white arrow) in the descending aorta. (**b**) Final deployment of first Sapien 3 valve. (**c**) Second balloon-expandable THV positioned over the AV annulus (yellow arrow) and successfully inflated

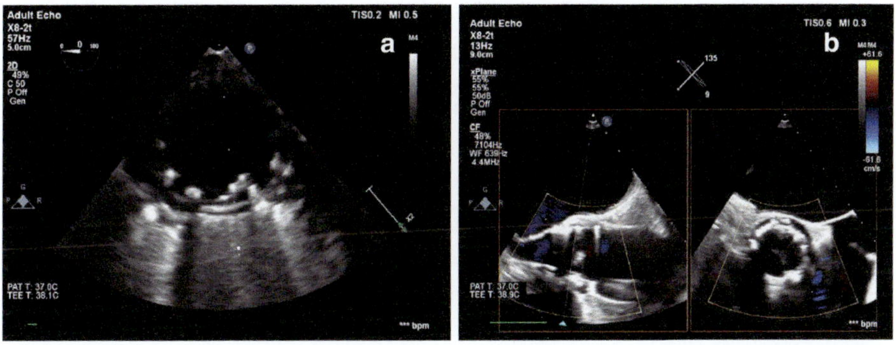

Fig. 7 Balloon-expandable THV positioning in the descending aorta using TEE guidance. (**a**) The metallic THV struts seen on descending aorta SAX TEE view. (**b**) Second balloon-expandable THV successfully deployed over the AV annulus

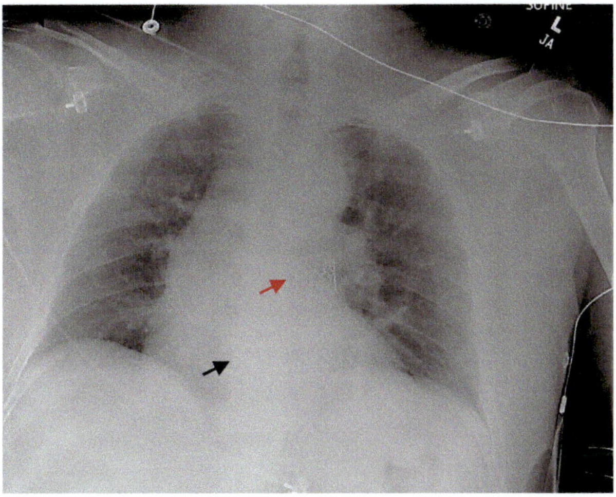

Fig. 8 Chest X-ray after the deployment of the THVs at the AV annulus (black arrow) and the descending aorta (red arrow)

4 Discussion

Valve embolization is a relatively rare but potentially life-threatening complication of transcatheter heart valve implantation, with studies estimating an incidence rate of approximately 1% [1]. Potential causes of valve embolization include using an inappropriately sized prosthesis, presence of severe left ventricular hypertrophy, prematurely stopping pacing, and failing to inflate the balloon [2–4] adequately. Studies suggest that patients with bicuspid aortic valves are at increased risk of embolization when undergoing transcatheter aortic valve implantation [1, 5]. To reduce the probability of embolization, the provider must select an appropriately sized prosthesis, ensure precise positioning, and deliver effective rapid pacing. The majority of embolization events occur immediately at the time of implantation.

Nevertheless, delayed embolization has been described in the literature to occur up to 43 days postoperatively [6–8]. Implantation of a second transcatheter heart valve is considered a first-line treatment for embolization [9–12]. Treatment strategies depend on the location of the prosthesis. For example, embolization of the aorta has been successfully treated with a percutaneous approach in which coaxial guide wires were used to prevent blood flow obstruction. In comparison, embolization to the left ventricle most often requires open-heart surgery [13].

Key Points

- Effective rapid pacing is essential for the safe delivery of balloon-expandable TAVR devices.
- Peri-procedural device embolization can occur due to sizing mismatch, inappropriate placement, insufficient calcium, or failure of rapid pacing.
- If embolization occurs, it is essential not to lose wire access through the embolized valve to prevent the device from flipping and impeding blood flow.
- Repositioning the embolized valve in the descending aorta away from major branches where there is an appropriate diameter for device anchoring.
- Post-dilatation should be pursued to ensure valve stability.
- Safe valve delivery through the embolized valve can be performed.

References

1. Kim WK, Schäfer U, Tchetche D, Nef H, Arnold M, Avanzas P, Rudolph T, Scholtz S, Barbanti M, Kempfert J, Mangieri A. Incidence and outcome of peri-procedural transcatheter heart valve embolization and migration: the TRAVEL registry (TranscatheteR HeArt Valve EmboLization and Migration). Eur Heart J. 2019;40(38):3156–65.
2. Masson JB, Kovac J, Schuler G, Ye J, Cheung A, Kapadia S, Tuzcu ME, Kodali S, Leon MB, Webb JG. Transcatheter aortic valve implantation: a review of the nature, management, and avoidance of procedural complications. J Am Coll Cardiol Interv. 2009;2(9):811–20.
3. Binder RK, Webb JG. Transcatheter heart valve migration and embolization: rare and preventable? Eur Heart J. 2019;40(38):3166–8.

4. Giannini F, Montorfano M, Romano V, Ruparelia N, Jabbour RJ, Benincasa S, Latib A, Colombo A. Valve embolization with a second-generation fully-retrievable and repositionable transcatheter aortic valve. Int J Cardiol. 2016;223:867–9.
5. Cimci M, Roffi M, Noble S. Embolization to two different vascular territories in a patient with bicuspid aortic stenosis undergoing transcatheter aortic valve implantation. CJC Open. 2020;2(5):432–4.
6. Nkomo VT, Suri RM, Pislaru SV, Greason KL, Sinak LJ, Holmes DR, Mathew V, Rihal CS. Delayed transcatheter heart valve migration and failure. JACC Cardiovasc Imaging. 2014;7(9):960–2.
7. Clavel MA, Dumont E, Pibarot P, Doyle D, De Larochellière R, Villeneuve J, Bergeron S, Couture C, Rodés-Cabau J. Severe valvular regurgitation and late prosthesis embolization after percutaneous aortic valve implantation. Ann Thorac Surg. 2009;87(2):618–21.
8. Pang PY, Chiam PT, Chua YL, Sin YK. A survivor of late prosthesis migration and rotation following percutaneous transcatheter aortic valve implantation. Eur J Cardiothorac Surg. 2012;41(5):1195–6.
9. Radu C, Raffoul R, Brochet E, Himbert D. Delayed migration of a transfemorally implanted aortic bioprosthesis. J Thorac Cardiovasc Surg. 2012;143(1):e1–3.
10. Makkar RR, Jilaihawi H, Chakravarty T, Fontana GP, Kapadia S, Babaliaros V, Cheng W, Thourani VH, Bavaria J, Svensson L, Kodali S. Determinants and outcomes of acute transcatheter valve-in-valve therapy or embolization: a study of multiple valve implants in the US PARTNER trial (Placement of AoRTic TraNscathetER Valve Trial Edwards SAPIEN Transcatheter Heart Valve). J Am Coll Cardiol. 2013;62(5):418–30.
11. Ussia GP, Barbanti M, Ramondo A, Petronio AS, Ettori F, Santoro G, Klugmann S, Bedogni F, Maisano F, Marzocchi A, Poli A. The valve-in-valve technique for treatment of aortic bioprosthesis malposition: an analysis of incidence and 1-year clinical outcomes from the Italian CoreValve registry. J Am Coll Cardiol. 2011;57(9):1062–8.
12. Moreno-Samos JC, Vidovich MI. Device embolization in transcatheter aortic valve procedures: expect the unexpected. JACC Case Rep. 2019;1(2):105–7.
13. Tay EL, Gurvitch R, Wijeysinghe N, Nietlispach F, Leipsic J, Wood DA, Yong G, Cheung A, Ye J, Lichtenstein SV, Carere R. Outcome of patients after transcatheter aortic valve embolization. J Am Coll Cardiol Interv. 2011;4(2):228–34.

Bailout Solution in a Case of an Embolized Balloon Expanding THV

Ofir Koren, Rafael Skorka, and Mamoo Nakamura

1 Clinical Presentation

An 87-year-old obese male with a past medical history of emphysema from extensive tobacco use, thrombocytopenia, hypertension and hyperlipidemia has had progressive dyspnea with minimal exertion, bilateral lower extremity edema, and fatigue. He also reported multiple syncopal episodes and chest pain and is now wheelchair-bound. Cardiac workup at an outside facility demonstrated severe aortic stenosis and coronary artery disease with high-grade stenosis in the mid-left anterior descending (LAD) artery. He was referred for treatment evaluation of aortic stenosis and coronary artery disease.

2 Images and Supported Data

Transthoracic echocardiogram revealed hyperdynamic left-ventricular systolic function with an ejection fraction of 78%, aortic valve area of 0.7 cm^2, mean peak gradients of 48 and 69 mmHg, respectively. Pre-TAVR reconstructed CT of

Supplementary Information The online version contains supplementary material available at [https://doi.org/10.1007/978-3-031-05965-0_9].

O. Koren (✉)
Smidt Heart Institute, Cedars-Sinai Medical Center, Los Angeles, CA, USA

Faculty of Medicine, Technion, Israel Institute of Technology, Haifa, Israel
e-mail: Ofir.Koren@cshs.org

R. Skorka
Smidt Heart Institute, Cedars-Sinai Medical Center, Los Angeles, CA, USA

M. Nakamura
Cedars Sinai Medical Center, Los Angeles, California, USA

O. Koren et al. (eds.), *Complex Cases in Structural Heart Intervention*,
https://doi.org/10.1007/978-3-031-05965-0_9

periaortic valve anatomy demonstrated the following key annular measurements; the mean internal diameter of 22.5 mm, the area of 399.8 mm^2, and the perimeter of 71.7 mm. Mean diameters of the Sinus of Valsalva, the STJ, and the LVOT were 35.7, 33.7, and 20.9 mm, respectively (Fig. 1). The maximal diameter of the ascending aorta was 39.7 mm, with angulation between the aortic root and left ventricle of 67°. The coronary ostia originated above the annular plane, and the distance from the annulus level to the ostium was 20.1 mm for the RCA and 14.5 mm for the LCA. Using 850 Hounsfield units as a threshold, the aortic root calcium was quantified at 287.7 mm^3 (Fig. 2). Reconstructed CT angiogram of the aorta to femoral artery demonstrated a right-side aortic arch with an abnormal take of the left subclavian artery. Minimal calcification was observed, but there was significant tortuosity of the entire aorta. There is moderate tortuosity in the right innominate artery, the left subclavian artery, and the bilateral iliofemoral arteries without stenosis (Figs. 3, 4, and 5, Videos 1, 2 and 3).

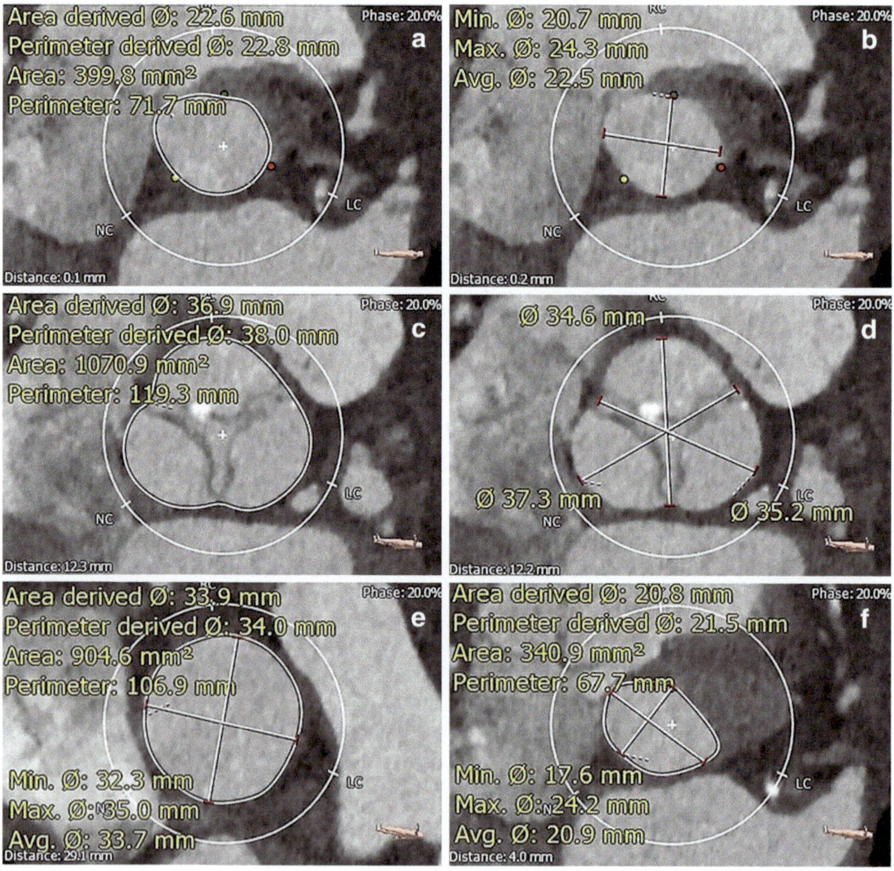

Fig. 1 Reconstructed CT analysis pre-TAVR. (**a**, **b**) Area, perimeter, and diameter measurement of the AV annulus. (**c**, **d**) SOV. (**e**) The sinotubular junction. (**f**) The LVOT

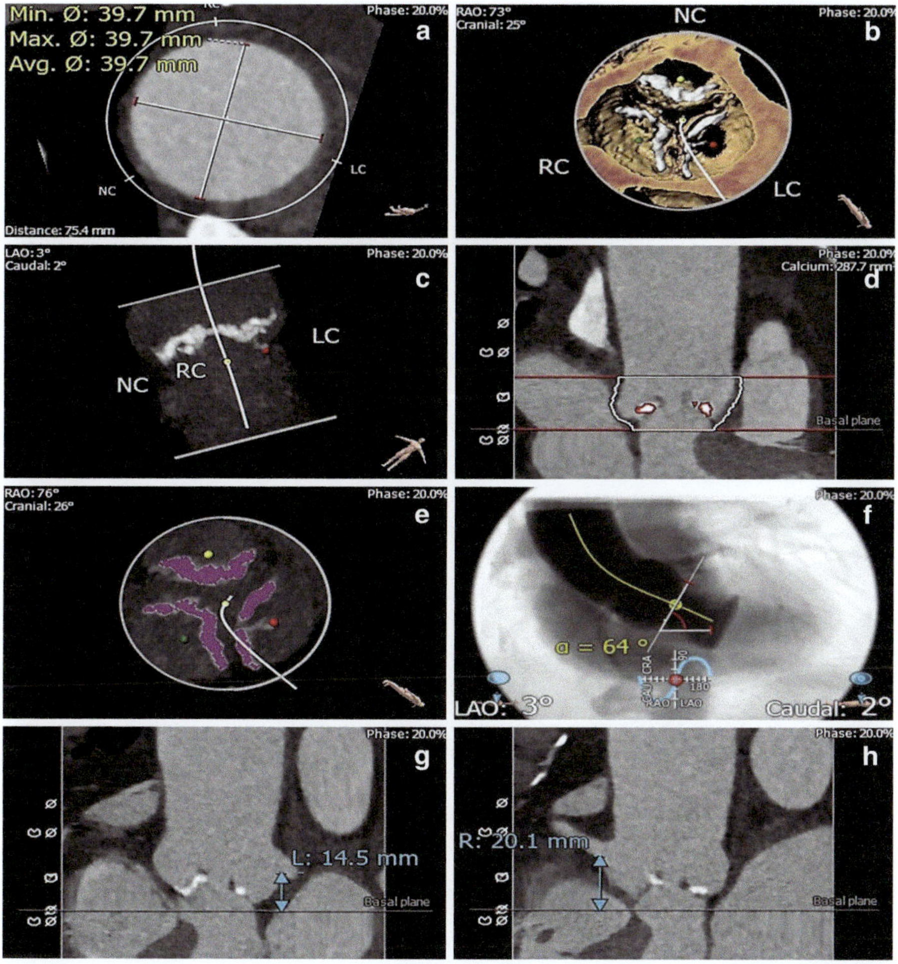

Fig. 2 Reconstructed CT analysis pre-TAVR. (**a**) Maximal diameter of the ascending aorta. (**b**) Hockey puck VR view of the aortic annulus. (**c**) Long axis hockey puck MIP view of aortic valve. (**d**) The aneurysmal region near the right coronary cusps. (**e**) Aortic root calcification assessment using a HU850 threshold. (**f**) Co-planar angle between the LV and aortic root. (**g**, **h**) Coronary artery height above the annular plane

3 Pre-Procedural Consideration: Pitfalls, Dilemmas, and Challenges

The heart team evaluated the patient and decided that the patient was an appropriate candidate for TAVR and concomitant percutaneous coronary intervention. Due to excessive tortuosity of the entire aorta, favorable trajectory, and acceptable vessel caliber, the right subclavian was chosen as the access site for TAVR. Based on reconstructed CT measurements, we decided to use a 23-mm Sapien-3 Ultra transcatheter heart valve.

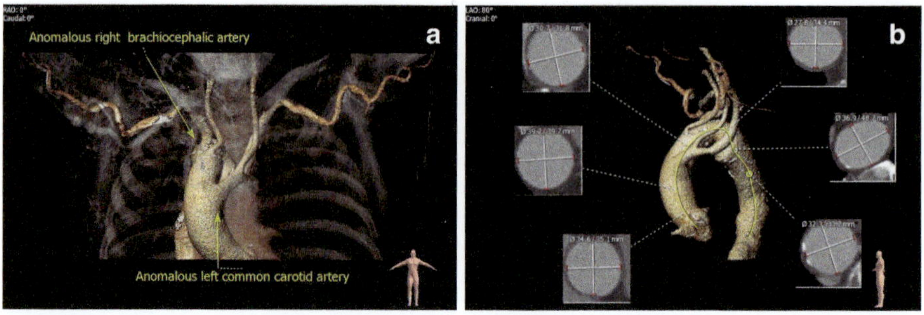

Fig. 3 Aortic arch CT analysis. (**a**) The tortuosity and anomaly of the right brachiocephalic artery and the left common carotid artery. (**b**) The diameter of the ascending aorta

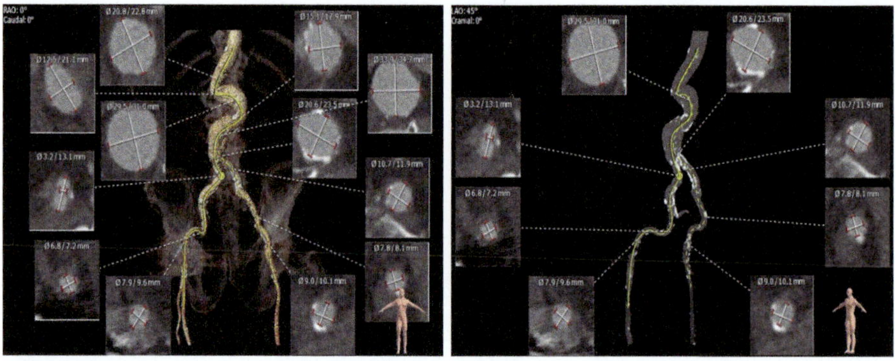

Fig. 4 Abdominal aorta and iliofemoral arteries CT analysis indicating a significant calcification and tortuosity

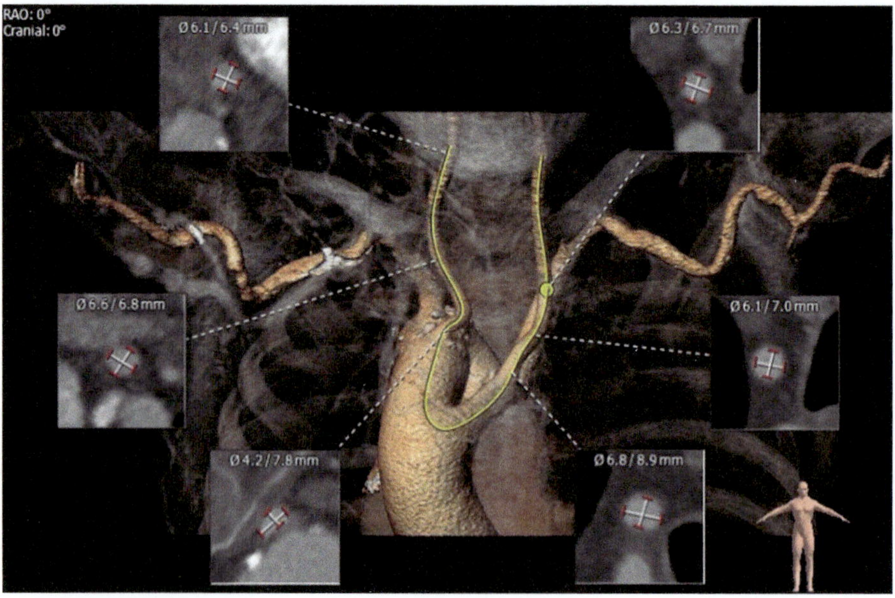

Fig. 5 Pre-procedural subclavian CT analysis

4 Procedure and Outcome

We initially performed coronary intervention and treated the LAD stenosis via the left femoral access using a 3.0 × 20 mm Synergy drug-eluting stent (Fig. 6). Subsequently, we attempted to advance the valve via the right subclavian approach through a 14-french e-sheath (Video 4). Despite multiple attempts, the valve deployment system could not be advanced across the native aortic valve. The valve delivery system was removed, and pre-dilation of the native aortic valve was then performed with a 22 mm × 5 mm Emerge balloon (Fig. 7).

Following this, the 23-mm Sapien 3 ultra-transcatheter heart valve was advanced and deployed under rapid RV pacing at 180 bpm using a nominal balloon inflation volume. Immediately following valve deployment, TEE demonstrated the ventricular edge of the transcatheter valve above the annular plane (Figs. 8 and 9, Videos 5, 6 and 7). Subsequent fluoroscopy showed an embolized transcatheter valve toward the ascending aorta (Fig. 10, Video 8).

We remeasured the aortic valve area using transesophageal echocardiography. TEE indicated an area of 450 mm^2, much higher than on CT. Based on this measurement, a 26-mm Sapien 3 ultra-transcatheter heart valve was advanced from the right subclavian and deployed across the aortic valve under rapid pacing at normal inflation volume (Fig. 11, Videos 9 and 10). The valve delivery system was then parked in the subclavian sheath.

Next, the focus shifted to managing the embolized aortic valve. A 6-French sheath was inserted in the left femoral artery following puncture of the artery with a micropuncture kit needle under ultrasound guidance. A 6-French multipurpose catheter was advanced over a J-wire into the abdominal aorta, advancing a 0.035-in. Terumo Glidewire into the ascending aorta. The multipurpose catheter was advanced into the thoracic aorta.

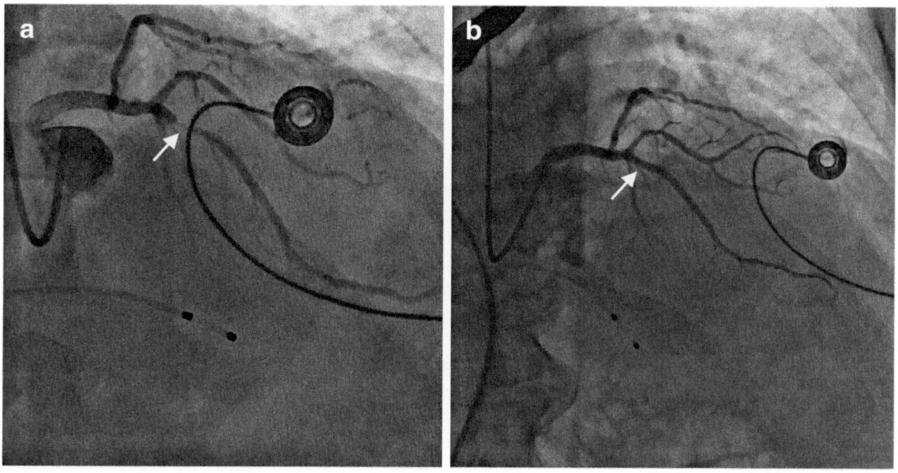

Fig. 6 Coronary angiography before the TAVR. (**a**) Significant lesion on mid LAD (white arrow). (**b**) After implantation of a drug-eluting stent (white arrow)

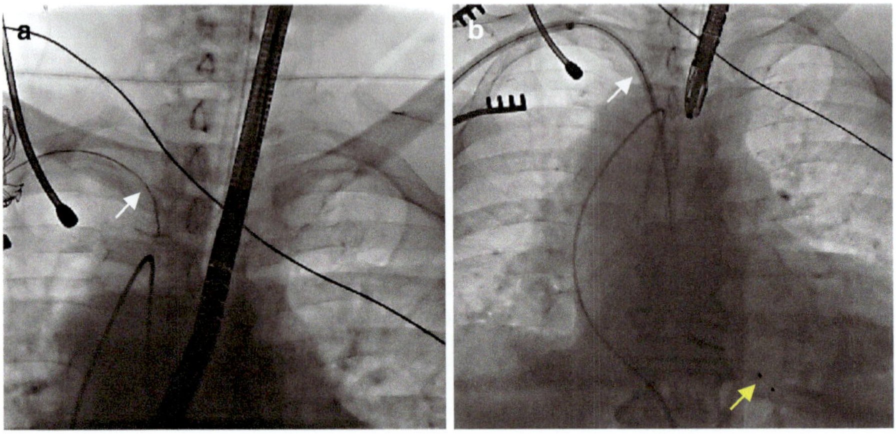

Fig. 7 Subclavian TAVR approach. (**a**) Initial attempts to cross the aortic annulus with the THV delivery system in the subclavian approach failed. (**b**) We successfully crossed the annulus using a pre-dilatation technique with a 22 mm × 5 mm Emerge balloon (yellow arrow)

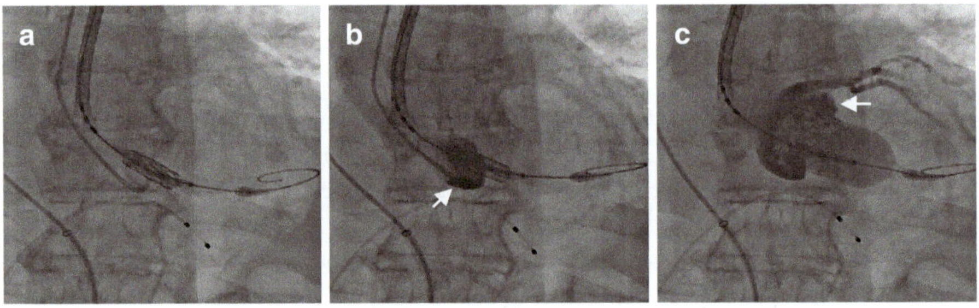

Fig. 8 A 23 mm balloon-expandable THV deployment via subcutaneous approach. (**a**) Positioning the THV over the AV annulus. (**b**) THV positioning with respect to right coronary cups (white arrow) demonstrated by contrast from a pigtail catheter. (**c**) THV post balloon inflation. Note the free space between the SOV and the THV (white arrow) indicating improper support

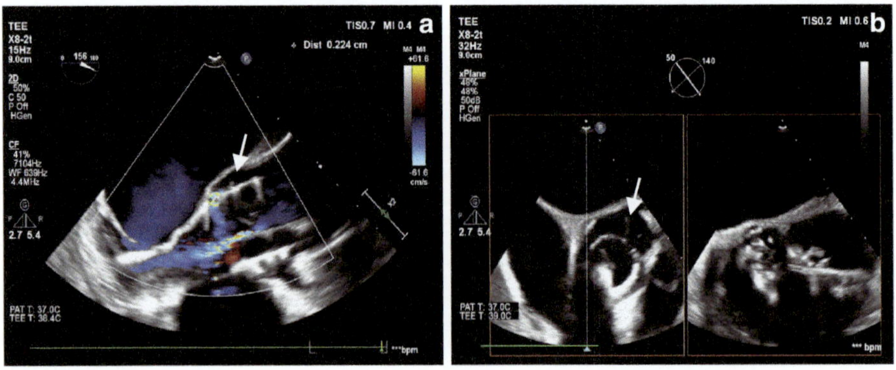

Fig. 9 Balloon-expandable THV post-deployment in LAX and SAX TEE modes. (**a**) Area between the SOV and the THV (white arrow). (**b**) Aneurysmal dilatation over the right coronary cusp (white arrow)

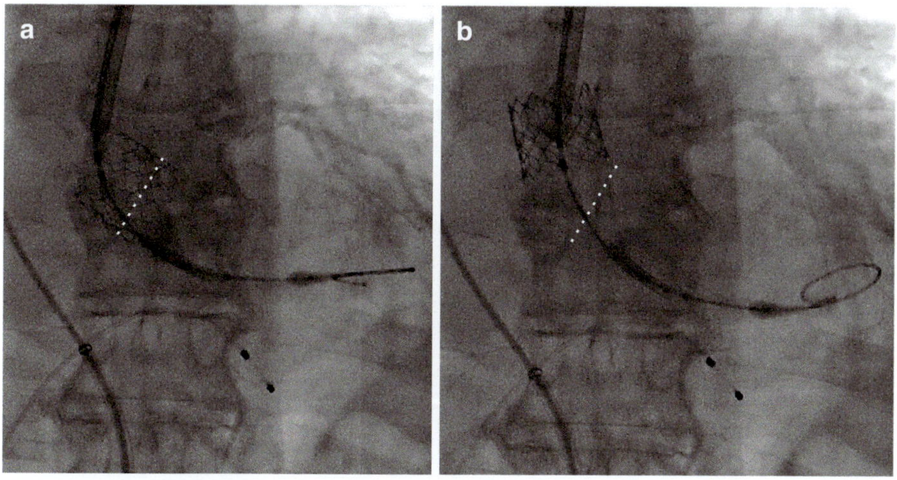

Fig. 10 THV embolization during deployment. (**a**) THV inflated over the AV annulus (white dashed line). (**b**) Displacement of the THV toward the ascending aorta following balloon inflation

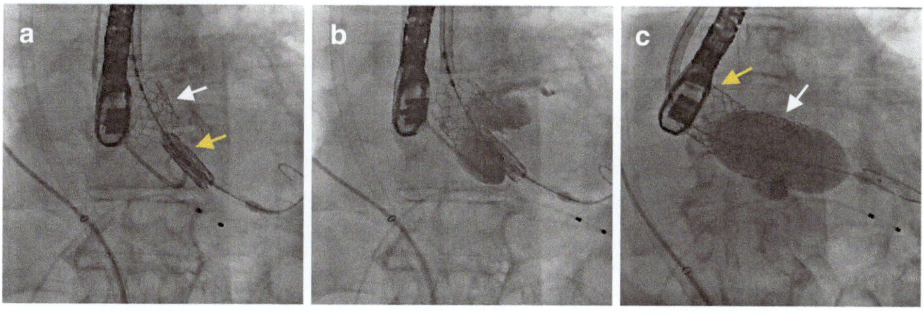

Fig. 11 Deployment of second Sapien 3 valve. (**a**) Crossing a 23 mm embolized THV (white arrow) with a 26 mm balloon-expandable THV (yellow arrow) and deploying it over the AV annulus. (**b**, **c**) Positioning of the second THV using fluoroscopy and contrast from a pigtail catheter to final inflation over the AV annulus (white arrow Figure **c**). Note the freely floating 23 mm THV at the ascending aorta (yellow arrow Figure **c**)

A 0.35-in. Lunderquist wire was advanced through the multipurpose catheter, followed by the insertion of a 12-French 80 cm Gore dry seal sheath into the thoracic aorta.

A 6-French multipurpose catheter was advanced across the embolized transcatheter heart valve through the Gore dry seal. We used an Amplatz extra-stiff wire to cross the embolized transcatheter heart valve. After that, multiple attempts were made to cross the transcatheter heart valve unsuccessfully. Then a 0.035-in. extra small curve safari wire was advanced across the embolized transcatheter heart valve into the ascending aorta. A Reliant balloon was advanced into the transcatheter heart valve and inflated, dragging the embolized valve into the aortic arch (Fig. 12). At that time, we decided to deploy a 34-mm Evolut valve to anchor the embolized valve in the ascending aorta. After resecting its leaflets outside the body, the Evolut valve was successfully deployed inside the embolized valve (Figs. 13 and 14, Video 11). The patient remained hemodynamically stable throughout the procedure. Unfortunately, the patient died several months following the procedure due to acute respiratory distress syndrome secondary to COVID-19 infection.

5 Discussion

Transcatheter valve embolization and migration (TVEM) is an unusual but potentially catastrophic complication. TVEM has been reported since the first TAVR experiences [1–3] and can happen as an acute or chronic sequela of TAVR. It was reported in 1% of TAVR cases and is associated with fourfold higher mortality and

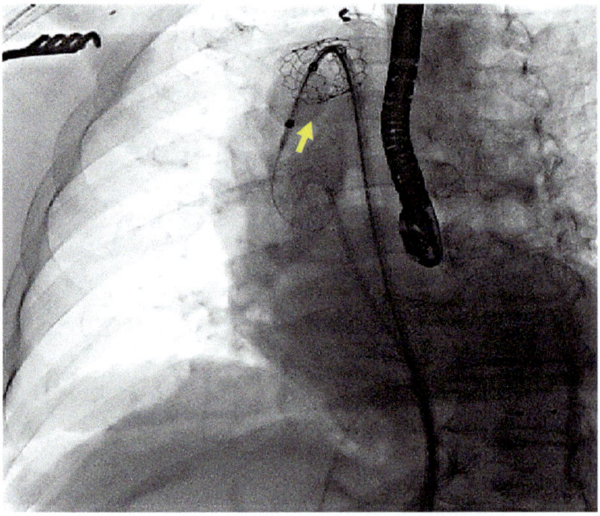

Fig. 12 A 23 mm embolized THV dragged to the aortic arch using a reliant balloon (yellow arrow)

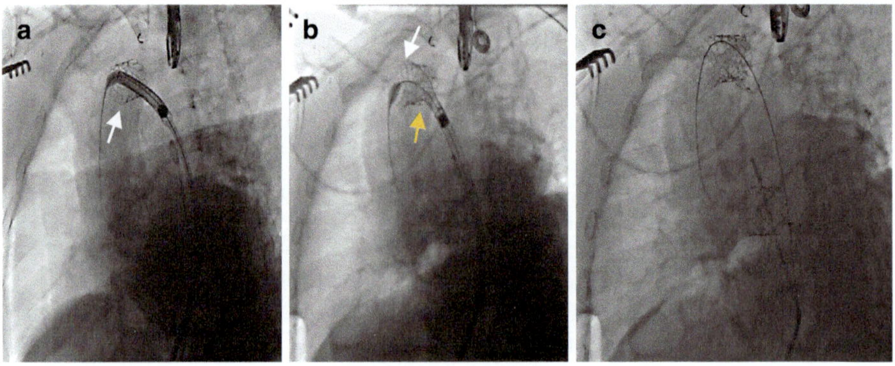

Fig. 13 Deployment of Evolut R over embolized Sapien 3 valve. (**a**) Evolut R position across Sapien 3 valve. (**b**) A "naked" 34 mm self-expandable Evolute R THV (yellow arrow) was advanced to the aortic arch. (**c**) Evoult R (over an embolized 23 mm balloon-expandable THV) (white arrows)

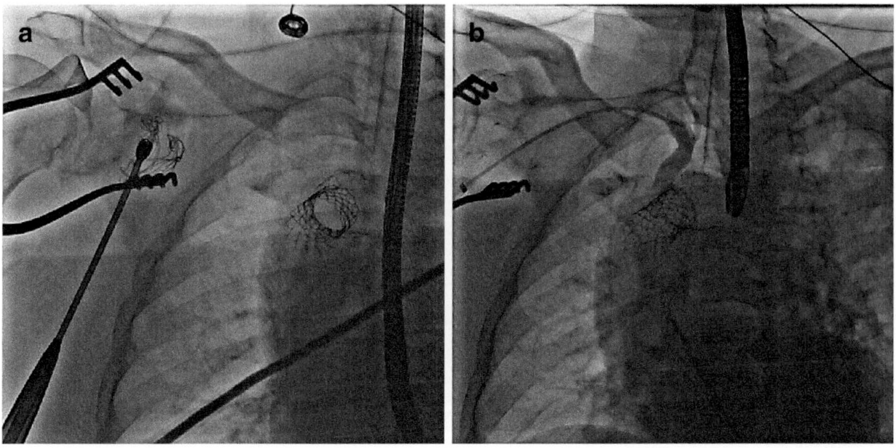

Fig. 14 A 34 mm self-expandable Evolute R THV deployed over a 23 mm balloon-expandable THV in different fluoroscopy view. (**a**) An LAO-CRA view. (**b**) RAO-CRA view

threefold higher stroke rate at 30 days [4]. Depending on its occurrence setting, clinical presentation varies from asymptomatic to acute unstable presentation that require surgical intervention [5].

6 Incidence and Causes

In a multicenter study based on outcome data from 26 centers and approximately 30,000 TAVR procedures, the incidence of TVEM was approximately 1%, with the vast majority of THV migrating to the ascending aorta with 20% embolizing into the left ventricle. Most cases were handled by implanting an additional THV, but 20% required open-heart surgery. Two independent predictors for TVEM were identified: the use of first-generation self-expanding prostheses and the use of bicuspid aortic valves [4]. The most common technical cause of TVEM is mispositioning, which is responsible for 50% of cases. Other potential causes include extensive THV manipulation, post-dilation, sizing error, and pacing failure during THV deployment [4].

The best approach to avoid TVEM is primary prevention. It has been previously estimated that one in three TVEM is preventable. Pre-procedural planning with the correct measurement of the aortic annulus, proper selection of prosthesis type and size, accurate deployment techniques, adequate temporary pacing, and proper communication with caregivers can further lessen the incidence of TVEM [4].

When TVEM occurs, initial assessment and management must be focused on hemodynamic stability. If the patient is hemodynamically unstable, immediate access to cardiac mechanical support and cardiac surgical intervention is crucial to salvage the patient life. Upon stabalization, management depends on the type, size, and location of the embolized device.

TVEM cases involving anterograde displacement toward the ascending aorta can be managed percutaneously by cautiously pulling the dislodged valve to a steady position, avoiding side branch occlusion. Aggressive manipulation (pulling large devices beyond the aortic arch) is not recommended and should be avoided due to the risk of aortic dissection [4, 6–8]. The embolized valves may remain stable without strut fractures in the perioperative period. Securing the wire to the left ventricle through embolized THV is another crucial step to avoid flipping the position of the embolized THV and maintain hemodynamic stability. Immediate implantation of a second THV, was successful in most of the patients and is be a suitable treatment strategy [4].

Key Points

- Strongly consider alternative access when the transfemoral access site is challenging. Before starting the case, confirm aortic valve area by both CT and TEE when available.
- The strategy of pre-dilatation of the aortic valve should be discussed before engaging the procedure.
- The incidence of TVEM is less than 1%, but the priority should be hemodynamic stabilization using the second THV.
- The embolized THV can be stabilized in the aortic arch by the placement of a modified self-expanding Evolut valve without its leaflets inside the embolized Sapien valve.
- Three main criteria should be considered to prevent TVEM: appropriate positioning of the THV in the co-planar view, correct alignment to LVOT and ascending aorta, and choosing the proper THV size based on the annulus, LVOT, and STJ areas.

References

1. Gaede L, Blumenstein J, Liebetrau C, Dörr O, Kim WK, Nef H, Husser O, Elsässer A, Hamm CW, Möllmann H. Outcome after transvascular transcatheter aortic valve implantation in 2016. Eur Heart J. 2018;39(8):667–75.
2. Makkar RR, Jilaihawi H, Chakravarty T, Fontana GP, Kapadia S, Babaliaros V, Cheng W, Thourani VH, Bavaria J, Svensson L, Kodali S. Determinants and outcomes of acute transcatheter valve-in-valve therapy or embolization: a study of multiple valve implants in the US PARTNER trial (Placement of AoRTic TraNscathetER Valve Trial Edwards SAPIEN Transcatheter Heart Valve). J Am Coll Cardiol. 2013;62(5):418–30.
3. Ibebuogu UN, Giri S, Bolorunduro O, Tartara P, Kar S, Holmes D, Alli O. Review of reported causes of device embolization following trans-catheter aortic valve implantation. Am J Cardiol. 2015;115(12):1767–72.
4. Kim WK, Schäfer U, Tchetche D, Nef H, Arnold M, Avanzas P, Rudolph T, Scholtz S, Barbanti M, Kempfert J, Mangieri A. Incidence and outcome of peri-procedural transcatheter heart valve embolization and migration: the TRAVEL registry (TranscatheteR HeArt Valve EmboLization and Migration). Eur Heart J. 2019;40(38):3156–65.
5. Hein R, Abdel-Wahab M, Sievert H, Kuck KH, Voehringer M, Hambrecht R, Sack S, Hauptmann KE, Senges J, Zahn R, Mudra H. Outcome of patients after emergency conversion from transcatheter aortic valve implantation to surgery. EuroIntervention. 2013;9(4):446–51.

6. Tay EL, Gurvitch R, Wijeysinghe N, Nietlispach F, Leipsic J, Wood DA, Yong G, Cheung A, Ye J, Lichtenstein SV, Carere R. Outcome of patients after transcatheter aortic valve embolization. J Am Coll Cardiol Interv. 2011;4(2):228–34.
7. Ali AM, Altwegg L, Horlick EM, Feindel C, Thompson CR, Cheung A, Carere RG, Humphries K, Ye J, Masson JB, Webb JG. Prevention and management of transcatheter balloon-expandable aortic valve malposition. Catheter Cardiovasc Interv. 2008;72(4):573–8.
8. Masson JB, Kovac J, Schuler G, Ye J, Cheung A, Kapadia S, Tuzcu ME, Kodali S, Leon MB, Webb JG. Transcatheter aortic valve implantation: review of the nature, management, and avoidance of procedural complications. J Am Coll Cardiol Interv. 2009;2(9):811–20.

Displacement of a THV Toward Ascending Aorta Due to Premature Ventricular Contraction

Ofir Koren, Elli Izrailov, and Ahmed Al Badri

1 Clinical Presentation

A 75-year-old Caucasian man with a history of hypertension, coronary artery disease, heart failure with preserved ejection fraction, and NYHA class III symptoms was found to have severe aortic stenosis.

2 Images and Supported Data

TTE revealed normal left ventricular systolic function, LV ejection fraction of 60%, moderate diastolic dysfunction, and normal right ventricular systolic function. Aortic cusps appeared severely calcified, revealing severe aortic valve stenosis with a peak transaortic gradient of 64 mmHg (Fig. 1, Videos 1 and 2). The aortic valve area of 0.9 cm^2 was determined by VTI's continuity equation and was verified by reconstructed gated CT (Video 3). Mild aortic valve regurgitation was present.

Supplementary Information The online version contains supplementary material available at [https://doi.org/10.1007/978-3-031-05965-0_10].

O. Koren (✉)
Smidt Heart Institute, Cedars-Sinai Medical Center, Los Angeles, CA, USA

Faculty of Medicine, Technion, Israel Institute of Technology, Haifa, Israel
e-mail: Ofir.Koren@cshs.org

E. Izrailov
Bendigo Health, Bendigo, VIC, Australia

A. Al Badri
Cedars Sinai Medical Center, Los Angeles, CA, USA

O. Koren et al. (eds.), *Complex Cases in Structural Heart Intervention*,
https://doi.org/10.1007/978-3-031-05965-0_10

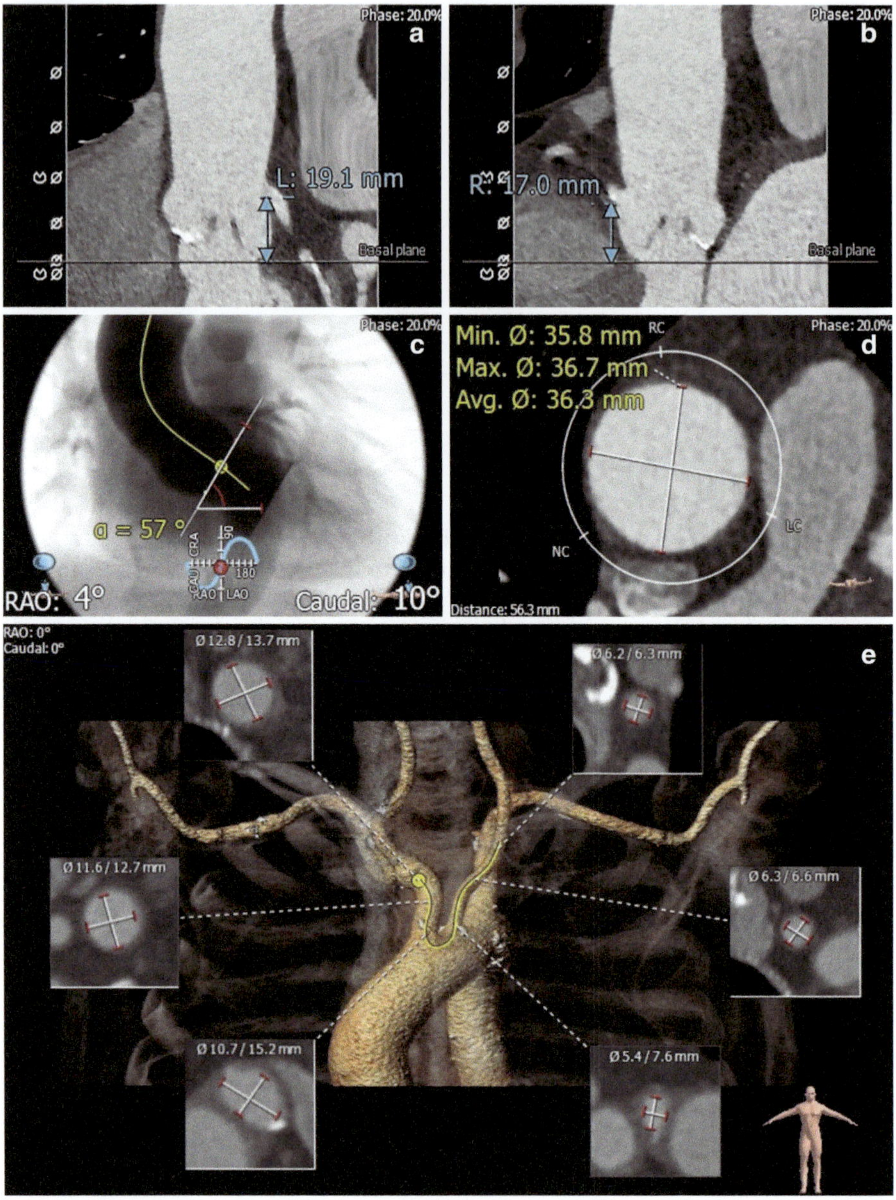

Fig. 1 Left (**a**) and right (**b**) coronary ostium height in respect to annular plane, the coplanar view angle (**c**), the maximal aortic diameter of the ascending aorta (**d**), and the aortic anatomy with its corresponding branches (**e**)

Cardiac reconstructed CT indicated an annular mean internal diameter of 24.2 mm, area of 452.9 mm^2, and a perimeter of 76.3 mm (Fig. 2). The coronary arteries were high above the annular plane (Figs. 3 and 4). A coronary angiogram before the TAVR indicated patent arteries with no significant obstructive lesions (Fig. 5).

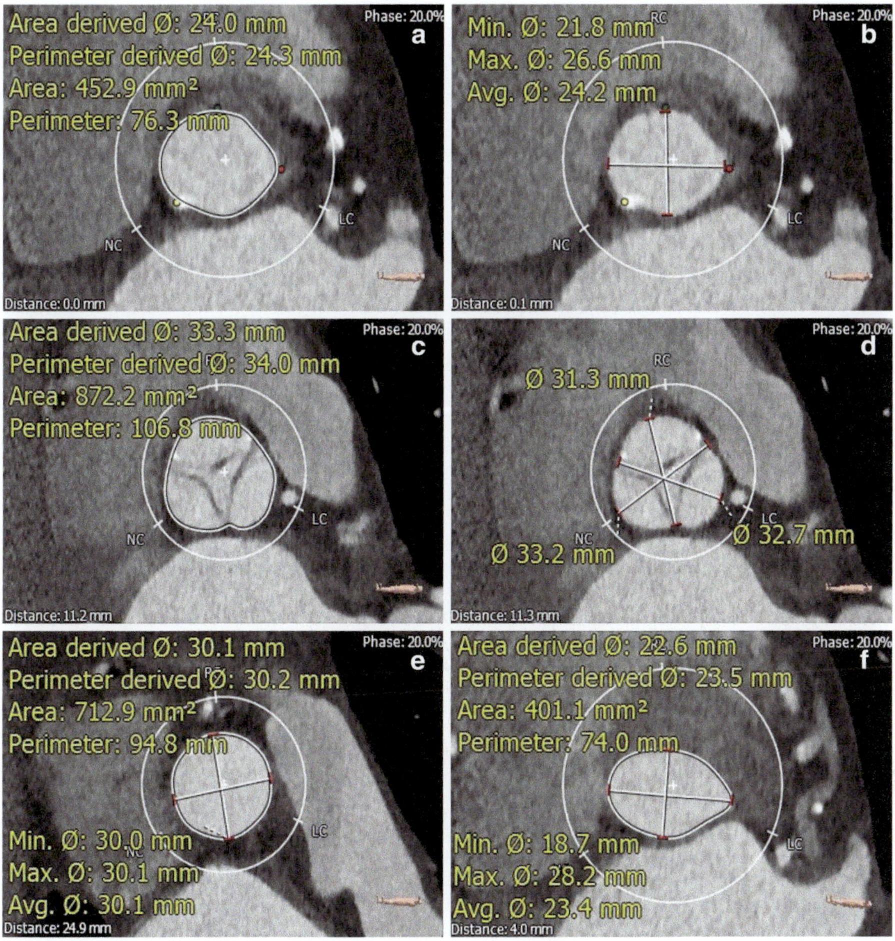

Fig. 2 Reconstructed CT analysis pre-TAVR. Area, perimeter, and diameter measurement of the AV annulus (Figures **a**, **b**), the SOV (**c**, **d**), the STJ (**e**), and the LVOT (**f**)

3 Procedure and Outcome

A 26-mm Edwards Sapien Ultra valve delivery system was positioned across the stenotic aortic valve. The valve was deployed using the standard technique with rapid pacing, of 180 bpm (Video 4). There was a loss of capture during deployment as the patient developed a premature ventricular contraction (PVC). This led to embolization of the valve before full deployment (Fig. 6). Subsequently, the valve was deployed into the descending aorta (Fig. 7, Video 5). There was good hemodynamic recovery without any issues.

After placing the first valve in the descending aorta, a new 26-mm Edwards Sapien Ultra valve delivery system was positioned across the stenotic aortic valve.

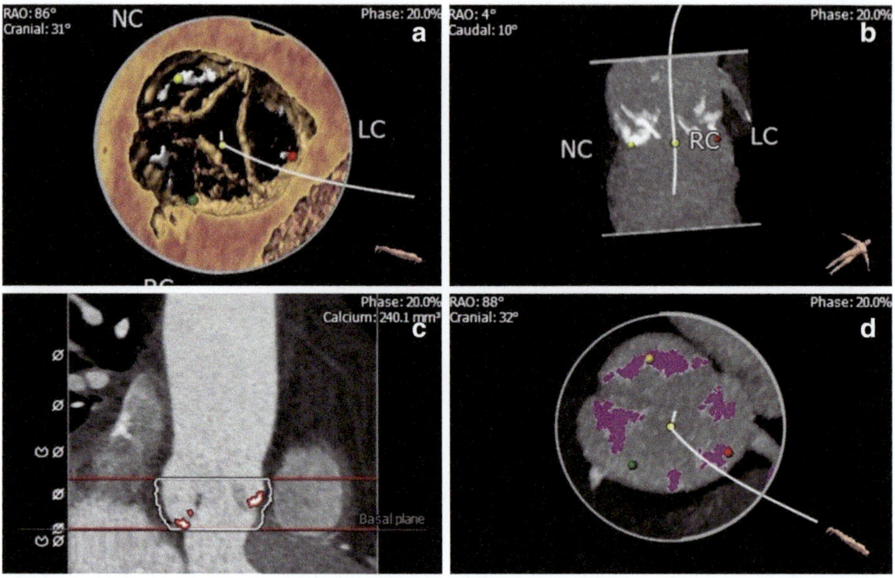

Fig. 3 Calcium deposition over the AV annulus in various CT views. (**a**) Hockey puck VR view of aortic annulus. (**b**) Hockey puck MIP view. (**c**) Ascending aorta longitudinal (**c**) and cross-sectional annulus (**d**) view using a HU850 threshold

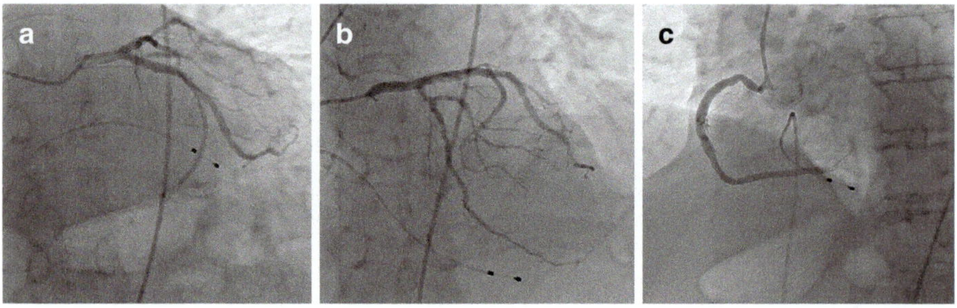

Fig. 4 Angiography of (**a**, **b**) the left and (**c**) the right coronary arteries prior to the TAVR procedure

With rapid pacing at 180 beats per minute, the valve was deployed in the standard technique (Fig. 8, Videos 6 and 7). A post-procedure TTE revealed no central aortic regurgitation and trace perivalvular regurgitation (Fig. 9).

The patient tolerated the procedure well without any immediate post-procedural complications. He was monitored overnight under routine post-operative protocols. He remained hemodynamically stable, afebrile, and normotensive throughout his hospital stay. Telemetry revealed no significant arrhythmias, and a post-TAVR echocardiogram showed no acute findings. The patient was discharged home in stable condition.

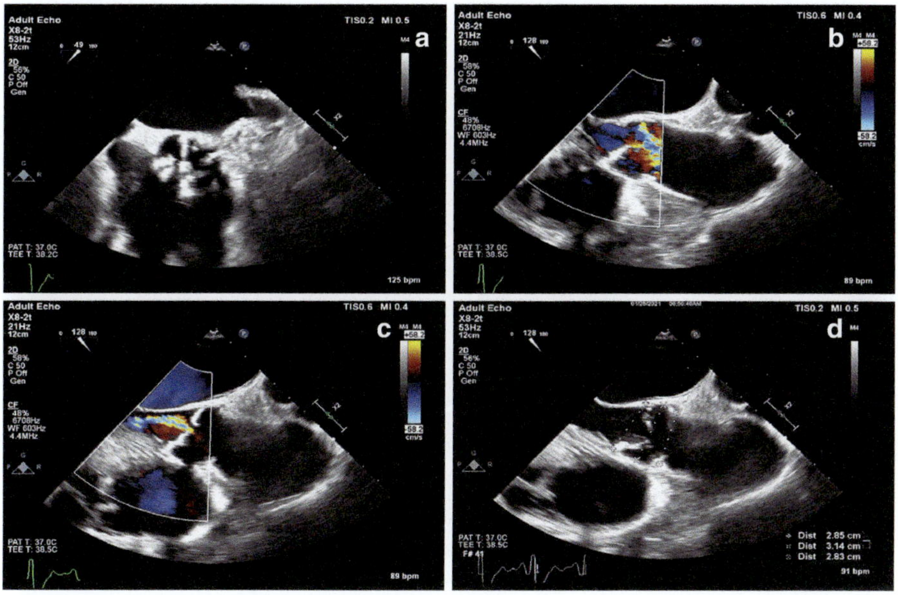

Fig. 5 Pre-procedure TEE indicating a severely calcified (**a**) and stenotic AV (**b**) with mild aortic regurgitation (**c**) and normal diameters of aortic root (**d**)

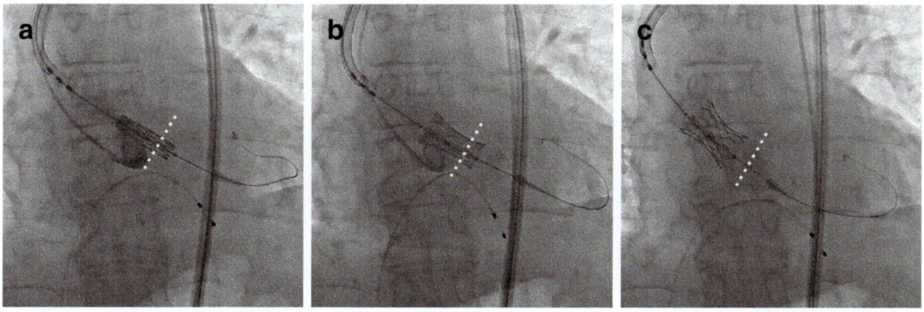

Fig. 6 Deployment of a 26 mm balloon expandable THV. (**a**) Positioning of the THV over the AV annulus (white dashed line). (**b**) Balloon inflation. (**c**) Displacement of the THV toward the ascending aorta (**c**)

4 Discussion

Transcatheter valve embolization and migration (TVEM) is a rare complication, occurring in 1% of transcatheter aortic valve implantation (TAVI). It entails potentially grim outcomes, such as fourfold higher mortality and threefold higher stroke rate at 30 days [1].

TVEM has been reported since the first TAVI experiences and varies between asymptomatic presentations and more acute ones requiring surgery [2].

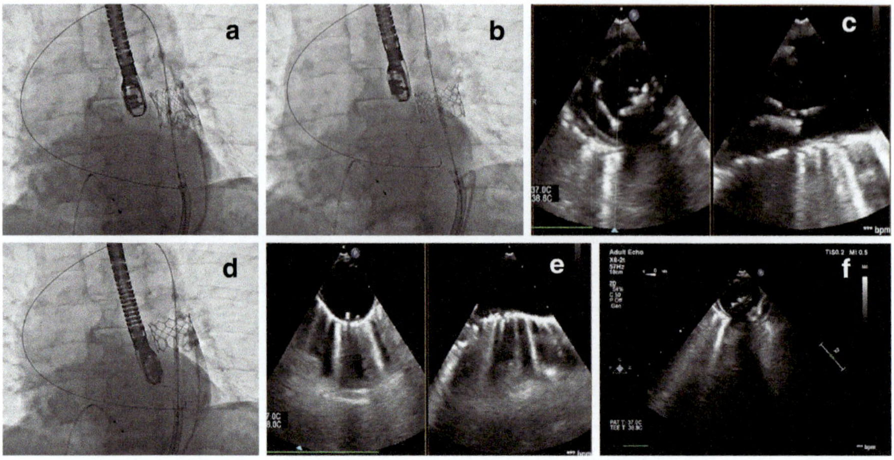

Fig. 7 TEE images showing relocation and deployment of a displaced THV to a proper diameter site on the descending aorta. (**a**) Removing the non-deployed, partialy inflated THV toward the descending aorta. (**b**) FFinal positioning, considering THV size and expansion diameter (**c**) Guidance. (**d–f**) Full inflation and final deployment

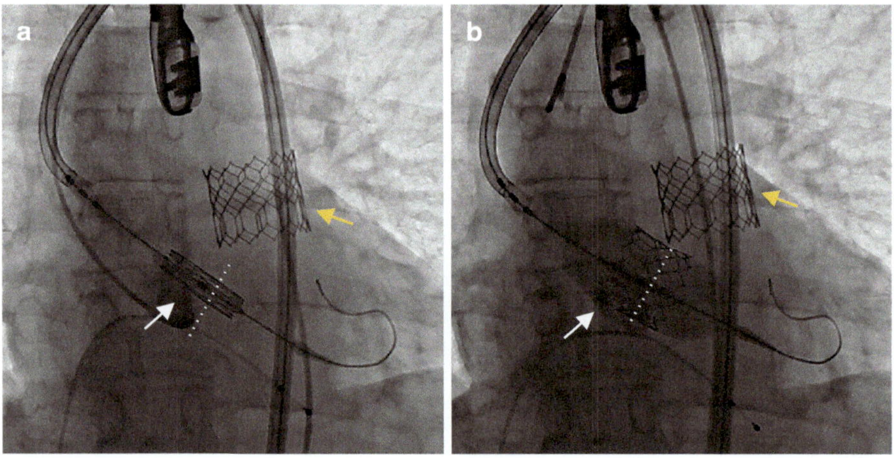

Fig. 8 (**a**) Positioning and (**b**) deployment of a second 26 mm balloon expandable THV (white arrow) over the AV annulus (white dashed line). Note the 26 mm balloon expandable THV in the descending aorta (yellow arrow)

In a multicenter report based on data from 26 centers and approximately 30,000 TAVI procedures, the incidence of TVEM was close to 1%, with the vast majority migrating to the ascending aorta. In contrast, 20% of THVs advanced to the left ventricle. Most cases were handled by implanting an additional THV, and 20% required open-heart surgery. Moreover, two independent predictors have been identified: the use of self-expanding first-generation prostheses and bicuspid aortic valves [2].

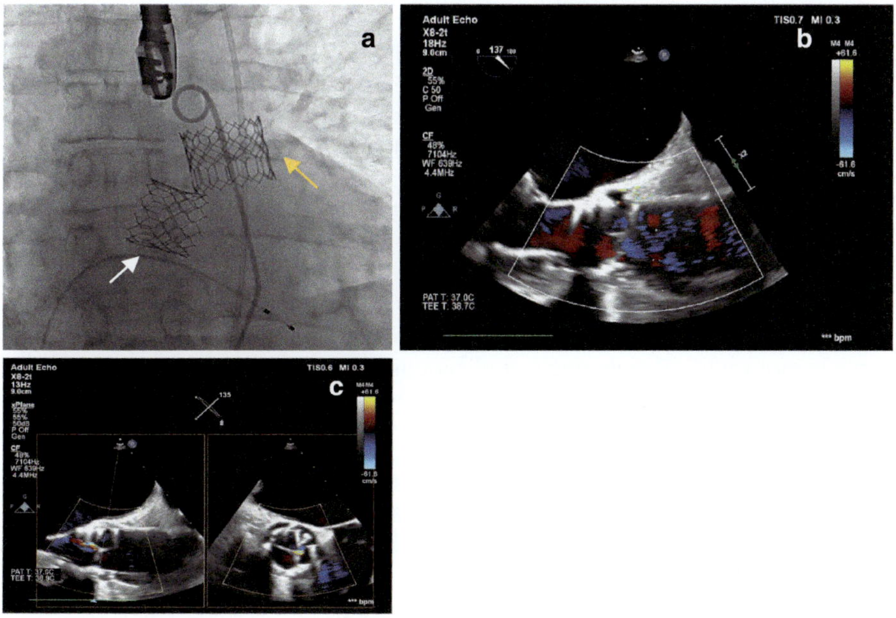

Fig. 9 Successful deployment of a second THV over the AV annulus with trivial aortic regurgitation. (**a**) Fluoroscopy view of the two THVs at the AV annulus (white arrow) and the descending aorta (yellow arrow). ME LAX (**b**) and SAX (**c**) TEE views of a balloon expandable THV at the aortic position

The most common cause of TVEM is mispositioning, responsible for 50% of cases. Manipulation, post-dilation, sizing errors, and fast rate pacing failures were other leading causes [1].

The best therapeutic approach is primary prevention. It has been previously estimated that one in three THV Embolization and Migration (TVEM) are preventable. Pre-procedural planning with the correct measurement of the aortic annulus, proper selection of prosthesis type and size, accurate deployment techniques, adequate temporary pacing, and proper communication between caregivers can help minimize TVEM [1].

In anticipation of this unwanted outcome, the availability of cardiothoracic surgery should be taken into consideration when performing TAVI. In addition, we must ensure the operating team is experienced and aware of this uncommon complication and how to manage it properly.

The initial evaluation has to be of hemodynamic stability and assess the need for surgical intervention to avoid uncommon yet detrimental outcomes. If the latter is unnecessary, strategies are related to the type, the size and location of the embolized device, the timing of diagnosis, and the patient's clinical presentation.

In most cases of TVEM, the transcatheter valve is displaced toward ascending aorta and can be managed percutaneously by pulling the valve to a steady position within the lumen while cautiously avoiding tears or obstruction of vascular branches. Aggressive manipulation (pulling large devices beyond the aortic arch) *is not recommended and should be avoided* due to the risk of aortic dissection [3].

It is important to remember that outcomes are favorable when proper management is undertaken, and the embolized valves may remain stable without strut fractures at follow-up [4].

Implantation of a second THV while avoiding the prior errors was successful in the vast majority of patients and should be the first-line treatment strategy [1].

Our case emphasizes the importance of pre-procedural planning in identifying possible rare yet life-threatening complications of TAVR, enabling us to avoid these situations and managing them when they occur.

Key Points

- Transcatheter valve embolization is a rare yet serious complication.
- The availability of cardiothoracic surgery is crucial when performing TAVI.
- Long term outcome of deploying the embolized valve in the descending aorta is still unknown.

References

1. Kim WK, Schäfer U, Tchetche D, Nef H, Arnold M, Avanzas P, Rudolph T, Scholtz S, Barbanti M, Kempfert J, Mangieri A. Incidence and outcome of peri-procedural transcatheter heart valve embolization and migration: the TRAVEL registry (TranscatheteR HeArt Valve EmboLization and Migration). Eur Heart J. 2019;40(38):3156–65.
2. Makkar RR, Jilaihawi H, Chakravarty T, Fontana GP, Kapadia S, Babaliaros V, Cheng W, Thourani VH, Bavaria J, Svensson L, Kodali S. Determinants and outcomes of acute transcatheter valve-in-valve therapy or embolization: a study of multiple valve implants in the US PARTNER trial (Placement of AoRTic TraNscathetER Valve Trial Edwards SAPIEN Transcatheter Heart Valve). J Am Coll Cardiol. 2013;62(5):418–30.
3. Généreux P, Head SJ, Van Mieghem NM, Kodali S, Kirtane AJ, Xu K, Smith C, Serruys PW, Kappetein AP, Leon MB. Clinical outcomes after transcatheter aortic valve replacement using valve academic research consortium definitions: a weighted meta-analysis of 3,519 patients from 16 studies. J Am Coll Cardiol. 2012;59(25):2317–26.
4. Pelliccia F, Cianfrocca C, Rosano G, Mercuro G, Speciale G, Pasceri V. Role of endothelial progenitor cells in restenosis and progression of coronary atherosclerosis after percutaneous coronary intervention: a prospective study. J Am Coll Cardiol Interv. 2010;3(1):78–86.

Coronary Access Protection Technique (The Chimney Procedure) During TAVR

Ofir Koren, Asaf Israeli, and Danon Kaewkes

1 Clinical Presentation

An 87-year-old male was admitted to our center with acute dyspnea and signs of decompensated heart failure. His past medical history was notable for chronic kidney disease (stage III), complete heart blockage, which required pacemaker implantation, atrial fibrillation complicated by hemorrhagic stroke, and coronary artery disease (CAD) with multiple stenting of the left main (LM), left anterior descending artery (LAD), and the right coronary artery (RCA). Ten years ago, the patient had a bioprosthetic AVR with a 25 Mitroflow valve (Sorin Group USA Inc., Arvada, CO) and a coronary artery bypass surgery with anastomosis of the left internal mammary artery to LAD and the saphenous vein graft to a left circumflex artery.

Supplementary Information The online version contains supplementary material available at [https://doi.org/10.1007/978-3-031-05965-0_11].

O. Koren (✉)
Smidt Heart Institute, Cedars-Sinai Medical Center, Los Angeles, CA, USA

Faculty of Medicine, Technion, Israel Institute of Technology, Haifa, Israel
e-mail: Ofir.Koren@cshs.org

A. Israeli
Technion, Israel Institute of Technology, Haifa, Israel

D. Kaewkes
Department of Medicine, Faculty of Medicine, Khon Kaen University, Khon Kaen, Thailand

O. Koren et al. (eds.), *Complex Cases in Structural Heart Intervention*,
https://doi.org/10.1007/978-3-031-05965-0_11

2 Images and Supported Data

Transthoracic and transesophageal echocardiography (TTE and TEE) showed a new and severe bioprosthetic aortic regurgitation (AR) with an eccentric and anteriorly directed jet (Fig. 1), moderate to severe mitral regurgitation (MR) from the restriction of the P2 mitral scallop, and severe tricuspid regurgitation (TR) with two discrete jets. Left ventricular ejection fraction (LVEF) was mildly reduced with no apparent wall motion abnormalities. Cardiac reconstructed computed tomography (CT) indicated a prosthetic aortic valve annular mean internal diameter of 19.8 mm, area of 312.1 mm^2, and perimeter of 63.0 mm. The following means diameters were measured: 26 mm at the sinus of Valsalva, 23.8 mm at the sinotubular junction (STJ), and 21.5 mm at the left ventricular outflow tract (LVOT) (Fig. 2). The coronary ostia originated at low height regarding the annular plane. The RCA ostium was 9.2 mm, and the left coronary artery (LCA) ostium was estimated 4.4 mm above the annular plane (Fig. 3). The right femoral access was feasible with a minimal lumen diameter of 6.1 × 7.6 mm measured at the right external iliac artery.

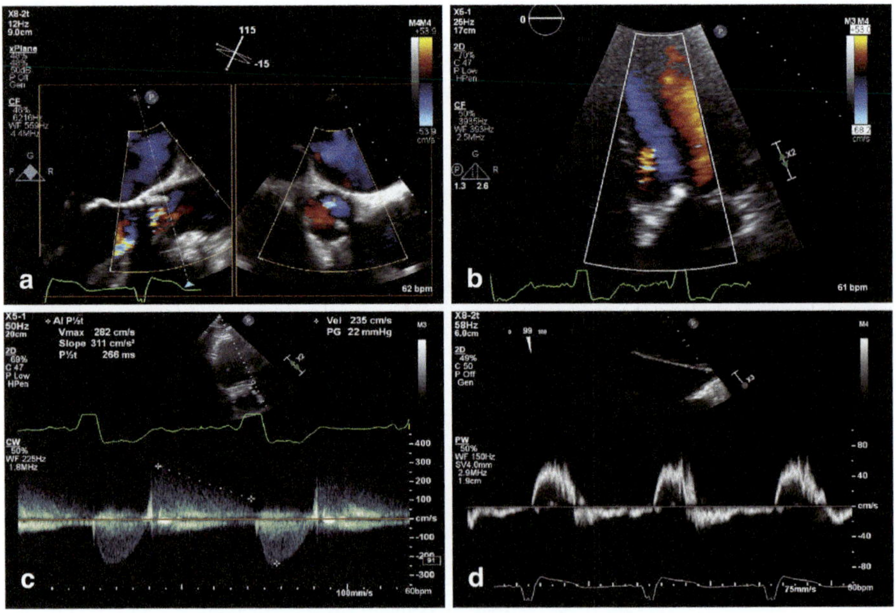

Fig. 1 Bioprosthetic aortic insufficiency on different echocardiographic views. (**a**) Aortic valve in long axis view (TEE); (**b**, **c**) five-chamber view (TTE) with continuous wave Doppler mode. (**d**) Diastolic flow reversal in descending aorta (TEE)

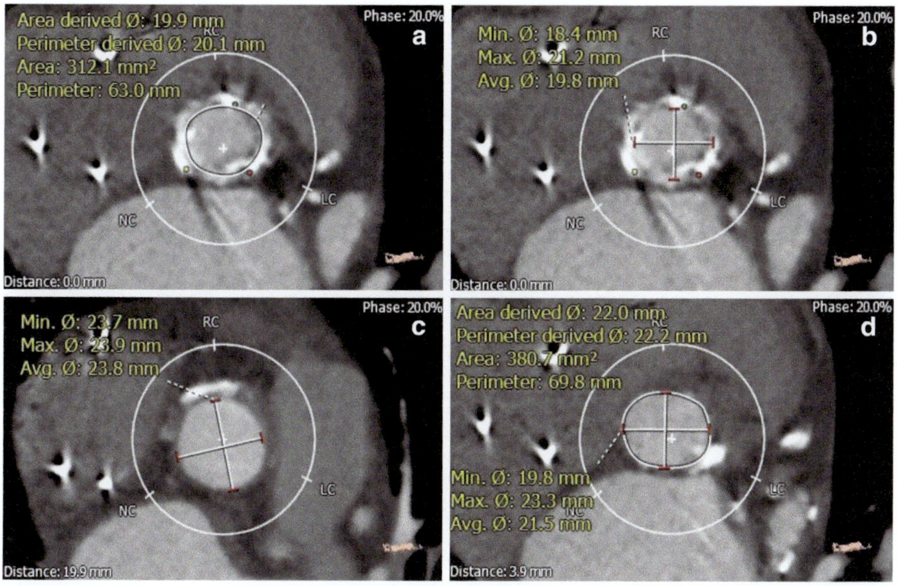

Fig. 2 CT analysis pre-TAVR. (**a**) Inflow area of a bioprosthetic aortic valve. (**b**) Inflow diameter of a bioprosthetic aortic valve. (**c**) STJ diameter. (**d**) LVOT measurements

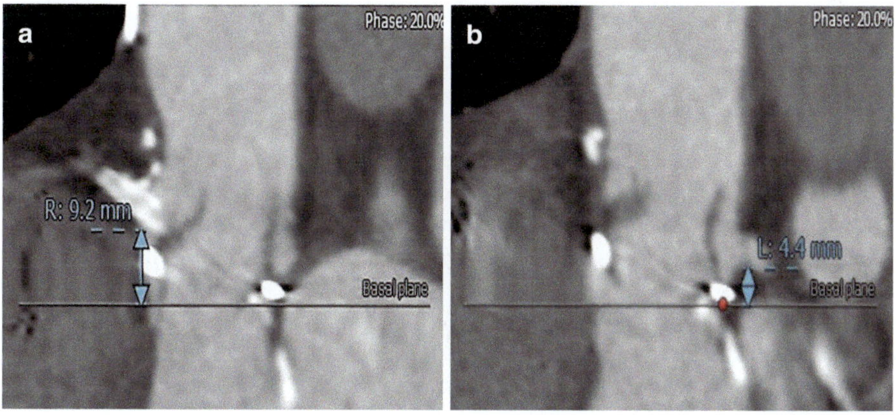

Fig. 3 Coronary height from the aortic prosthetic valve inflow on pre-TAVR CT. (**a**) Right coronary artery height, (**b**) left coronary artery height

3 Pre-Procedural Consideration: Pitfalls, Dilemmas, and Challenges

Pre-procedure dilemmas were focused on choosing the largest transcatheter heart valve (THV) possible for a larger orifice area and better gradient after the procedure without compromising future coronary access and avoiding intraoperative coronary

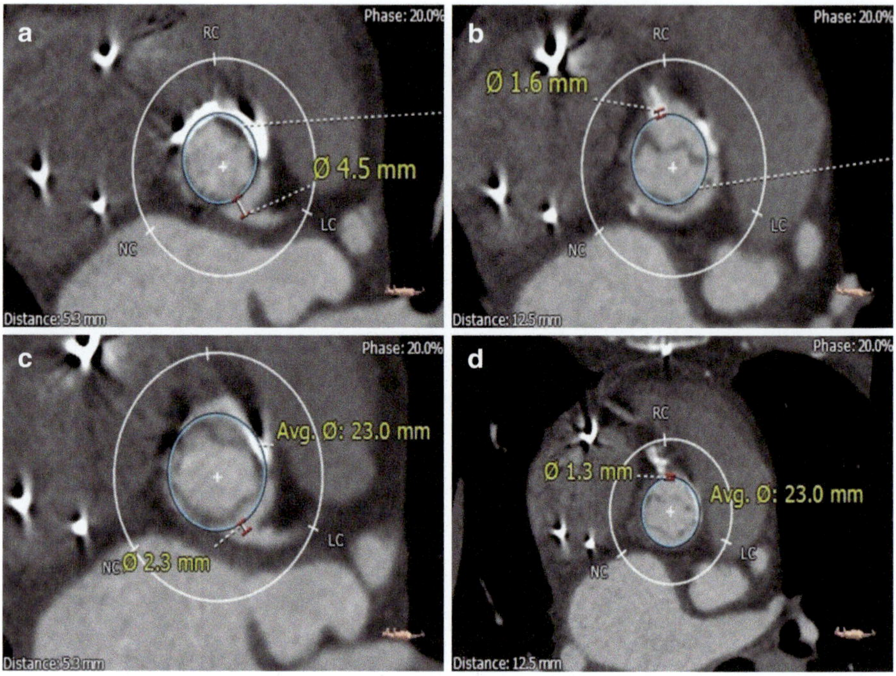

Fig. 4 Pre-procedural CT analysis. The distance from the virtual THV to coronary ostia. (**a**) The distance from 20 mm virtual THV to LCA ostium; (**b**) the distance from 20 mm virtual THV to RCA ostium, (**c**) the distance from 23 mm virtual THV to LCA ostium; (**d**) the distance from 23 mm virtual THV to RCA ostium

obstruction. The actual internal diameter of the Mitroflow is 21 mm. Therefore, either the 20 mm or the 23 mm balloon-expandable Sapien-3 valve was considered. CT analysis of the distance between a virtual 20 mm Sapien-3 THV and the coronary ostia was 1.6 mm for the RCA and 4.5 mm for LCA, while the distance between a 23 mm Sapien-3 was 1.3 and 2.3 mm, respectively (Fig. 4). There was an increase risk of coronary obstruction in both the 20 mm and the 23 mm THV. Thus, we decided to proceed with the highest diameter possible and use devices to protect the coronary access. Preprocedural coronary angiogram revealed no significant lesions (Fig. 5, Videos 1, 2, 3 and 4).

4 Technique

The left and right coronary arteries were protected with a deflated third-generation (Xience, Abbott, USA) drug-eluting stents (DES; 4.0 × 15 mm stent in the LCA and 3.0 × 15 mm stent in the RCA) (Videos 5, 6 and 7). Transcatheter aortic valve

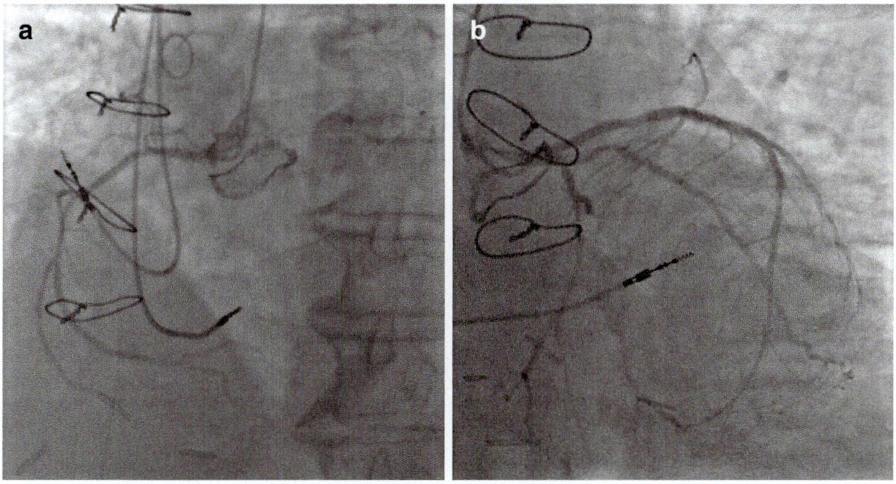

Fig. 5 Coronary angiography before the TAVR procedure. (**a**) Right coronary artery, (**b**) left coronary artery

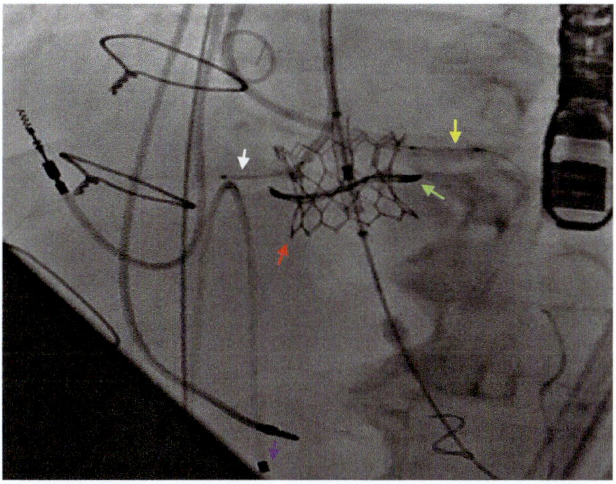

Fig. 6 Transcatheter aortic valve deployment. Balloon-expandable Sapien-3 deployment (red arrow) over a previous bioprosthetic valve (green arrow) with protection wires in the right (white arrow) and left coronary arteries (yellow arrow) during rapid RV pacing (purple arrow)

replacement (TAVR) was performed using the balloon-expandable 23 mm Sapien-3 ultra (Edwards Lifesciences, Irvine, CA), deployed inside the Mitroflow bioprosthetic valve with a standard valve-in-valve technique (Fig. 6). After deployment, the patient developed ST elevation on EKG in the RCA territory and significant hypotension (Fig. 7). Thus, both stents were deployed (Fig. 8, Videos 8 and 9) at the ostial portion of the LM and RCA with immediate normalization of the ECG changes and hemodynamic stabilization.

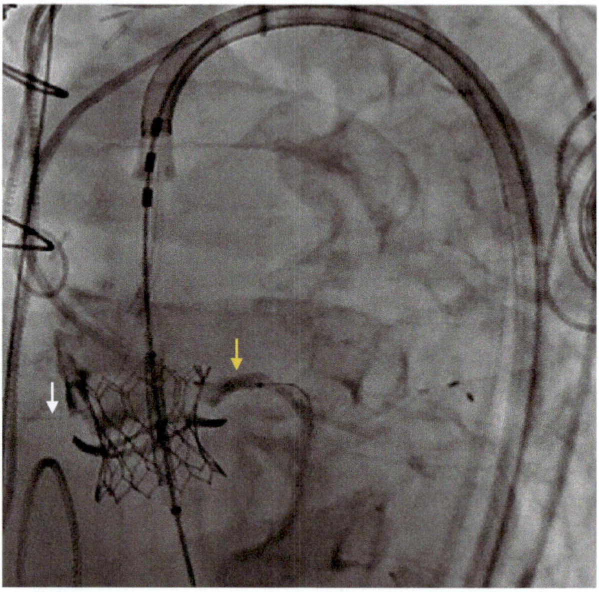

Fig. 7 Coronary obstruction after THV deployment. The deployment of a Sapien-3 THV over a bioprosthetic valve resulted in compromised coronary flow to the right (white arrow) and left coronary arteries and necessitated urgent stenting to the left main artery (yellow arrow). Noted contrast flow across the left coronary artery (yellow arrow)

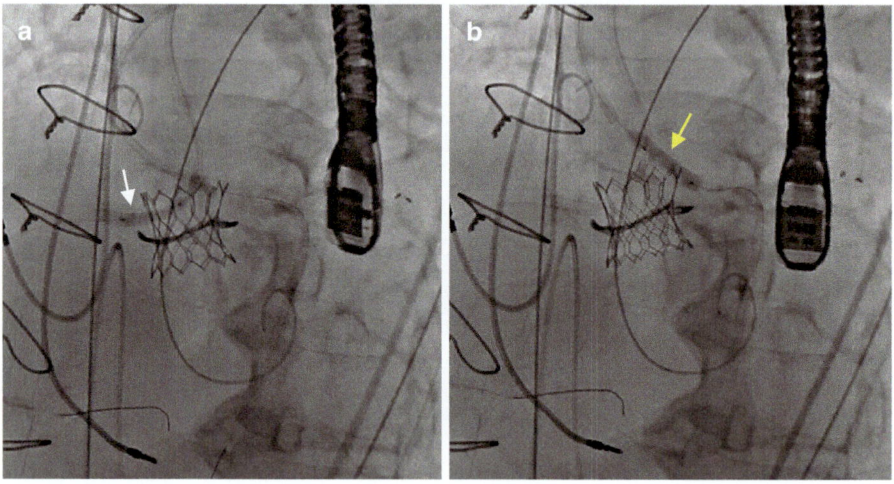

Fig. 8 Coronary arteries stenting (Chimney stenting) following abrupt obstruction during valve-in-valve TAVR procedure. (**a**) RCA stenting (white arrow). (**b**) LCA stenting (yellow arrow)

5 Outcomes and Follow-Up

A post-procedure TEE revealed no central AR and no paravalvular regurgitation. The THV was well-seated in the aortic position with normal leaflet motion. 30-days and 1-year follow-ups were unremarkable. The patient was on a maximally tolerated heart failure regimen and well compensated despite a significant MR and TR. However, the patient died 1.5 years later from sepsis related to COVID-19.

6 Discussion

The abrupt closure of the coronary ostium during TAVR may be a devastating event and leads to poor outcomes. The incidence seems to be as low as <1% in the standard TAVR procedure. However, it is more prevalent with valve-in-valve procedures (2.3%) [1, 2], especially when coronary height <10 mm, the sinus of Valsalva diameter <30 mm, the distance between a virtual THV to the coronary ostium <4 mm, and when an externally mounted stented bioprosthetic valve is involved [3]. Patients presented with one or more of the above criteria were traditionally referred to surgical AVR. The chimney technique was adapted from endovascular interventions and served as a bailout technique for over a decade [4–6]. The procedure involved the placement of a deflated stent over a wire in one or both coronary arteries before THV deployment. In acute coronary obstruction, the stent is immediately withdrawn to the ostium and inflated parallel to the THV and along the aortic wall to create a chimney-like structure allowing coronary reperfusion [7, 8]. The procedure was found to be a good bailout technique for coronary artery obstruction (CAO) and significantly reduced catastrophic events such as acute myocardial infarction and cardiogenic shock [9]. Our case emphasizes the need for proper periprocedural planning and equipment preparation which can significantly reduce undesired outcomes immediately following CAO.

Key Points

- CAO incidence after valve-in-valve is relatively high compared to native-valve TAVR.
- Coronary artery protection might be necessary and lifesaving in TAVR cases with increased risk of CAO.
- Be familiar with the chimney technique commonly used for coronary artery protection during TAVR procedures.
- Know the risk factors predicting CAO following TAVR.

References

1. Ribeiro HB, Webb JG, Makkar RR, Cohen MG, Kapadia SR, Kodali S, Tamburino C, Barbanti M, Chakravarty T, Jilaihawi H, Paradis JM. Predictive factors, management, and clinical outcomes of coronary obstruction following transcatheter aortic valve implantation: insights from a large multicenter registry. J Am Coll Cardiol. 2013;62(17):1552–62.
2. Ribeiro HB, Rodés-Cabau J, Blanke P, Leipsic J, Kwan Park J, Bapat V, Makkar R, Simonato M, Barbanti M, Schofer J, Bleiziffer S. Incidence, predictors, and clinical outcomes of coro-

nary obstruction following transcatheter aortic valve replacement for degenerative bioprosthetic surgical valves: insights from the VIVID registry. Eur Heart J. 2018;39(8):687–95.
3. Dvir D, Leipsic J, Blanke P, Ribeiro HB, Kornowski R, Pichard A, Rodés-Cabau J, Wood DA, Stub D, Ben-Dor I, Maluenda G. Coronary obstruction in transcatheter aortic valve-in-valve implantation: preprocedural evaluation, device selection, protection, and treatment. Circ Cardiovasc Interv. 2015;8(1):e002079.
4. Adamo M, Fiorina C, Curello S, Chizzola G, Pezzotti E, Gavazzi E, Branca L, Chiari E, Quinzani F, Rinaldi M, Metra M. Self-expanding transcatheter aortic valve implantation for degenerated small Mitroflow bioprosthesis: early and midterm outcomes. EuroIntervention. 2017;13(9):e1032–9.
5. Banno H, Cochennec F, Marzelle J, Becquemin JP. Comparison of fenestrated endovascular aneurysm repair and chimney graft techniques for pararenal aortic aneurysm. J Vasc Surg. 2014;60(1):31–9.
6. Spaziano M, Akodad M, Hovasse T, Lefèvre T, Bouvier E, Chevalier B. Simultaneous TAVR and left main "chimney" stenting in a patient with low left main height. J Am Coll Cardiol Interv. 2017;10(20):e185–7.
7. Abramowitz Y, Chakravarty T, Jilaihawi H, Kashif M, Kazuno Y, Takahashi N, Maeno Y, Nakamura M, Cheng W, Makkar RR. Clinical impact of coronary protection during transcatheter aortic valve implantation: first reported series of patients. EuroIntervention. 2015;11(5):572–81.
8. Yamamoto M, Shimura T, Kano S, Kagase A, Kodama A, Koyama Y, Watanabe Y, Tada N, Takagi K, Araki M, Shirai S. Impact of preparatory coronary protection in patients at high anatomical risk of acute coronary obstruction during transcatheter aortic valve implantation. Int J Cardiol. 2016;217:58–63.
9. Mercanti F, Rosseel L, Neylon A, Bagur R, Sinning JM, Nickenig G, Grube E, Hildick-Smith D, Tavano D, Wolf A, Colonna G. Chimney stenting for coronary occlusion during TAVR: insights from the chimney registry. JACC Cardiovasc Interv. 2020;13(6):751–61.

Left Main Coronary Artery Obstruction Following Valve-in-Valve TAVR Procedure Involving Mitroflow Valve

Vivek Patel, Edmund Naami, and Muhammad Zubair

1 Clinical Background

The patient is a 74-year-old female with a history of dyslipidemia, obesity, congestive heart failure NYHA class III, and previous surgical bioprosthetic aortic valve replacement in October 2013 using a 21 mm Mitroflow pericardial valve. A complete heart block complicated the patient's prior surgical aortic valve replacement and she was treated with a permanent pacemaker. The patient has suffered from increased shortness of breath with minimal exertion, intermittent episodes of chest pain with exertion, and lower extremity edema in recent months. Echocardiography revealed new and severe stenosis of the patient's aortic bioprosthesis, and she was therefore treated with increased Lasix by her primary cardiologist. Nevertheless, the patient was hospitalized for acute-on-chronic decompensated heart failure, requiring intubation in September 2016. She was subsequently transferred to our center for further evaluation.

Supplementary Information The online version contains supplementary material available at [https://doi.org/10.1007/978-3-031-05965-0_12].

V. Patel (✉)
Smidt Heart Institute, Cedars-Sinai Medical Center, Los Angeles, CA, USA
e-mail: vivek.patel@cshs.org

E. Naami
University of Illinois College of Medicine, Chicago, IL, USA

M. Zubair
Cedars Sinai Medical Center, Los Angeles, CA, USA

O. Koren et al. (eds.), *Complex Cases in Structural Heart Intervention*,
https://doi.org/10.1007/978-3-031-05965-0_12

2 Imaging

Transthoracic echocardiogram (TTE) revealed severe prosthetic aortic stenosis with a mean gradient of 44 mmHg, mildly reduced left ventricular systolic function (ejection fraction 50%), moderate mitral regurgitation, and severe mitral stenosis (Fig. 1a–c, Videos 1 and 2). Cardiac reconstructed computed tomogram (CT)

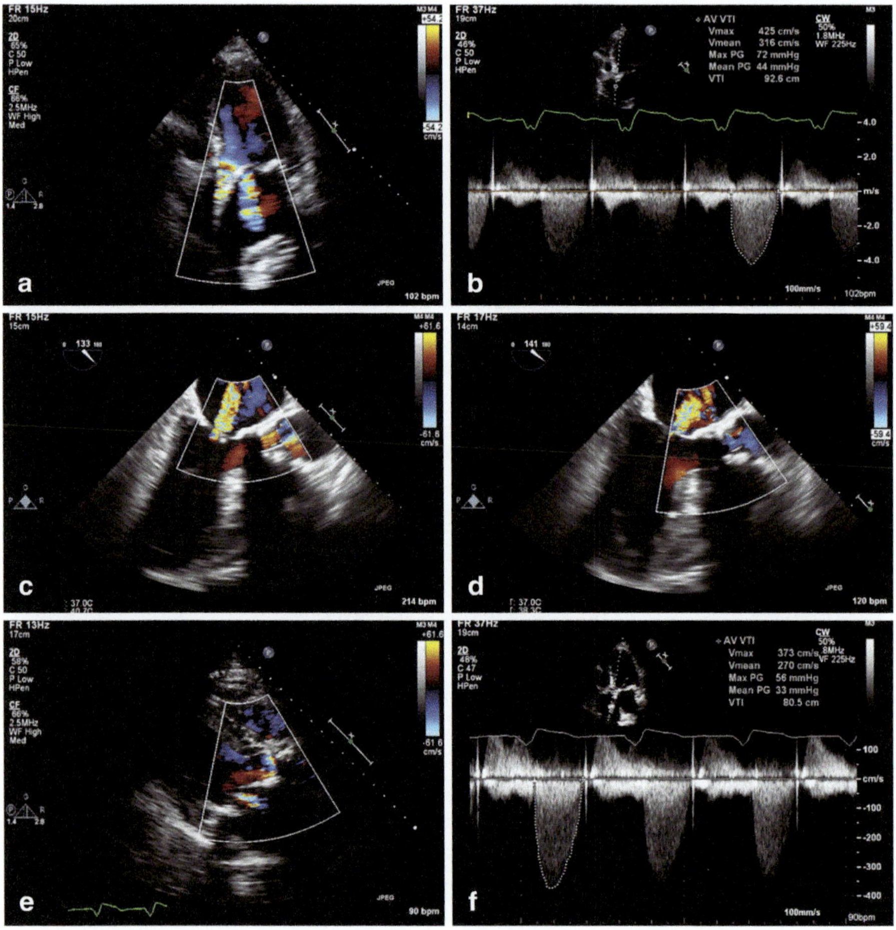

Fig. 1 ECHO imaging. (**a**) Pre-procedural TTE 3 chamber view shows moderate Mitral regurgitation and severe mitral stenosis. (**b**) Aortic valve mean gradient of 44 mmHg measured in 5 chamber TTE view. (**c**) Procedural TEE LVOT outflow tract view before TAVR valve implantation shows severe aortic stenosis and moderate Mitral regurgitation. (**d**) Procedural TEE LVOT outflow tract view after TAVR valve implantation shows reduction in aortic stenosis. (**e**) 30 days follow-up TTE shows moderate aortic stenosis with a mean gradient of 33 mmHg (**e**, **f**)

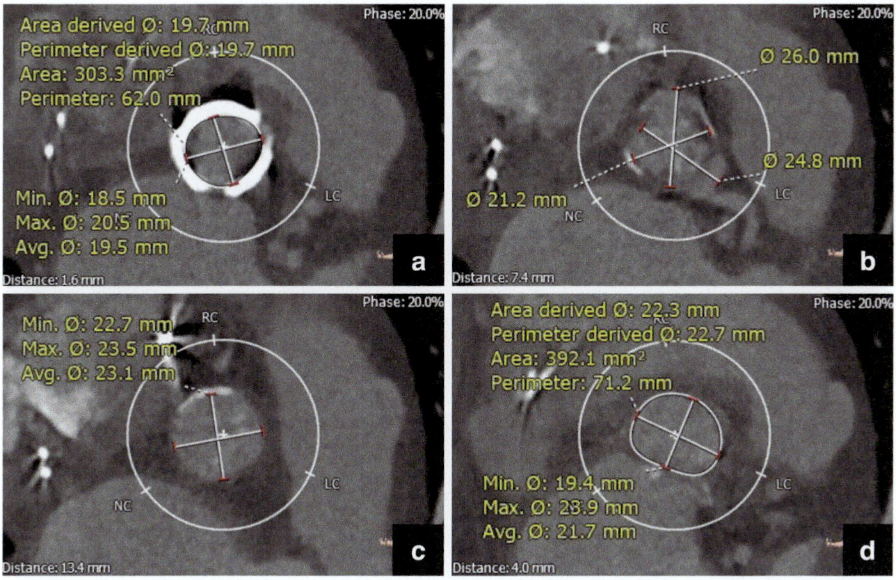

Fig. 2 Pre-TAVR CT analysis. (**a**) Annular measurements. (**b**) SOV measurements. (**c**) Sinotubular junction measurements. (**d**) Left ventricular outflow tract measurement (4 mm below annulus plane)

indicated an annular mean internal diameter of 19.5 mm, area of 303.3 mm^2, and perimeter of 62.0 mm. The following mean diameters were measured: 24.0 mm at the Sinus of Valsalva, 23.1 mm at the STJ, and 21.7 mm at the LVOT (Fig. 2). The coronary ostia originated at 7.8 and 7.1 mm (LCA and RCA, respectively) above the annular plane (Figs. 3a, b and 4a, b). The distance between a virtual 20-mm transcatheter heart valve (THV) and LCA, RCA ostium was 5.0 and 3.4 mm, respectively. A similar calculation was made for a 23-mm THV and found to be 3.5 and 2.5 mm, respectively (Fig. 3c–f).

3 Pre-Procedural Considerations, Dilemmas, and Challenges

The patient was evaluated by cardiothoracic (CT) surgery and deemed a high-risk surgical candidate. Therefore, the patient was approved for transfemoral transcatheter aortic valve replacement (TAVR) using a 23-mm Edwards Sapien 3 valve. Measures were employed to prevent post-deployment coronary obstruction due to the low coronary height and the inherent high risk of coronary occlusion associated with the location of the Mitroflow valve leaflets outside the stent frame.

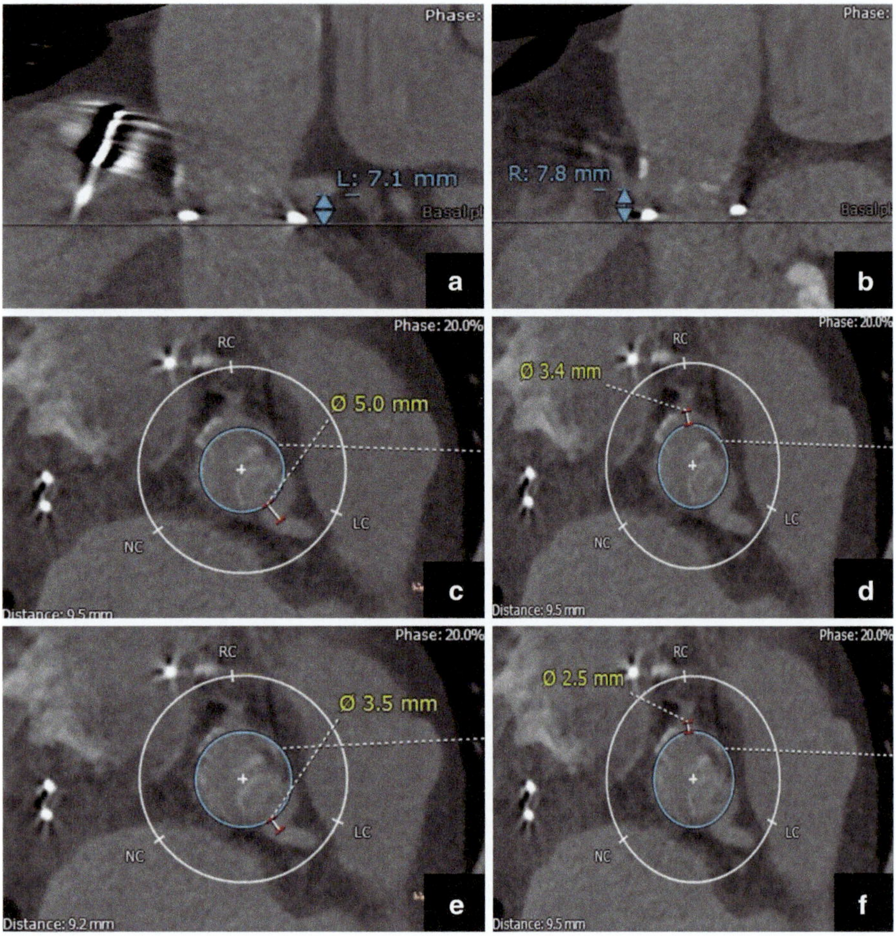

Fig. 3 Pre-TAVR CT analysis. (**a**) Left coronary artery height. (**b**) Right coronary artery height. (**c**) The distance from 20 mm virtual THV to LCA ostium. (**d**) The distance between 20 mm THV to RCA ostium. (**e**) The distance from 23 mm virtual THV to LCA ostium. (**f**) The distance from 23 mm virtual THV to LCA ostium

4 Procedure, Outcome, and Follow-Up

Coronary protection was first established with a 4.0 × 12 mm Xience Alpine DES positioned in the LAD and a 3.5 × 12 mm Xience Alpine DES positioned in the RCA. After obtaining femoral access, the valve delivery system and THV were positioned across the stenotic aortic valve (Fig. 5a–c). With rapid pacing at 180 beats per minute (Video 3), the valve delivery system was then taken out. A post-procedure TEE revealed no central aortic regurgitation, mild paravalvular regurgitation, and reduced aortic stenosis (Fig. 1d).

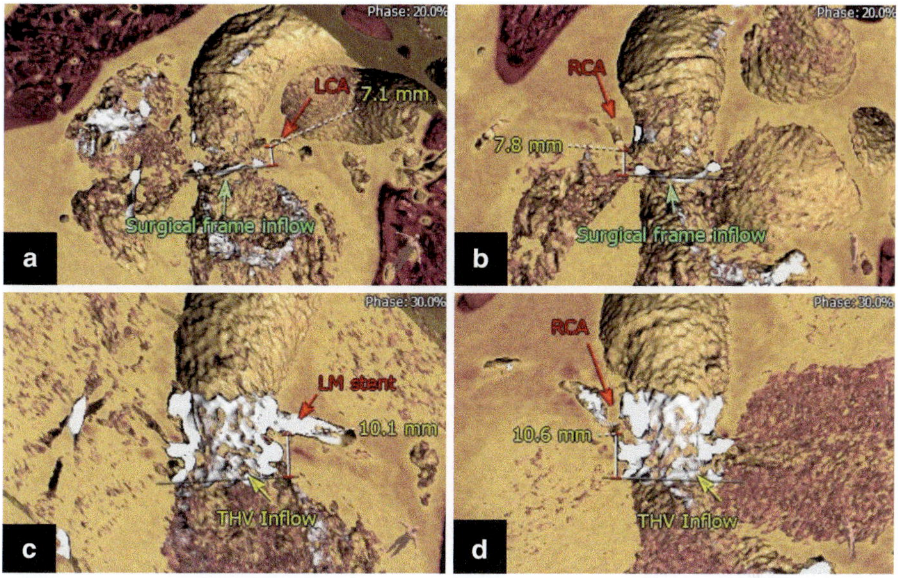

Fig. 4 Pre and post-TAVR Cardiac CT volume rendered image analysis: (**a**) LCA height from surgical valve inflow before the procedure. (**b**) RCA height from surgical valve inflow before the procedure. (**c**) LCA height from THV inflow (left main stent present) after procedure. (**d**) RCA height from the THV inflow after the procedure

The patient was noted to have persistent hypotension immediately following valve deployment, followed by cardiopulmonary arrest requiring initiation of CPR. TEE revealed a significant reduction in LV function with akinesis of the anterior wall (Videos 4, 5, 6 and 7). An indirect coronary angiogram revealed patent RCA and LM occlusion (Video 8), and the LAD stent was pulled back and deployed across the ostium of the LM. The patient continued to have persistent cardiac arrest despite ostial LM stenting (Fig. 5d–f). The right femoral venous access was immediately obtained. The patient was placed on cardiopulmonary bypass by inserting the venous cannula into the right femoral vein and arterial cannula through the 14-French Edwards sheath.

Repeat left coronary angiogram revealed complete occlusion of the LM due to the Mitroflow valve leaflets (Video 9). A 6 French XB LAD 3.0 guide catheter engaged the LM ostium. A 0.014-in. Ultimate Bro, Confianza Pro guidewires failed to puncture the bioprosthetic valve leaflet into the LM. A 0.018 in. Astute 30 peripheral guidewire was then used to puncture the bioprosthetic valve leaflet, and the guidewire was exchanged for a 0.014-in. Grandslam wire through a corsair catheter. Following balloon angioplasty, a 4.0 × 15 mm Xience Alpine drug-eluting stent was deployed, extending from the TAVR stent frame into the ostium of the LM (Fig. 6a–f, Videos 10 and 11). IVUS was used to confirm that the Xience stent was extending into the TAVR valve frame (Video 12).

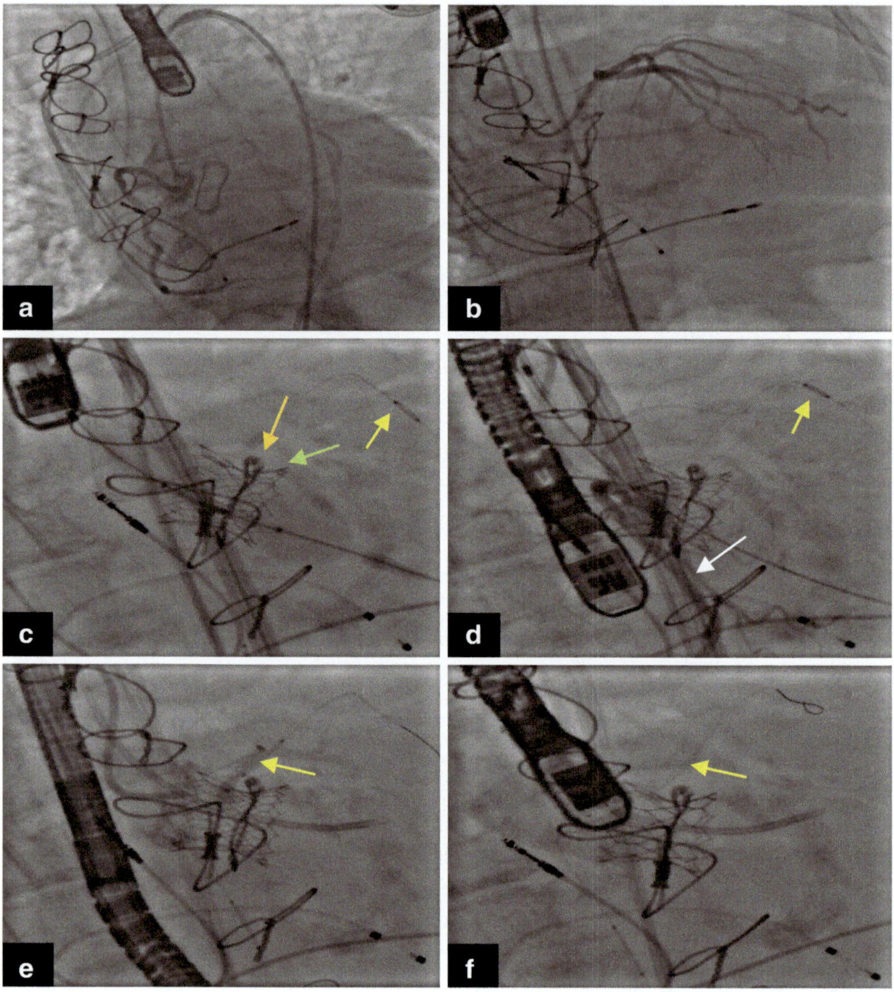

Fig. 5 Procedural fluoroscopic imaging: (**a**) Pre-procedural right coronary artery. (**b**) Left coronary artery. (**c**) Xience Alpine DES was placed in both coronaries considering low coronary height: Xience Alpine DES IN LAD (yellow arrow) Sapien 3. (**d**) Balloon-expandable Sapien-3 deployment (green arrow) over bioprosthetic stented valve (yellow arrow) with coronary protection wire in the left coronary artery (yellow arrow). Occlusion of the left coronary artery (yellow arrow) following the deployment of the Sapien-3 THV over a bioprosthetic stented valve. Note contrast flow across the right coronary artery (white arrow). (**e**) LAD stent was pulled back over left main coronary artery (yellow arrow). (**f**) Deployment of the stent across the ostium of the LM (yellow arrow)

The patient was in ventricular fibrillation for a significant time while on cardiopulmonary bypass and was defibrillated several times. Following successful recanalization of the LM, the patient returned into sinus rhythm following defibrillation. Over the next 30–60 min, the patient was weaned from cardiopulmonary bypass,

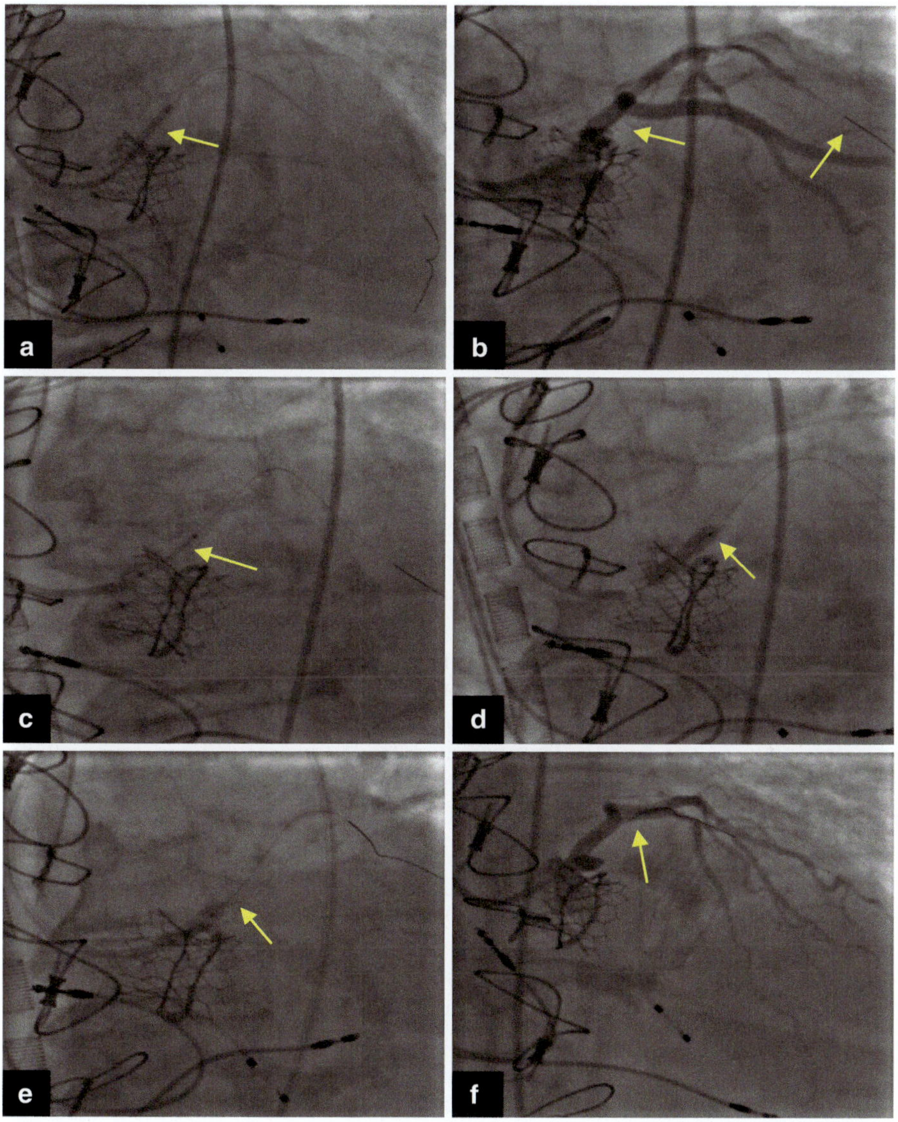

Fig. 6 Procedural fluoroscopic imaging: (**a**) Repeat left coronary angiogram revealed complete occlusion of the LM due to the Mitroflow valve leaflets (yellow arrow). (**b**) Successful puncture of Mitroflow valve leaflet: Corsair catheter present in LAD (yellow arrow). (**c**) Stent was placed across LM (yellow arrow). (**d**) Predilation of the balloon was performed (yellow arrow). (**e**) Xience Alpine drug-eluting stent was pulled into the transcatheter aortic valve frame and deployed. (**f**) Left coronary flow achieved: Contrast can be seen in the left coronary artery (yellow arrow)

and eventually, the cardiopulmonary bypass was discontinued. Post-TAVR echocardiogram showed a mean transaortic gradient of 28 mmHg. The remainder of the patient's hospitalization was uneventful as the patient remained hemodynamically stable.

At 30 days follow-up, the patient continued to have exertional dyspnea, chest discomfort, and volume overload, requiring escalation of diuretic therapy.

Coronary angiography was recommended to evaluate LM obstruction and demonstrate left main coronary artery patency. TTE revealed moderately depressed left ventricular systolic function (EF 40%) and moderate prosthetic aortic stenosis with an aortic valve area of 1.0 cm^2, peak transaortic gradient of 63.0 mmHg, and mean transaortic gradient of 33.0 mmHg (Fig. 1d–f, Videos 13 and 14). At a 6-month follow-up, the patient showed clinical improvement and normalized ejection fraction (56%). However, her mean transaortic gradient increased to 60 mmHg with an AV peak velocity of 487 cm/s, suggesting narrowing of the THV. The patient, therefore, underwent redo surgical aortic valve replacement 6 months following TAVR.

5 Discussion

Over the past two decades, there has been an ever-increasing use of bioprosthetic valves for aortic valve replacement [1]. The use of biological valves increased from 37.7% to 63.3% in an analysis from the National Inpatient Sample done in the USA between two study periods (1998–2001; 2007–2011). This increase in the utilization of biological valves was most seen in patients between ages 55 and 64 years [2]. This may be explained by the modification of consensus guidelines which now recommends patients the choice of not being anticoagulated as a class I indication to use prosthetic valves [3, 4]. This paradigm shift toward utilizing bioprosthetic valves has also been heralded by the increasing use of transcatheter therapies for aortic valve replacement (TAVR). A valve-in-valve (ViV) replacement using a minimally invasive technique is a practical alternative should the initial bioprosthetic valve fail. Bio-prosthetic surgical valves (BPV) are prone to deterioration and degeneration. In a meta-analysis conducted by Etnel et al. [5], the median time to structural BPV deterioration was 17.3 years, and the time for re-intervention was found to be 16.9 years. This meta-analysis looked at the BPV non-elderly (mean age 50.7 years). Young age, hypertension, diabetes, end-stage renal disease, metabolic syndrome, and porcine tissue valve are risks associated with early valve degeneration [6].

Coronary obstruction is a devastating complication that can occur after TAVR in a failing surgically replaced aortic valve. A report from the VIVID registry showed an incidence of 2.7% for coronary obstruction when a TAVR valve was deployed for a degenerative bio-prosthetic surgical valve (BPV) [7]. Incidence of coronary obstruction was also determined for ViV in various degenerating BPV types. The highest incidence was found to be in stentless BPV (48.6%), followed by stented valves with externally mounted leaflets such as Mitroflow valve (32.4%) [7]. Coronary obstruction after ViV results from displacement of the bioprosthetic valve leaflets against the coronaries' ostia. This complication (seen in stented valves with externally mounted leaflets) results from longer leaflets that obstruct the coronary ostia. Supra annular placement of the stentless valve results in a shorter distance between the coronary ostia, explains the obstruction associated with these ViV procedures [7, 8]. A higher rate of post-dilation and VTC <4 mm (distance between a virtual transcatheter ring at the size of the implanted device at the level of each coronary ostium) has been associated with higher rates of coronary obstruction [7]. Various strategies can be used as a bailout when a coronary obstruction in TAVR occurs. These include our above mentioned salvage technique, the open conversion while initiating cardiopulmonary bypass, percutaneous interventions, emergent coronary artery bypass grafting, mechanical circulatory support, and rotational atherectomy in case of calcium embolization. All of these have been successfully described [7, 9].

Key Points

- Bioprosthetic valves are increasingly used for aortic valve replacement.
- Valve-in-valve (ViV) TAVR procedure is a practical option for a degenerative bioprosthetic valve for selected patients.
- Coronary obstruction is rare but a devastating complication of ViV replacement.
- Coronary obstruction can be accurately predicted using reconstructed CT by measuring the distance of a virtual valve to the coronary ostia.
- Various percutaneous techniques are known to protect and treat coronary obstructions.

References

1. Tam DY, Dharma C, Rocha RV, Ouzounian M, Wijeysundera HC, Austin PC, Chikwe J, Gaudino M, Fremes SE. Transcatheter ViV versus redo surgical AVR for the management of failed biological prosthesis: early and late outcomes in a propensity-matched cohort. JACC Cardiovasc Interv. 2020;13(6):765–74.
2. Isaacs AJ, Shuhaiber J, Salemi A, Isom OW, Sedrakyan A. National trends in utilization and in-hospital outcomes of mechanical versus bioprosthetic aortic valve replacements. J Thorac Cardiovasc Surg. 2015;149(5):1262–9.
3. Nishimura RA, Otto CM, Bonow RO, Carabello BA, Erwin JP, Fleisher LA, Jneid H, Mack MJ, McLeod CJ, O'Gara PT, Rigolin VH. 2017 AHA/ACC focused update of the 2014 AHA/ACC guideline for the management of patients with valvular heart disease: a report of the American College of Cardiology/American Heart Association Task Force on Clinical Practice Guidelines. J Am Coll Cardiol. 2017;70(2):252–89.
4. Baumgartner H, Falk V, Bax JJ, De Bonis M, Hamm C, Holm PJ, Iung B, Lancellotti P, Lansac E, Munoz DR, Rosenhek R. 2017 ESC/EACTS Guidelines for the management of valvular heart disease. Kardiol Pol. 2018;76(1):1–62.
5. Etnel JR, Huygens SA, Grashuis P, Pekbay B, Papageorgiou G, Roos Hesselink JW, Bogers AJ, Takkenberg JJ. Bioprosthetic aortic valve replacement in nonelderly adults: a systematic review, meta-analysis, and microsimulation. Circ Cardiovasc Qual Outcomes. 2019;12(2):e005481.
6. Nitsche C, Kammerlander AA, Knechtelsdorfer K, Kraiger JA, Goliasch G, Dona C, Schachner L, Öztürk B, Binder C, Duca F, Aschauer S. Determinants of bioprosthetic aortic valve degeneration. JACC Cardiovasc Imaging. 2020;13(2):345–53.
7. Ribeiro HB, Rodés-Cabau J, Blanke P, Leipsic J, Kwan Park J, Bapat V, Makkar R, Simonato M, Barbanti M, Schofer J, Bleiziffer S. Incidence, predictors, and clinical outcomes of coro-

nary obstruction following transcatheter aortic valve replacement for degenerative bioprosthetic surgical valves: insights from the VIVID registry. Eur Heart J. 2018;39(8):687–95.
8. Dvir D, Webb JG, Bleiziffer S, Pasic M, Waksman R, Kodali S, Barbanti M, Latib A, Schaefer U, Rodés-Cabau J, Treede H. Transcatheter aortic valve implantation in failed bioprosthetic surgical valves. JAMA. 2014;312(2):162–70.
9. Choudhury T, Bakar SN, Kiaii B, Teefy P. Emergent percutaneous rotational atherectomy to bailout surgical transapical aortic valve implantation: a successful case of heart team turnaround. Arq Bras Cardiol. 2019;113:1151–4.

Reduction in Left Coronary Artery Flow After Valve-in-Valve TAVR Procedure

Ofir Koren, Daniel Benhamou, and Jubin Joseph

1 Clinical Presentation

The patient is a 74-year-old female with a history of aortic stenosis secondary to the bicuspid aortic valve, status-post surgical aortic-valve replacement using 21 mm Trifecta valve (2012), congestive heart failure (NYHA Class III–IV), liver cirrhosis, diabetes mellitus type 2, hypertension, hyperlipidemia, coronary artery disease, and chronic thrombocytopenia. She has complained of fatigue, dyspnea with minimal exertion, intermittent, non-radiating, midsternal, exertional chest pain for the past year. The patient was referred for an evaluation as well as a discussion of treatment options for her severe, symptomatic aortic stenosis.

2 Images and Supported Data

Prior to the procedure, TTE revealed EF 61%, severe AS (mean transaortic gradient 42 mmHg, peak transaortic gradient 72 mmHg, AV area 0.7 cm^2), trivial mitral regurgitation, and trivial tricuspid regurgitation. Cardiac reconstructed CT indicated

Supplementary Information The online version contains supplementary material available at [https://doi.org/10.1007/978-3-031-05965-0_13].

O. Koren (✉)
Smidt Heart Institute, Cedars-Sinai Medical Center, Los Angeles, CA, USA

Faculty of Medicine, Technion, Israel Institute of Technology, Haifa, Israel
e-mail: Ofir.Koren@cshs.org

D. Benhamou
Technion, Israel Institute of Technology, Haifa, Israel

J. Joseph
Smidt Heart Institute, Cedars-Sinai Medical Center, Los Angeles, CA, USA

O. Koren et al. (eds.), *Complex Cases in Structural Heart Intervention*,
https://doi.org/10.1007/978-3-031-05965-0_13

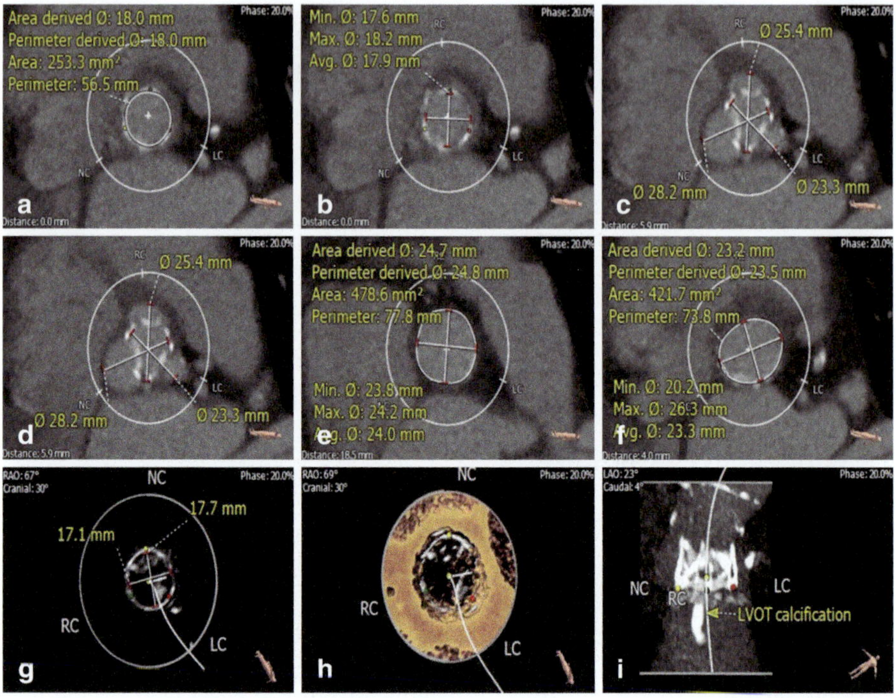

Fig. 1 Reconstructed CT analysis pre-TAVR. (**a**) Bioprosthetic annulus area. (**b**) Bioprosthetic internal annular diameter. (**c**) The area and the perimeter of sinus of valsalva (SOV). (**d**) SOV diameters. (**e**) Sinotubular junction dimensions. (**f**) Left ventricular outflow tract measurement. (**g**) Internal diameter of the bioprosthetic valve using a Hockey puck MIP view. (**h**) Aortic valve view using a hockey puck VR view. (**i**) Aortic root calcification using Hockey puck MIP view

the existing bioprosthetic valve mean internal diameter of 17.9 mm, an area of 253.3 mm^2, and a perimeter of 56.5 mm. The following mean diameters were measured: 25.6 mm at the Sinus of Valsalva, 24.0 mm at the STJ, and 23.3 mm at the LVOT. Significant calcium deposition was noticed mainly on the aortic root (Fig. 1). The coronary ostia originated at 8.2 and 5.5 mm (for the RCA and LCA) above the annular plane. The distance of a virtual 20 and 23 mm Sapien-3 valve THV to the LCA ostium was measured at 4.3 and 2.9 mm, respectively. The distance of a virtual 20 and 23 mm Sapien-3 THV to the RCA ostium was 4.1 and 2.7 mm, respectively (Fig. 2). Coronary angiography before the TAVR procedure illustrated narrowing of >80% of the lumen in the second diagonal and the mid LAD artery (Fig. 3).

3 Procedure and Outcome

The heart team deemed the patient at high surgical risk for repeat SAVR due to the patient's underlying liver disease, along with the need for a repeat sternotomy. Therefore, the patient was selected for transfemoral TAVR using a 20-mm Edward

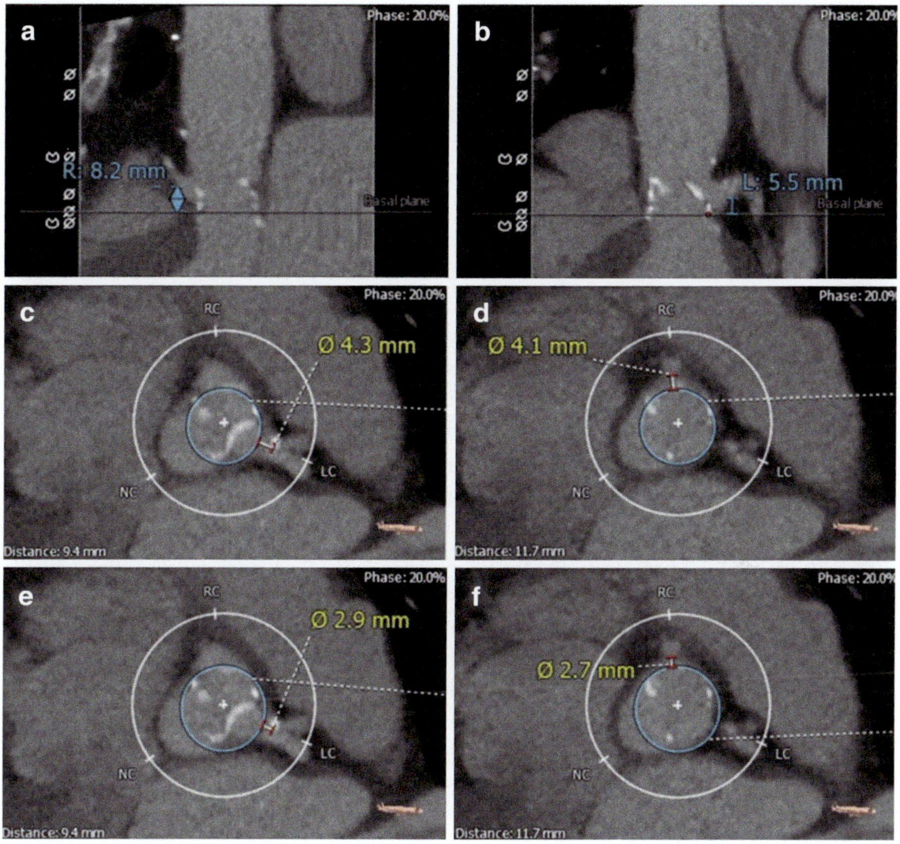

Fig. 2 Reconstructed CT analysis for anticipating coronary obstruction using a virtual valve. (**a**) Right coronary artery (RCA) height from the annular plane. (**b**) Left coronary artery (LCA) height from the annular plane. (**c**) The distance of a virtual 20 mm Sapien-3 valve to the LCA ostium. (**d**) The distance of a virtual 20 mm Sapien-3 valve to the RCA ostium. (**e**) The distance from a virtual 23 mm Sapien-3 valve to the LCA. (**f**) The distance from a virtual 23 mm Sapien-3 valve to the RCA

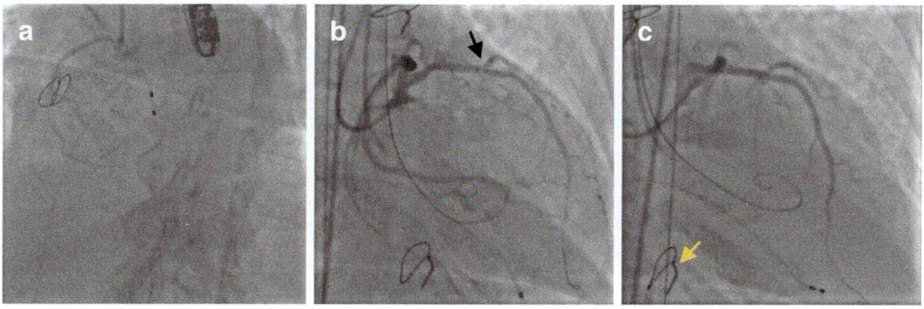

Fig. 3 Coronary angiography before the TAVR procedure. (**a**) Right coronary angiography shows patent artery, (**b**) narrowing of >80% of the lumen in the second diagonal and the mid-LAD artery involving the bifurcation region (black arrow). (**c**) LAD flow following multiple drug-eluting stenting in D2 and LAD arteries. Note the previous surgical sutures (yellow arrow)

Sapien S3 bioprosthesis. After reviewing the coronary angiogram prior to the procedure and anticipating difficulty engaging the left coronary artery following valve-in-valve, we decided to proceed with a percutaneous coronary intervention of the LAD and the diagonal. The mid LAD was treated with a 3.5 × 16 mm Synergy drug-eluting stent, and the diagonal branch was treated with a 2.5 × 12 mm Synergy DES (Fig. 3, Videos 1 and 2). Given the prior SAVR with #21 Trifecta and the proximity to the ostium of the left main artery, an XB-LAD 3.5 guide catheter was left intubated in the LMS. A Balance wire was placed in the distal LAD, and a 4.0 × 18 mm Xience DES was positioned in the mid-LAD for possible obstruction of the LMS via TAVR. A 20-mm Edwards Sapien Ultra valve delivery system was positioned across the stenotic aortic valve. The valve was deployed in the standard technique while using rapid pacing, at 180 beats per minute (Fig. 4, Videos 3 and 4). A post-procedure TEE revealed no central aortic regurgitation and perivalvular regurgitation (Fig. 5, Video 5). The valve delivery system was then taken out. There was concern of obstruction for flow into the LMS (Video 6). Therefore, the 4.0 × 18 mm Xience DES was retracted to the LMS and positioned with significant extrusion into the aorta and deployed up to 18 atm. The delivery balloon was pulled and re-inflated up to 20 atm. Then, a 4.5 × 12 mm NC balloon was placed in the DES and inflated to 20 atm. Subsequently, another 4.0 × 8 mm Xience DES was placed at the bend outside the TAVR to provide extra radial strength. This DES was deployed up to 16 atm, and the delivery balloon was re-inflated up to 22 atm. There was good flow into the LCA without evidence of dissection or plaque shift in the LCA system (Fig. 6, Videos 7, 8 and 9). The patient remained hemodynamically stable, afebrile, and normotensive throughout the rest of the hospital stay. On a 30-day follow-up, the patient had improved symptoms, including decreased dyspnea on exertion.

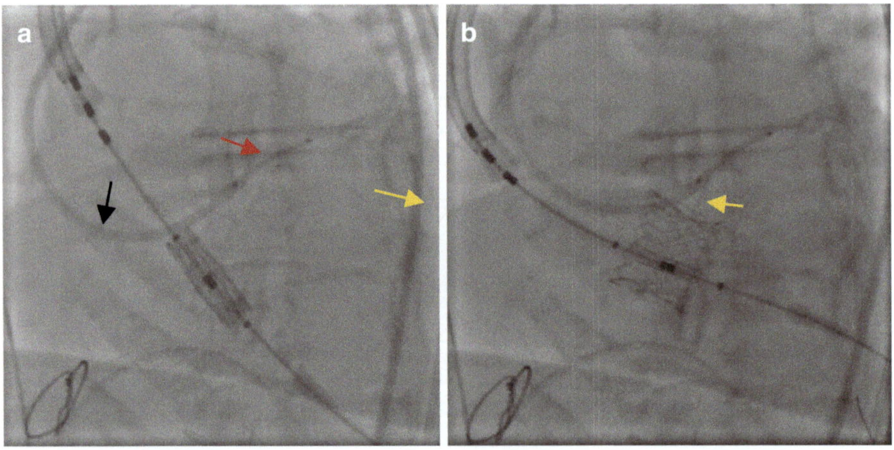

Fig. 4 Fluoroscopy views of the coronary protection technique. (**a**) Guiding catheter (black arrow) with a balance wire (yellow arrow) and deflated drug-eluting stent (red arrow) is placed in the left coronary artery before the procedure. (**b**) Drug-eluting stent in the LCA after the THV deployment. Note the proximity of the THV to the LCA ostium (yellow arrow)

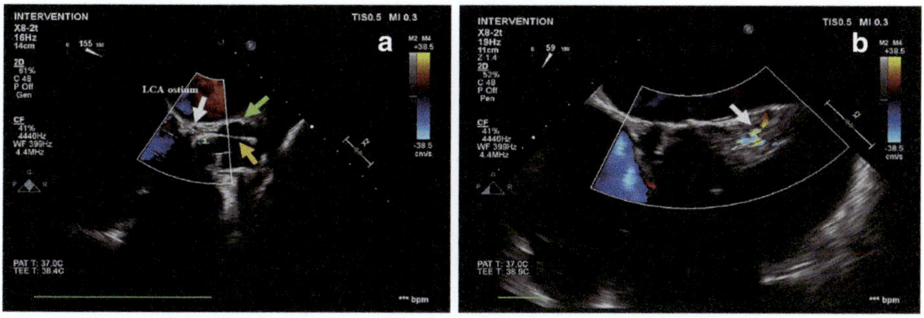

Fig. 5 Transesophageal echocardiography during the TAVR procedure. (**a**) Sapien-3 THV (yellow arrow) successfully deployed over a prior surgical bioprosthetic valve (green arrow) with a significant reduction in flow to the LCA (white arrow). Note the proximity of the THV to the left coronary ostium and the reduction in the coronary flow (white arrow). (**b**) Improvement in LCA flow (white arrow) following inflation of a pre-inserted stent (Chimney procedure)

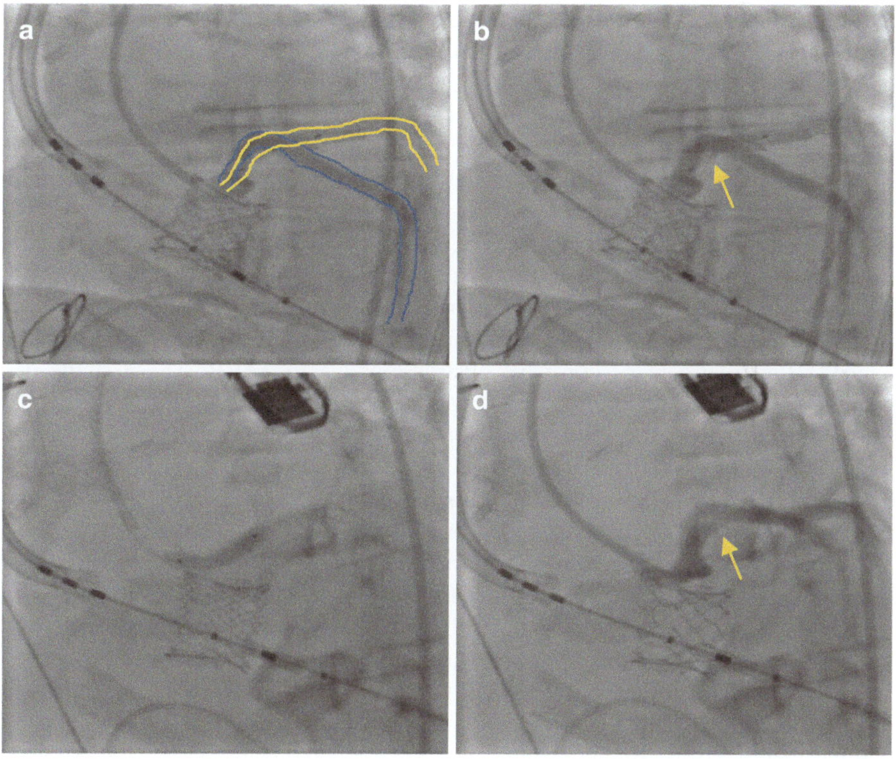

Fig. 6 Fluoroscopy views of the left coronary artery following THV deployment. (**a**) Coronary flow in the LCA (yellow lines) and the Circumflex artery (Blue lines) after THV deployment. (**b**) Reduction of coronary flow in the proximal segment of the LCA (yellow arrow) following valve deployment. (**c**) Inflation of a pre-inserted drug-eluting stent in LCA. (**d**) Stent dilatation using non-compact balloon with a significant improvement in the LCA flow (yellow arrow)

4 Discussion

Coronary obstruction in TAVR is a rare and serious complication occurring in up to 1.6% of procedures, with an associated increase in mortality [1]. Risk factors for coronary obstruction in native anatomy include short coronary height of the annulus, long valve leaflets (i.e., bicuspid valves), and small aortic sinus dimensions [2, 3] The most common pathogenesis of coronary obstruction is obstruction by native cusps. Risk for this phenomena is particularly high with annulus to coronary height distances of 10 mm and 15 mm in tricuspid and bicuspid valve anatomy, respectively. In patients undergoing valve-in-valve procedures, careful consideration needs to be given to the anatomy of the ascending aorta, the type of the surgical prosthesis (Supra vs. Intra-annular position), and leaflet profile. Valves with internal stent frames such as MitroFlow and Trifecta pose a higher risk of coronary obstruction. Furthermore, when considering valve-in-valve TAVR, measurements of the virtual distance to the coronary (VTC) ostia should be made pre-procedurally and values < 4 mm are at particularly increase risk for obstruction. Many experts believe these factors to be recommendations rather than strict guidelines and highlight the importance of patient-specific determination of TAVR safety. Factors of patients at higher risk of coronary obstruction during TAVR intervention include extreme calcification of the valve, AF, BAV, poor mobility, oxygen dependency, GFR <30 mL/min, and frailty [4–7].

In terms of management, the origin of the obstruction will determine the therapeutic approach. In the case of obstruction by the native cusp, approximately 80% of patients can be managed by PCI alone. However, 30-day outcomes for successful PCI showed a 22% mortality, 100% mortality for those with an unsuccessful PCI. Conversely, there was a 50% mortality for those who underwent CABG [4]. Prophylactic guidewire, catheter, or stenting of at-risk arteries can be considered to expedite the treatment of coronary obstruction due to TAVR. These stents can become entrapped and frequently utilized despite a lack of necessity. Additionally, the pinning of these catheter tools between the TAVR implant and the aortic root can make PCI unsuccessful as anatomical access becomes increasingly difficult [8].

Additionally, the repetitive compression of these stents can lead to their deformation or thrombosis providing risks for ischemic complications. Various new technology currently exists to help minimize or prevent risk of coronary obstructive during TAVR. For instance, the use of retrievable or repositionable devices, a method of acutely relieving obstruction intra-operatively. These include devices such as Evolut R (Medtronic, Minneapolis, MN), Lotus (Boston Scientific, Natick, MA), and Portico (Abbott St. Jude, Santa Clara, CA) [9, 10]. The BASILICA procedure involves intentional laceration of the bioprosthetic or native aortic scallop to prevent coronary artery obstruction in patients with a sequestered sinus. Recent data showed acceptable safety and no instances of coronary obstruction when performing TAVR. However, this may be expected given the low incidence of coronary obstruction, larger studies are required. To better assess its place as a preventive measure to coronary obstruction in physicians looking to avoid long-term complications of stenting [11].

Key Points

- Coronary obstruction following TAVR deployment is an uncommon but serious complication.
- Obstruction is commonly due to prolapse of the existing valve leaflet over the ostia—therefore, risk can be predicted by considering leaflet length, sinus size, and coronary height.
- In patients undergoing valve-in-valve TAVR, the risk is higher when treating surgical valves with leaflets sewn outside the posts (i.e., MitroFlow and Trifecta).
- Management of patients at high risk of coronary obstruction includes either peri-procedural coronary protection with a guide catheter or coronary stent ready to be deployed in the coronary ostia ("snorkel stenting") or pre-TAVR radiofrequency laceration of the valve leaflets to reduce the risk of leaflet prolapse over the ostia (BASILICA procedure).

References

1. Arai T, Lefèvre T, Hovasse T, Garot P, Benamer H, Unterseeh T, Roy AK, Romano M, Hayashida K, Watanabe Y, Bouvier E. Incidence and predictors of coronary obstruction following transcatheter aortic valve implantation in the real world. Catheter Cardiovasc Interv. 2017;90(7):1192–7.
2. Achenbach S, Delgado V, Hausleiter J, Schoenhagen P, Min JK, Leipsic JA. SCCT expert consensus document on computed tomography imaging before transcatheter aortic valve implantation (TAVI)/transcatheter aortic valve replacement (TAVR). J Cardiovasc Comput Tomogr. 2012;6(6):366–80.
3. Holmes DR, Mack MJ, Kaul S, Agnihotri A, Alexander KP, Bailey SR, Calhoon JH, Carabello BA, Desai MY, Edwards FH, Francis GS. 2012 ACCF/AATS/SCAI/STS expert consensus document on transcatheter aortic valve replacement. J Am Coll Cardiol. 2012;59(13):1200–54.
4. Ribeiro HB, Webb JG, Makkar RR, Cohen MG, Kapadia SR, Kodali S, Tamburino C, Barbanti M, Chakravarty T, Jilaihawi H, Paradis JM. Predictive factors, management, and clinical outcomes of coronary obstruction following transcatheter aortic valve implantation: insights from a large multicenter registry. J Am Coll Cardiol. 2013;62(17):1552–62.
5. Osnabrugge RL, Speir AM, Head SJ, Fonner CE, Fonner E, Kappetein AP, Rich JB. Performance of EuroSCORE II in a large US database: implications for transcatheter aortic valve implantation. Eur J Cardiothorac Surg. 2014;46(3):400–8.
6. Barili F, Pacini D, Capo A, Rasovic O, Grossi C, Alamanni F, Di Bartolomeo R, Parolari A. Does EuroSCORE II perform better than its original versions? A multicentre validation study. Eur Heart J. 2013;34(1):22–9.
7. Vahanian A, Baumgartner H, Bax J, Butchart E, Dion R, Filippatos G, Flachskampf F, Hall R, Iung B, Kasprzak J, Nataf P. Guidelines on the management of valvular heart disease: the Task Force on the Management of Valvular Heart Disease of the European Society of Cardiology. Eur Heart J. 2007;28(2):230–68.
8. Lederman RJ, Babaliaros VC, Rogers T, Khan JM, Kamioka N, Dvir D, Greenbaum AB. Preventing coronary obstruction during transcatheter aortic valve replacement: from computed tomography to BASILICA. J Am Coll Cardiol Interv. 2019;12(13):1197–216.

9. Ribeiro HB, Rodés-Cabau J, Blanke P, Leipsic J, Kwan Park J, Bapat V, Makkar R, Simonato M, Barbanti M, Schofer J, Bleiziffer S. Incidence, predictors, and clinical outcomes of coronary obstruction following transcatheter aortic valve replacement for degenerative bioprosthetic surgical valves: insights from the VIVID registry. Eur Heart J. 2018;39(8):687–95.
10. Jabbour RJ, Tanaka A, Finkelstein A, Mack M, Tamburino C, Van Mieghem N, de Backer O, Testa L, Gatto P, Purita P, Rahhab Z. Delayed coronary obstruction after transcatheter aortic valve replacement. J Am Coll Cardiol. 2018;71(14):1513–24.
11. Khan JM, Greenbaum AB, Babaliaros VC, Dvir D, Reisman M, McCabe JM, Satler L, Waksman R, Eng MH, Paone G, Chen MY. BASILICA trial: one-year outcomes of transcatheter electrosurgical leaflet laceration to prevent TAVR coronary obstruction. Circ Cardiovasc Interv. 2021;14(5):e010238.

Acute Embolic Occlusion of the Left Coronary Artery Following TAVR

Ofir Koren, Addee Lerner, and Hasan Jilaihawi

1 Clinical Presentation

An 89-year-old female patient who appeared considerably younger than her stated age presented for the evaluation of symptomatic aortic stenosis. She had a history of coronary artery disease (status post left circumflex and second obtuse marginal stenting), minor CVA more than 9 years ago with chronic paresthesia in her left hand, hypertension, hyperlipidemia, diabetes mellitus, osteoporosis, and atrial fibrillation treated with oral anticoagulation (Xarelto). Her primary complaints were chest pressure, lightheadedness, dizziness, and shortness of breath at rest over the prior year (NYHA III–IV). She had frequently been brought to the emergency room due to tingling and numbness in her left hand. However, sequential MRIs were negative for any acute strokes.

Supplementary Information The online version contains supplementary material available at [https://doi.org/10.1007/978-3-031-05965-0_14].

O. Koren (✉)
Smidt Heart Institute, Cedars-Sinai Medical Center, Los Angeles, CA, USA

Faculty of Medicine, Technion, Israel Institute of Technology, Haifa, Israel
e-mail: Ofir.Koren@cshs.org

A. Lerner
David Geffen School of Medicine, University of California, Los Angeles, Los Angeles, CA, USA

H. Jilaihawi
Heart Valve Center, NYU Langone Health, New York, NY, USA

O. Koren et al. (eds.), *Complex Cases in Structural Heart Intervention*, https://doi.org/10.1007/978-3-031-05965-0_14

2 Images and Supported Data

TEE before the procedure indicated good left ventricular function and severe calcific AS (Video 1). Pulmonary artery pressure and RV function were intact. Cardiac CT reconstructions indicated an annular mean internal diameter of 21.9 mm, area of 389.8 mm^2, and perimeter of 72.3 mm. AVA area by CT was 0.74 cm^2. The following mean diameters were measured: 31.9 mm at the Sinus of Valsalva, 23.8 mm at the STJ, and 29.1 mm at the LVOT. The coronary ostia originated at 16.3 and 14.6 mm (for the RCA and LCA) above the annular plane (Fig. 1). Significant calcium deposition was noticed mainly on the non-coronary cusp (NCC) and the left coronary cusp (LCC). Quantification of the calcium using 850 Hounsfield units as a threshold indicated 222.1 mm^3 volume of calcium over the AV annulus (Fig. 2).

3 Procedure and Outcome

The heart team's evaluation was that the patient would not be suitable for surgery due to her multiple comorbidities. They proceeded with a transfemoral TAVR using a 23-mm Edward Sapien S3 bioprosthesis. The THV was positioned across the stenotic aortic valve with rapid pacing at 180 beats per minute and deployed using standard technique (Fig. 3, Video 2). An immediate post-procedure TEE revealed no central aortic regurgitation and traced paravalvular regurgitation. The delivery system was removed, and a 6F multipurpose catheter was inserted into the LV to measure post-valve deployment hemodynamics. Upon removing the multipurpose catheter, the patient became unstable with a significant reduction in blood pressure

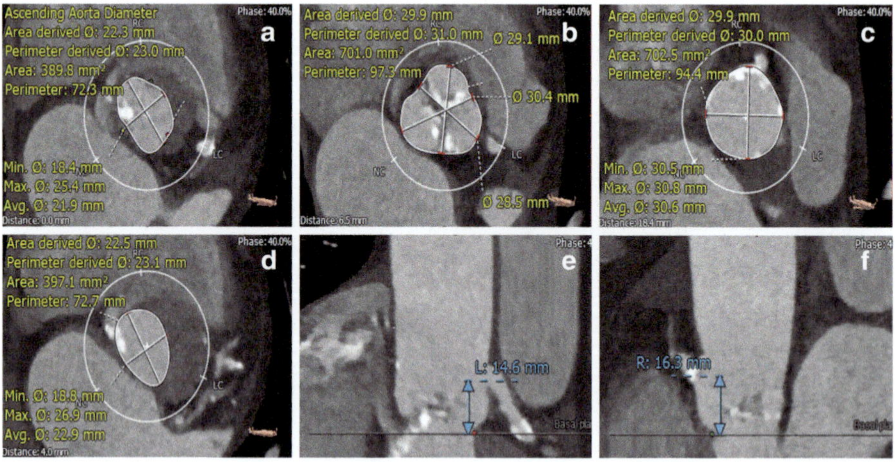

Fig. 1 Reconstructed CT analysis pre-TAVR. (**a**) AV annulus. (**b**) Sinus of Valsalva. (**c**) Sinotubular junction. (**d**) Left ventricular outflow tract. (**e**) Height of the LCA from the annular plane. (**f**) Height of the RCA from the annular plane

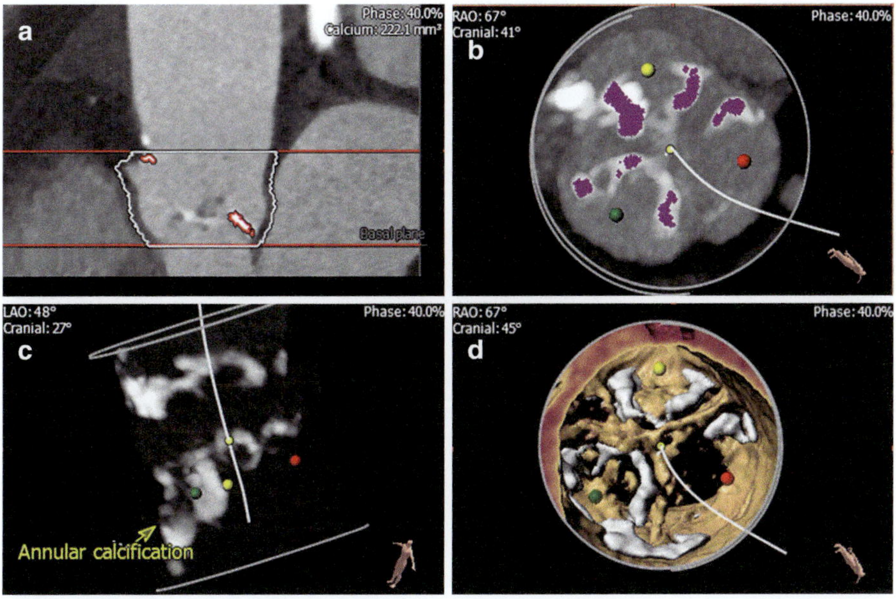

Fig. 2 Reconstructed CT of calcium quantification and distribution before TAVR. (**a**) Significant AV calcification of 222.1 mm^3 measured with an HU850 threshold. (**b**) Calcium deposition on the NCC and RCC (cross section at the SOV level). (**c**) Hockey Puck MIP view of significant leaflets and STJ calcification. (**d**) Hockey Puck VR view of the leaflet's calcification

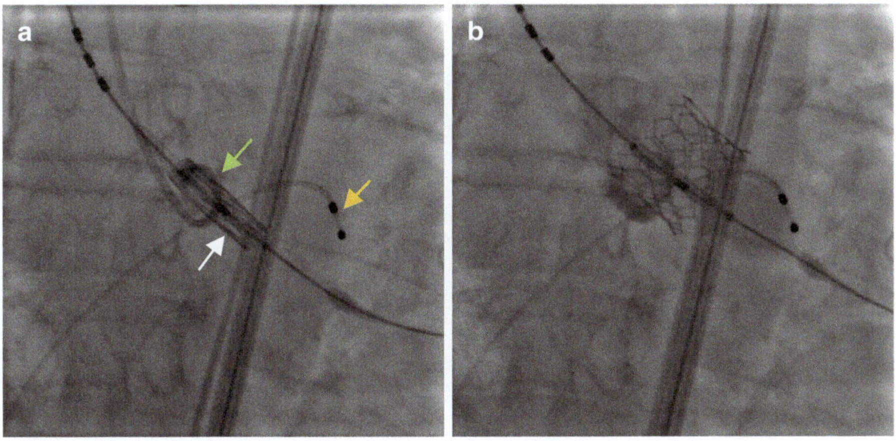

Fig. 3 Fluoroscopy views of the TAVR procedure. TAVR procedure before (**a**) and after (**b**) THV deployment. Note the non-inflated THV at the AV position (white arrow), RV pacemaker lead (yellow arrow), and the pigtail catheter over the AV sinuses (green arrow)

(BP), heart block, and eventually cardiac arrest. CPR was immediately initiated. TEE indicated a severe reduction in LV function and an estimated LVEF of 10% with regional wall motion abnormalities involving predominantly the septum, anterior, and anterolateral walls (Video 3) and mild to moderate pericardial effusion

(Video 4). We used the already placed pigtailed catheter to demonstrate the aortic root and the coronary flow. We noticed a significant reduction in blood flow to the left coronary artery (LCA) (Video 5, Fig. 4). Selective angiography using an XB guiding catheter indicated interruptions of coronary flow affecting the ostial LAD, the first diagonal branch, and the LCx (Video 6, Fig. 5). A series of sequential

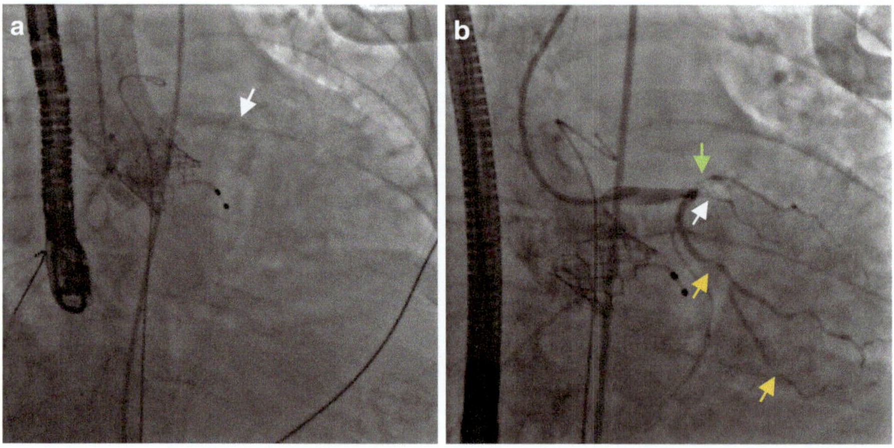

Fig. 4 (**a**) Fluoroscopy views of acute coronary obstruction during balloon-expandable THV deployment. Note, the lack of contrast perfusion in left coronary artery (white arrow). (**b**) Note the cutoff lesion of the Ostial LAD (green arrow), significant lesion at the mid and distal LCx (yellow arrows), and the ostium of the ramus intermedius (green arrow)

Fig. 5 Left coronary angiogram, following multiple stent deployment and balloon inflation—fluoroscopy view. Note the restoration of flow across the left anterior descending artery (white arrow)

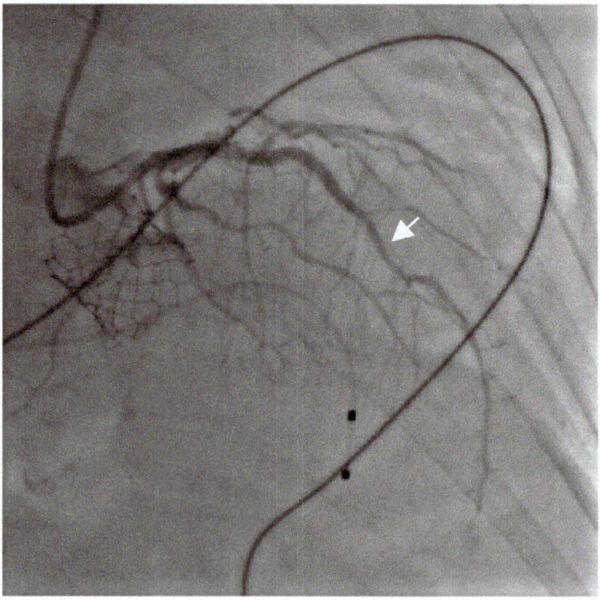

balloon dilatations and multiple drug-eluting stents were used to restore the blood flow to the LAD while partially restoring the blood flow to the LCx due to its proximal tortuosity (Fig. 5). An Impella assist device (Biomed, Danvers, MA) was then inserted in a percutaneous approach via the right femoral artery across the aortic valve (Video 7, Fig. 6). Impella flow was maintained at 5 L/min with improved hemodynamics, during the PCI procedure. Once the PCI was completed, a significant improvement in LV function was achieved, but the patient still required two different vasopressor medications to maintain an adequate BP (Video 8). A non-contrast brain CT demonstrated a large cerebrovascular infarct (Fig. 7). The patient deteriorated in the intensive care unit and died several days later.

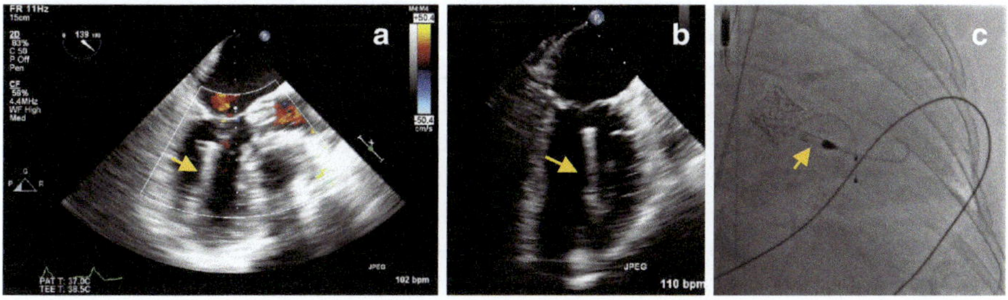

Fig. 6 Transesophageal echocardiography and fluoroscopy view during acute cardiogenic shock. Note the Impella device positioned in the LV apex (orange arrow) in the ME AV LAX view (**a**) and ME mitral commissural view (**b**) and on fluoroscopy view (**c**). An Impella device was inserted across the THV toward the LV apex (yellow arrow). *ME* mid-esophagus, *AV* aortic valve, *LAX* long-axis view, *TEE* transesophageal echocardiography

Fig. 7 Brain CT following TAVR. A large frontoparietal ischemic cerebrovascular infarct (orange arrow) following TAVR procedure (non-contrast brain CT)

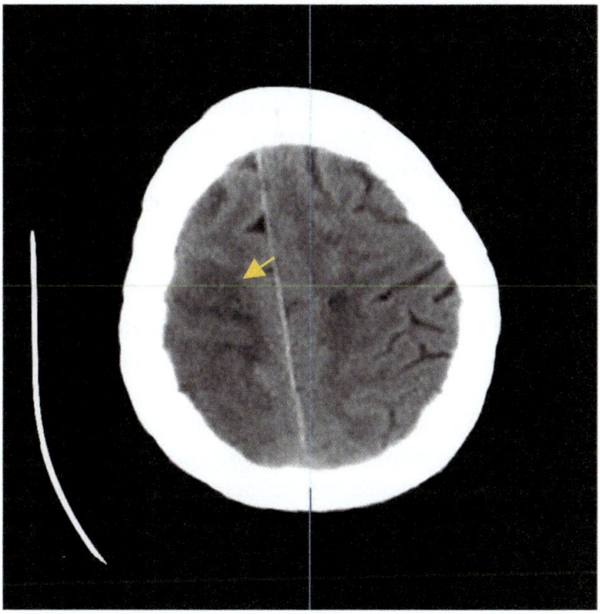

4 Discussion

Coronary obstruction after TAVR has a very poor outcome and occurs in up to 1.6% of cases [1]. It is associated with a high mortality rate as almost all obstructions occur in the LAD, with right coronary obstruction being much rarer. Important predictors of coronary obstruction include the annulus' distance to the coronary ostia on MSCT and sinus of Valsalva dimensions; the mechanisms underlying coronary obstruction include obstruction via native cusps, embolization, and prosthesis compression [2]. Obstruction by the native cusps is the most common cause, which explains why the distance of the annulus to the left main is the best predictor for coronary obstruction [1]. An expert consensus between the CT-TAVI, ACCF, AATS, SCAI, and the STS suggests a 10 mm cut-off between the annulus and the coronary ostium. It should be used as a rough estimate, and many patients require greater heights for the safe TAVR procedure, especially those with BAV [3, 4]. In terms of management, the etiology of the obstruction determines the therapy of choice.

In the case of a malpositioned valve, snaring of the valve is most effective. In the case of obstruction by the native cusp, approximately 80% of patients can be managed by PCI alone. However, 30-day outcomes for successful PCI demonstrated 22% mortality, whereas unsuccessful PCI was associated with a 100% mortality. Alternatively, there was a 50% mortality risk in those who underwent CABG [5]. Write in cases of high risk of coronary obstruction, it is essential to have a primed bypass circuit. A full sternotomy kit is available for the heart team during a TAVR, and the anesthesia team should be made aware of the possibility of conversion in cases of moderate sedation. For patients with an anatomical predisposition for coronary obstruction, guidewire insertion for coronary protection and utilization of a recapturable/repositionable valve should be considered. In the case of valve-in-valve operations, ensuring patency and stent access of the left main coronary ostium via wire placement is fairly common [6]. In one study of patients undergoing coronary protection with preventive coronary wiring, 60% eventually had stents placed across the coronary ostia after valve deployment. During a 3-year follow-up, cardiac death rates were 7.8% in patients who received stents and 15.7% for those who did not. In that patient population, stent thromboses occurred in 0.9% [2]. The BASILICA procedure involves intentional laceration of the bioprosthetic or native aortic scallop to prevent coronary artery obstruction and showed acceptable safety and no coronary obstruction during TAVR in 30 subjects. However, this is expected given the low incidence of coronary obstruction, so larger studies are needed to assess its place as a preventive measure to coronary obstruction in physicians looking to avoid long-term complications of snorkel stenting [7].

New cerebral ischemic events are a known embolic complication in TAVR patients. While many of these are so small that they clandestinely settle into a vessel with little consequence, stroke incidence following TAVR is significantly increased from baseline [8]. For this reason, stroke is a common barrier to both patients and physicians when considering aortic valve replacement or implantation. A diffusion-weighted MRI study of silent and apparent cerebral ischemia found cerebral ischemia more frequent in TAVR (84%) than in open surgery (48%, $P = 0.011$) [8]. The comorbidity of arrhythmias is also considerably higher in those who would be potential candidates for TAVR, and arrhythmia is a common side effect of TAVR [9]. These arrhythmias can increase a patient's risk for CVEs and produce sluggish intracardiac blood flow potentiating embolization risk. Prolonged device manipulation during implantation and severely calcified or stenotic aortic valves can further increase the risk of embolic CVEs [10]. Brain hypoperfusion is another potential complication of TAVR that can manifest due to obstruction or turbulent flow during device implantation.

As TAVR is offered to younger and lower-risk patients, the implementation of cerebral protection devices will become increasingly important. There are two principal categories of cerebral protective devices: filters and deflectors. Filters can capture embolic material within the device itself, while deflectors redirect debris into the descending aorta. Filters currently available include the Emblok (ICS, LLC.), Emboliner (Emboline, Inc.), and the Sentinel (Boston Scientific). Deflectors include the Triguard3 (Venus Medtech, Inc.), Point-guard (Transvers Medical, Inc.), ProtEmbo (Protembis GmbH), and the Umbrella (Edwards Lifesciences) [11]. The use of cerebral protection devices is relatively rare at present. Though there have been promising small single-center studies for reducing in-hospital mortality, their use did not alter the risk for stroke or delirium [12]. Faroux et al. describe three similar cases of coronary obstructions in their review of TAVR and coronary artery disease, but our patient's coronary event coupled with her CVE is exceedingly rare [13].

Key Points

- Coronary obstruction during TAVR is rare but may lead to a catastrophic cascade of events requiring urgent intervention.
- TAVR on highly calcified annulus have a higher risk for debris embolization which may cause acute cerebral infarct or coronary obstruction.
- Operators should be aware of predictors, preprocedural planning, protective devices, and bailout solutions against debris embolization.

References

1. Arai T, et al. Incidence and predictors of coronary obstruction following transcatheter aortic valve implantation in the real world. Catheter Cardiovasc Interv. 2017;90:1192–7.
2. Palmerini T, et al. Coronary protection to prevent coronary obstruction during TAVR. J Am Coll Cardiol Interv. 2020;13:739–47.
3. Achenbach S, et al. SCCT expert consensus document on computed tomography imaging before transcatheter aortic valve implantation (TAVI)/transcatheter aortic valve replacement (TAVR). J Cardiovasc Comput Tomogr. 2012;6:366–80.
4. Holmes DR, et al. 2012 ACCF/AATS/SCAI/STS expert consensus document on transcatheter aortic valve replacement. J Am Coll Cardiol. 2012;59:1200–54.

5. Ribeiro HB, et al. Predictive factors, management, and clinical outcomes of coronary obstruction following transcatheter aortic valve implantation: insights from a large multicenter registry. J Am Coll Cardiol. 2013;62:1552–62.
6. Sultan I, Siki M, Wallen T, Szeto W, Vallabhajosyula P. Management of coronary obstruction following transcatheter aortic valve replacement. J Card Surg. 2017;32:777–81.
7. Khan JM, et al. BASILICA trial: one-year outcomes of transcatheter electrosurgical leaflet laceration to prevent TAVR coronary obstruction. Circ Cardiovasc Interv. 2021;14:e010238.
8. Kahlert P, et al. Silent, and apparent cerebral ischemia after percutaneous transfemoral aortic valve implantation: a diffusion-weighted magnetic resonance imaging study. Circulation. 2010;121:870–8.
9. Vora AN, et al. Incidence, management, and associated clinical outcomes of new-onset atrial fibrillation following transcatheter aortic valve replacement: an analysis from the STS/ACC TVT registry. JACC Cardiovasc Interv. 2018;11:1746–56.
10. Cubero-Gallego H, Pascual I, Rozado J, et al. Cerebral protection devices for transcatheter aortic valve replacement. Ann Transl Med. 2019;7(20):584.
11. Gasior T, Mangner N, Bijoch J, Wojakowski W. Cerebral embolic protection systems for transcatheter aortic valve replacement. J Interv Cardiol. 2018;31:891–8.
12. Stachon P, et al. The use and outcomes of cerebral protection devices for patients undergoing transfemoral transcatheter aortic valve replacement in clinical practice. J Am Coll Cardiol Interv. 2021;14:161–8.
13. Faroux L, et al. Coronary artery disease and transcatheter aortic valve replacement: JACC state-of-the-art review. J Am Coll Cardiol. 2019;74(3):362–72.

Two-Valves Solution for Unstable Self-Expandable Valve and Aortic Root Aneurysm

Ofir Koren, Mattan Arazi, and Jubin Joseph

1 Clinical Presentation

The patient is an 84-year-old male with calcific aortic valve stenosis, aortic regurgitation secondary to aortic root aneurysmal dilatation (5.34 cm), and non-ischemic cardiomyopathy in the setting of heart failure with reduced ejection fraction (35%, NYHA Class III–IV). The patient also has moderate mitral and tricuspid regurgitation due to atria enlargement secondary to long-standing atrial fibrillation (Fig. 1). He comes for evaluation and surgical risk assessment for aortic root and valve repair. The patient complains of worsening fatigue, decreased stamina, and shortness of breath with minimal effort. The patient denies orthopnea, paroxysmal nocturnal dyspnea, chest palpitation, lower extremity edema, and syncope.

Supplementary Information The online version contains supplementary material available at [https://doi.org/10.1007/978-3-031-05965-0_15].

O. Koren (✉)
Smidt Heart Institute, Cedars-Sinai Medical Center, Los Angeles, CA, USA

Faculty of Medicine, Technion, Israel Institute of Technology, Haifa, Israel
e-mail: Ofir.Koren@cshs.org

M. Arazi
Goldschleger Eye Institute, Sheba Medical Center, Ramat Gan, Israel

J. Joseph
Smidt Heart Institute, Cedars-Sinai Medical Center, Los Angeles, CA, USA

O. Koren et al. (eds.), *Complex Cases in Structural Heart Intervention*,
https://doi.org/10.1007/978-3-031-05965-0_15

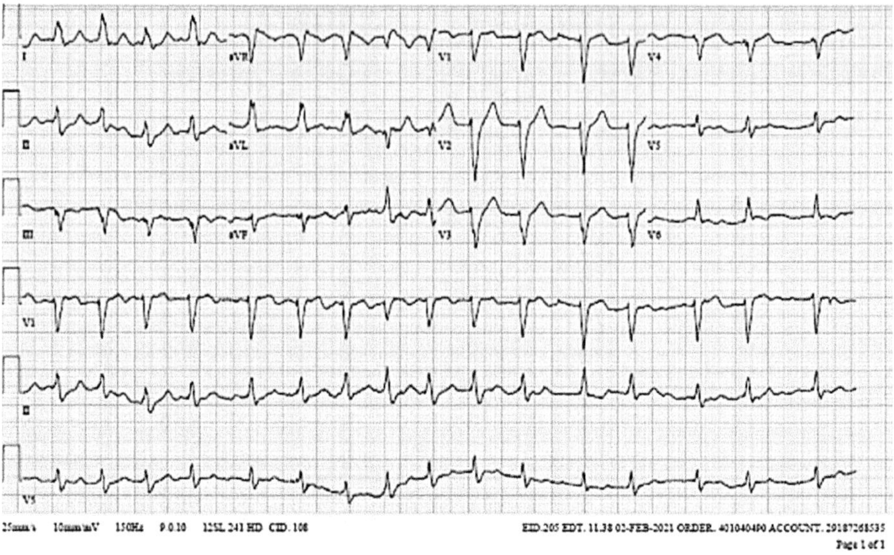

Fig. 1 ECG at admission, indicating atrial fibrillation and left bundle branch block

2 Images and Supported Data

TTE before intervention showed moderately depressed left LV function (38% EF), global left-ventricular hypokinesis, mild aortic stenosis (11 mm Hg mean transaortic gradient), severe ascending aortic dilation and severe aortic insufficiency. Cardiac reconstructed CT indicated an annular mean internal diameter of 27.8 mm, area of 668.8 mm^2 and a perimeter of 92.5 mm. The following mean diameters were measured: 51.1 mm at the Sinus of Valsalva, 41.1 mm at the STJ, 31.7 mm at the LVOT, and 43.2 mm at the ascending aorta (Fig. 2). The coronary ostia originated at 26.2 and 14.7 mm (for the RCA and LCA) above the annular plane. Quantitation of the calcium using 850 Hounsfield units as a threshold indicated 17.1 mm^3 at the aortic root. The angulation between the aortic root and left ventricle was measured at 58° (Fig. 3). Cardiac CT demonstrated substantial tortuosity of the brachiocephalic artery and abdominal aorta, as well as a severe calcific disease (Figs. 4 and 5). TEE illustrated aneurysmal dilation of the ascending aorta extending to the right coronary cusp (Fig. 6, Videos 1 and 2) and moderate mitral regurgitation with dilated left ventricle (Fig. 7).

3 Procedure and Outcome

Following heart team evaluation, the patient was considered high-risk for surgery; therefore, we decided to use a transfemoral TAVR to treat the regurgitant aortic valve. The patient was at increased risk of TVH embolization given aortic root

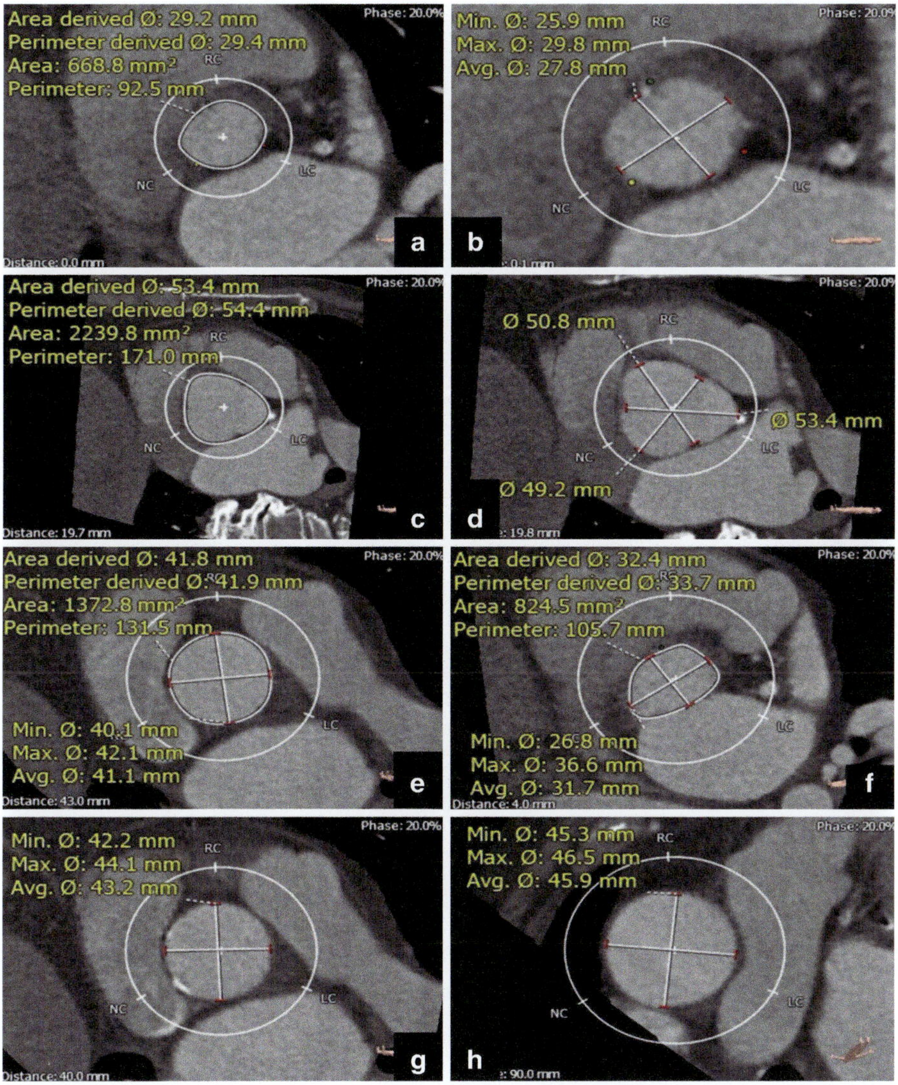

Fig. 2 Reconstructed CT measurements of aortic root components before TAVR. (**a**, **b**) The area, the perimeter, and the diameter of the AV annulus. (**c**, **d**) SOV area, perimeter, and diameter. (**e**) Sinotubular junction measurements. (**f**) LVOT measurement. (**g**) Ascending aorta diameter at the level of 40 mm. (**h**) Maximal diameter measured in ascending aorta

aneurysmal dilation and relatively low calcium burden, so a planned two-valve strategy was used. Using a Safari wire that was retrogradely placed in the left ventricle via transfemoral access using a 16F eSheath, a 34-mm self-expandable bioprosthetic Evolut R valve was advanced and positioned across the regurgitant aortic valve. With pacing at 120 bpm, the valve was partially deployed and recaptured multiple times until a suitable position was reached. At this point, the valve was

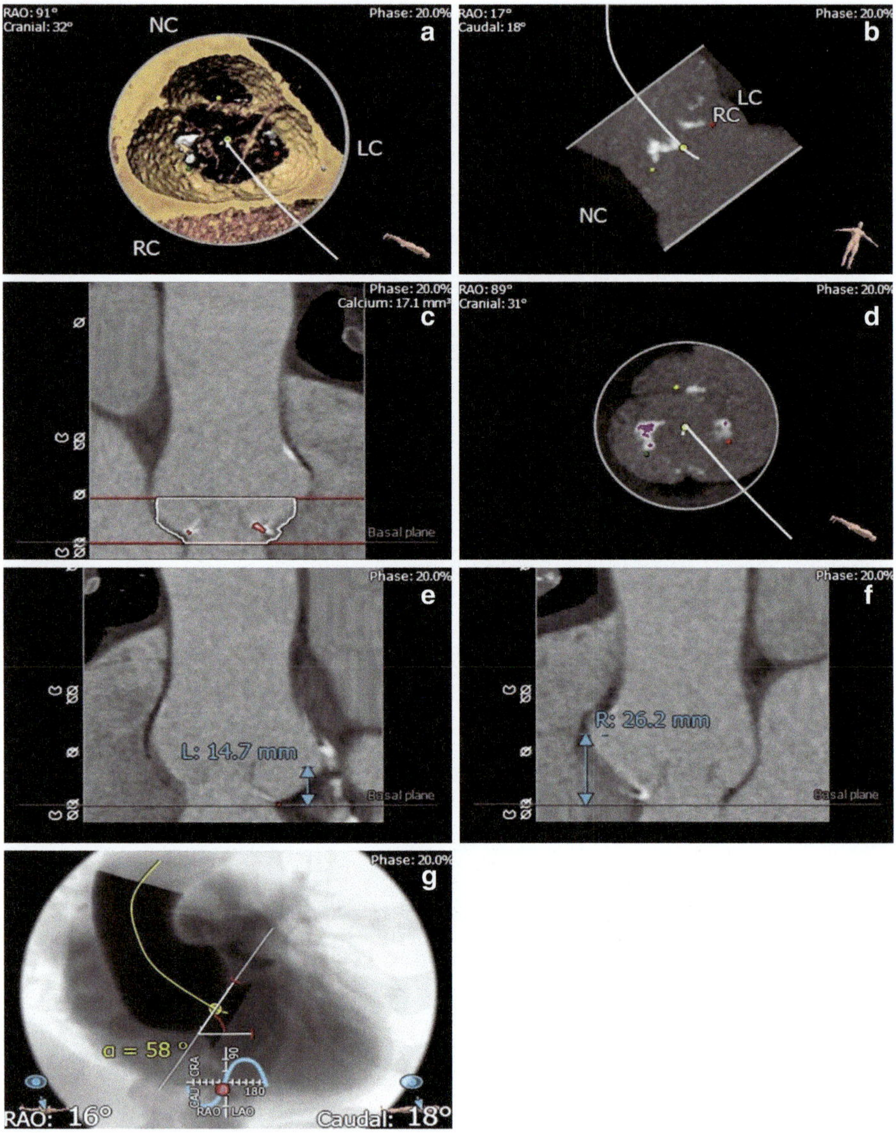

Fig. 3 Reconstructed CT analysis before TAVR. (**a**) Hockey puck VR view of the aortic analysis. Note the aneurismatic region near the right coronary cusps (green dot). (**b–d**) Aortic root calcification using a HU850 threshold. (**e**, **f**) Coronary artery height above the annular plane. (**g**) Co-planar angle between the LV and Aortic root

deployed and appeared relatively stable, without embolization to the aorta or LVOT (Figs. 8 and 9, Videos 3, 4 and 5) but with a mild to moderate paravalvular leak. Subsequently, a 29-mm Sapien 3 was deployed at the level of the native annulus within the Evolut valve to better anchor the initial prosthetic valvular apparatus to the aortic annulus (Fig. 10, Videos 6 and 7). A post-procedure TEE revealed no

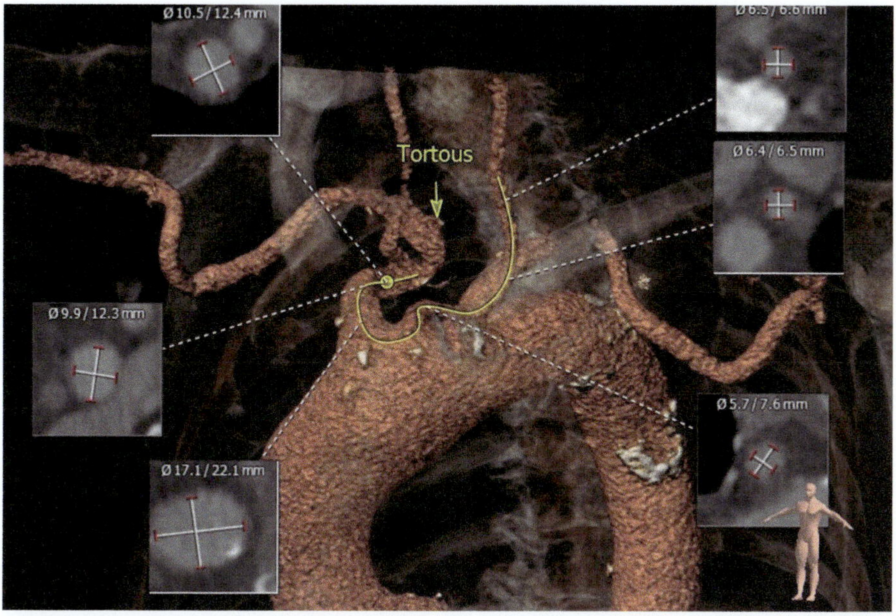

Fig. 4 Reconstructed 3D CT images of Aortic arch and its branches. Aortic arch diameter measurements. Note the tortuosity of the brachiocephalic trunk

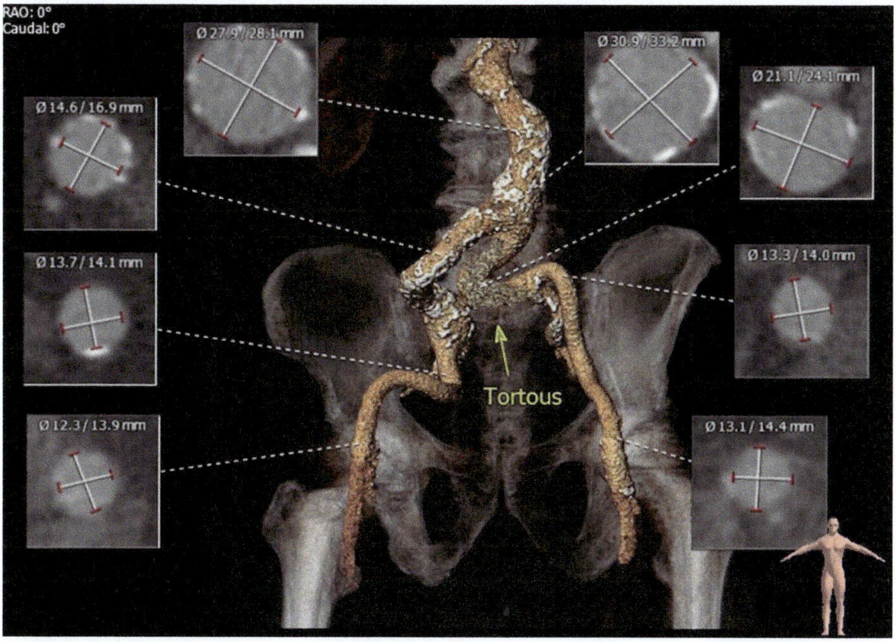

Fig. 5 Reconstructed 3D images of abdominal aorta and the iliofemoral arteries. Note the extensive calcification aortic arch diameter measurements. Note the tortuosity of the brachiocephalic trunk

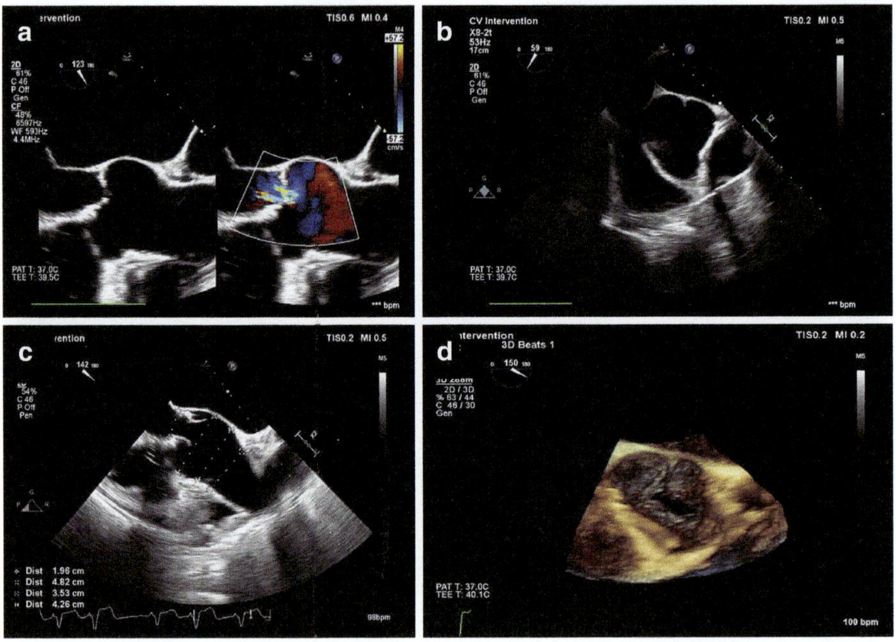

Fig. 6 Transesophageal echocardiography of the aortic root. Note the aneurysmatic dilatation seen on different echocardiographic views. (**a**) ME AV LAX TEE view. (**b**) ME AV SAX TEE view. (**c**) Aortic aneurysm diameter assessment in ME AV LAX TEE view. (**d**) Aortic valve annulus by 3D mode. Note the aneurysmatic dilatation in the right coronary cusp

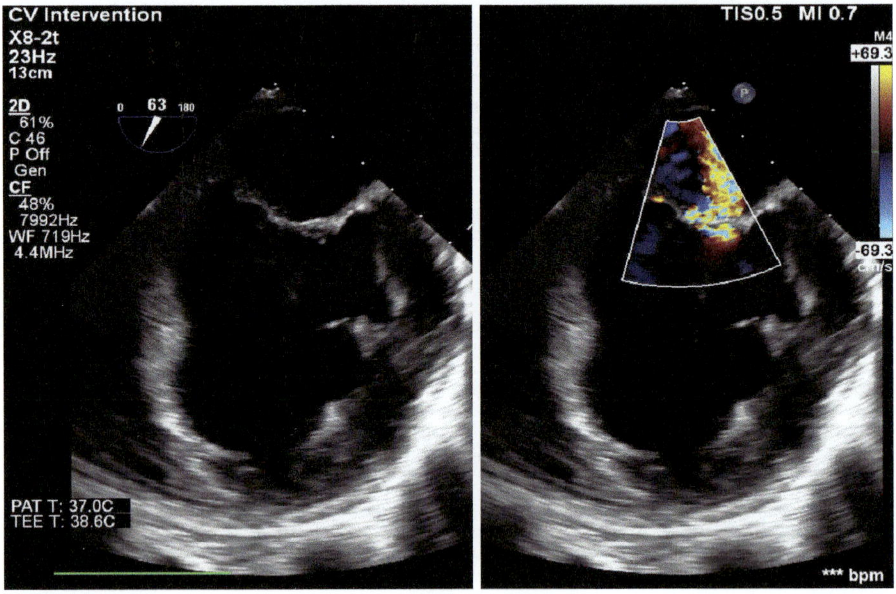

Fig. 7 Transesophageal echocardiography of left sided chambers. Note the moderate mitral regurgitation and dilated left ventricle (ME LAX TEE view)

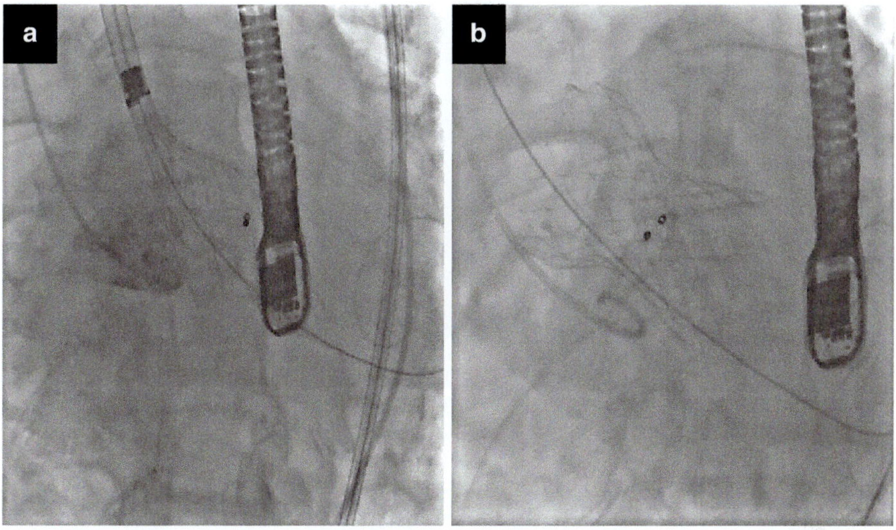

Fig. 8 Fluoroscopy views of the procedure. Positioning of a self-expandable Evolute-R THV over the AV annulus (**a**) to full deployment (**b**)

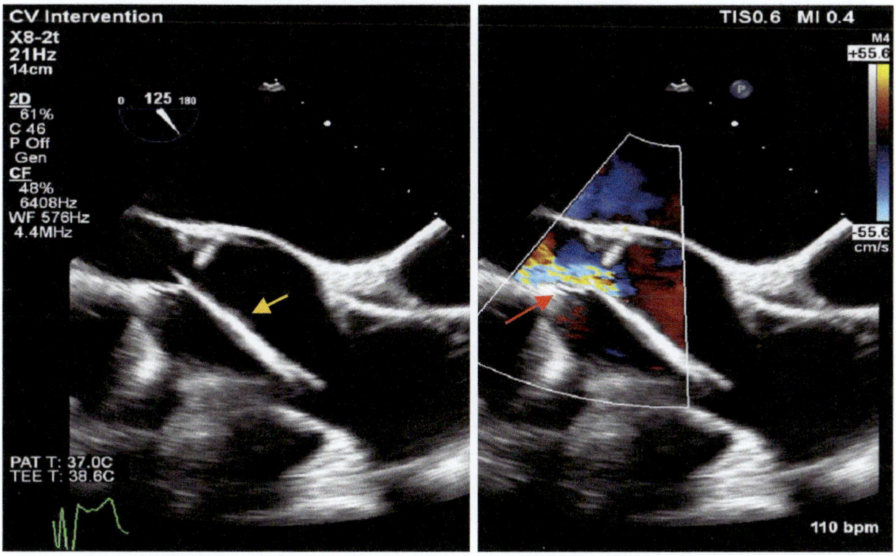

Fig. 9 Transesophageal echocardiography of the procedure. Deployment of a self-expandable Evolute-R THV (yellow arrow) over the AV annulus (ME AV LAX TEE View). Note the paravalvular leak after the THV deployment (red arrow)

central aortic regurgitation and only trace perivalvular regurgitation (Figs. 11 and 12, Videos 8 and 9). The patient remained hemodynamically stable, afebrile, and normotensive throughout the hospital stay. Telemetry revealed no significant arrhythmias. Post-TAVR TTE showed no paravalvular leak.

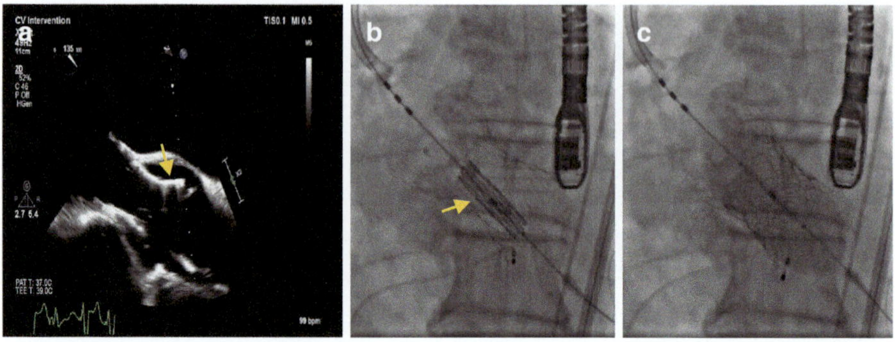

Fig. 10 Transesophageal echocardiography and fluoroscopy views of valve deployment. Deployment of a second balloon-expandable THV (yellow arrow) over a deployed self-expandable Evolute-R THV in ME AV LAX TEE view (**a**) and fluoroscopy (**b**, **c**)

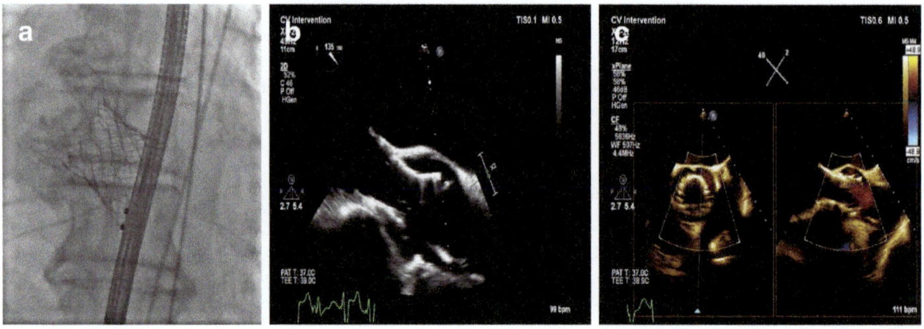

Fig. 11 Transesophageal echocardiography and fluoroscopy views during valve-in-valve procedure of valve deployment. Fluoroscopy view (**a**), ME AV LAX TEE view (**b**), and AV SAX TEE view (**c**)

4 Discussion

Ascending aortic dilation (AAD) may be associated with aortic valve disease. For example, ascending aortic dilation is seen in 20–25% of patients with aortic stenosis [1, 2]. Functional aortic regurgitation (AR), most commonly due to dilation of the sinotubular junction (STJ) in AAD patients, displaces the aortic commissures and impairs coaptation of the anatomically normal cusps [2–4]. Furthermore, up to 15% of patients with acute AAD have bicuspid aortic valves (BAV) linked to a deficiency in fibrillin-1 microfibrils, which causes detachment of smooth muscle cells from the extracellular matrix (ECM), increases matrix metalloproteinases, leads to loss of ECM integrity [5, 6].

Reported rupture or dissection of thoracic aortic aneurysms greater than 6.0 cm is roughly 7% per year, while death is roughly 12% per year [7, 8]. Therefore, ACC/AHA recommends surgical evaluation in patients with an ascending aorta or aortic sinus diameter 5.5 cm or greater, or an aneurysm growth rate of more than 0.5 cm/

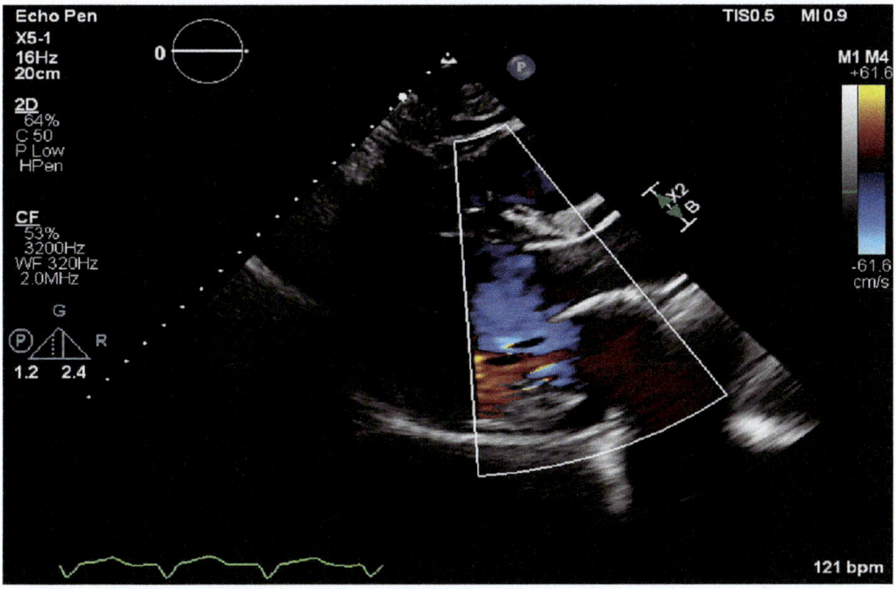

Fig. 12 Transthoracic echocardiography Doppler mode after the deployment of the second THV. Note the well seated valves, the lack of paravalvular leak, and aortic regurgitation

year in patients less than 5.5 cm in diameter [2, 6, 9]. Furthermore, patients scheduled for aortic valve surgery with an ascending aorta or aortic root greater than 4.5 cm should be considered for concomitant surgery of the valve and the aorta [6]. For example, the Bental procedure can correct aortic valve disease and ascending aortic aneurysm using a composite graft and prosthesis; however, long-term complications include embolism, valve dysfunction, prosthetic valve endocarditis, and risks of anticoagulation, especially among elderly patients and female patients planning pregnancy [3, 5].

Staged correction of the aortic valve and ascending aorta is viable in select patients. For example, the ACC/AHA guidelines recommend that elderly patients and younger patients with minimal dilatation of the aorta should be evaluated for separate valve and ascending aortic replacement [6]. However, progressive dilation of ascending aortic aneurysms following surgical AVR may occur, especially amongst BAV patients [2, 10]. Additionally, operative risks may render future surgical correction unfeasible.

While transcatheter aortic valve replacement (TAVR) is a well-established treatment for patients with symptomatic aortic valve disease, its usage in AAD patients is not well defined nor addressed in the current guidelines [6, 9, 11–13]. Rylski et al. in 2014 found that 22% of severe aortic stenosis patients that underwent TAVR were diagnosed with AAD of 4–5 cm; furthermore, these AAD patients demonstrated a low risk of peri-procedural adverse aortic events during TAVR with no effect on mid-term survival or in-hospital mortality and no increase AAD diameter at follow up [2]. However, TAVR in AAD patients may be complicated by prosthesis dislodgement and aneurysm rupture, for example, as demonstrated by an AAD patient who underwent TAVR for BAV stenosis, resulting in prosthesis dislocation and surgical intervention [12]. Overall, concomitant TAVR with other surgical or interventional procedures is an emerging field of discussion and research [11, 14].

This is a possible concern regarding TAVR in patients with an extra-large annulus of (ELA), especially in case of under-expansion causing valve embolization or paravalvular AV regurgitation (PAR). Masaki et al. reported that patients with an ELA of >683 mm^2 had the same rate of procedural complications and similar 1-year mortality [15]. The incidence of PAR of mild or great severity varies in different cohorts and is estimated to be up to 30%. Oversizing and calcified valves were identified as independent predictors for PAR [16].

Key Points
- Aortic dilatation often co-exists with aortic valve disease due to pathophysiological bicuspid valve disease, along with root dilation which causes functional aortic regurgitation.
- Using commercially available devices, TAVR can be performed in certain high-risk patients with large aortic root dimensions and low calcium burden using a planned two-valve strategy.
- Emerging therapies (i.e., JenaValve) may provide a reliable treatment option for patients with aortic regurgitation undergoing TAVR.

References

1. Son JY, Ko SM, Choi JW, Song MG, Hwang HK, Lee SJ, Kang JW. Measurement of the ascending aorta diameter in patients with severe bicuspid and tricuspid aortic valve stenosis using dual-source computed tomography coronary angiography. Int J Cardiovasc Imaging. 2011;27(1):61–71.
2. Rylski B, Szeto WY, Bavaria JE, Walsh E, Anwaruddin S, Desai ND, Moser W, Herrmann HC, Milewski RK. Transcatheter aortic valve implantation in patients with ascending aortic dilatation: safety of the procedure and mid-term follow-up. Eur J Cardiothorac Surg. 2014;46(2):228–33.
3. Al-Atassi T, Boodhwani M. Aortic valve insufficiency in aortic root aneurysms: consider every valve for repair. J Vis Surg. 2018;4:60.
4. La Canna G, Maisano F, De Michele L, Grimaldi A, Grassi F, Capritti E, De Bonis M, Alfieri O. Determinants of the degree of functional aortic regurgitation in patients with anatomically normal aortic valve and ascending thoracic aorta aneurysm. Transoesophageal Doppler echocardiography study. Heart. 2009;95(2):130–6.
5. Verma S, Siu SC. Aortic dilatation in patients with bicuspid aortic valve. N Engl J Med. 2014;370:1920–9.
6. American College of Cardiology Foundation, American Heart Association Task Force on Practice Guidelines, American Association for Thoracic Surgery, American College of Radiology, American Stroke Association, Society of Cardiovascular Anesthesiologists, Society for Cardiovascular Angiography and Interventions, Society of Interventional Radiology, Society of Thoracic Surgeons, Society for Vascular Medicine, North American Society for Cardiovascular Imaging. 2010 ACCF/AHA/AATS/ACR/ASA/SCA/SCAI/SIR/STS/SVM

guidelines for the diagnosis and management of patients with thoracic aortic disease. J Am Coll Cardiol. 2010;55(14):e27–129.
7. Kobayashi T, Mikamo A, Kurazumi H, Suzuki R, Shirasawa B, Hamano K. Secondary omental and pectoralis major double flap reconstruction following aggressive sternectomy for deep sternal wound infections after cardiac surgery. J Cardiothorac Surg. 2011;6(1):1–6.
8. Davies RR, Goldstein LJ, Coady MA, Tittle SL, Rizzo JA, Kopf GS, Elefteriades JA. Yearly rupture or dissection rates for thoracic aortic aneurysms: simple prediction based on size. Ann Thorac Surg. 2002;73(1):17–28.
9. Kobayashi A, Lazkani M, Moualla S, Orazio A, Tasset M, Morris M, Fang K, Pershad A. Impact of aortic aneurysms in trans-catheter aortic valve replacement: a single center experience. Indian Heart J. 2018;70:S303–8.
10. Yasuda H, Nakatani S, Stugaard M, Tsujita-Kuroda Y, Bando K, Kobayashi J, Yamagishi M, Kitakaze M, Kitamura S, Miyatake K. Failure to prevent progressive dilation of ascending aorta by aortic valve replacement in patients with bicuspid aortic valve: comparison with tricuspid aortic valve. Circulation. 2003;108(10_Suppl_1):II-291.
11. Tagliari AP, Taramasso M. Transcatheter aortic valve implantation combined with other heart interventions: current status and future perspectives. Vessel Plus. 2020;4:16.
12. Chen M, Feng Y, Mazzitelli D, Tang H, Wei X, Zhao ZG, Xu YN, Liao YB, Huang DJ. Transcatheter aortic valve implantation in a patient with severe bicuspid aortic valve stenosis and ascending aortic aneurysm. J Am Coll Cardiol Interv. 2014;7(7):e83–4.
13. Kassis N, Saad AM, Ahuja KR, Gad MM, Abdelfattah OM, Isogai T, Shekhar S, Krishnaswamy A, Svensson L, Unai S, Kapadia SR. Impact of thoracic aortic aneurysm on outcomes of transcatheter aortic valve replacement: a nationwide cohort analysis. Catheter Cardiovasc Interv. 2021;97(3):549–53.
14. Schroeter T, Subramanian S, Lehmann S, Kempfert J, Misfeld M, Mohr FW, Borger MA. Dislocation of a transapically implanted aortic valve prosthesis with a functionally bicuspid aortic valve and ascending aortic aneurysm. Thorac Cardiovasc Surg. 2011;59(08):503–6.
15. Miyasaka M, Yoon SH, Sharma RP, Maeno Y, Jaideep S, Taguri M, et al. Clinical outcomes of transcatheter aortic valve implantation in patients with extremely large annulus and SAPIEN 3 dimensions based on post-procedural computed tomography. Circ J. 2019;83(3):672–80. Epub 2019 Jan 30. PMID: 30700661. https://doi.org/10.1253/circj.CJ-18-1059.
16. Tang GHL, Zaid S, George I, Khalique OK, Abramowitz Y, Maeno Y, et al. Impact of aortic root anatomy and geometry on paravalvular leak in transcatheter aortic valve replacement with extremely large annuli using the Edwards SAPIEN 3 valve. JACC Cardiovasc Interv. 2018;11(14):1377–87. Epub 2018 Jun 27. PMID: 29960755. https://doi.org/10.1016/j.jcin.2018.03.034.

Bradycardia and Hypotension During TAVR Procedure

Ofir Koren, Mattan Arazi, and Danon Kaewkes

1 Clinical Background

This patient is a 92-year-old male with a history of diastolic heart failure with NYHA class III–IV symptoms, stable abdominal aortic aneurysm, alcohol abuse, myelodysplastic syndrome, hypertension, hyperlipidemia, chronic kidney disease, and atrial fibrillation without the use of anticoagulation due to repeated gastrointestinal bleeding. He was recently hospitalized for severe sepsis. While completing a course of antibiotics, he was assessed for valvular disease and found to have moderate to severe aortic stenosis. He was transferred to our center for further workup.

2 Imaging

Pre-procedural transthoracic echocardiography revealed an aortic valve area of 0.9 cm^2, mean gradient of 30 mmHg, peak gradient of 57 mmHg, and normal left ventricular systolic function (ejection fraction of 60%) (Fig. 1). Cardiac

Supplementary Information The online version contains supplementary material available at [https://doi.org/10.1007/978-3-031-05965-0_16].

O. Koren (✉)
Smidt Heart Institute, Cedars-Sinai Medical Center, Los Angeles, CA, USA

Faculty of Medicine, Technion, Israel Institute of Technology, Haifa, Israel
e-mail: Ofir.Koren@cshs.org

M. Arazi
Goldschleger Eye Institute, Sheba Medical Center, Ramat Gan, Israel

D. Kaewkes
Department of Medicine, Faculty of Medicine, Khon Kaen University, Khon Kaen, Thailand

O. Koren et al. (eds.), *Complex Cases in Structural Heart Intervention*,
https://doi.org/10.1007/978-3-031-05965-0_16

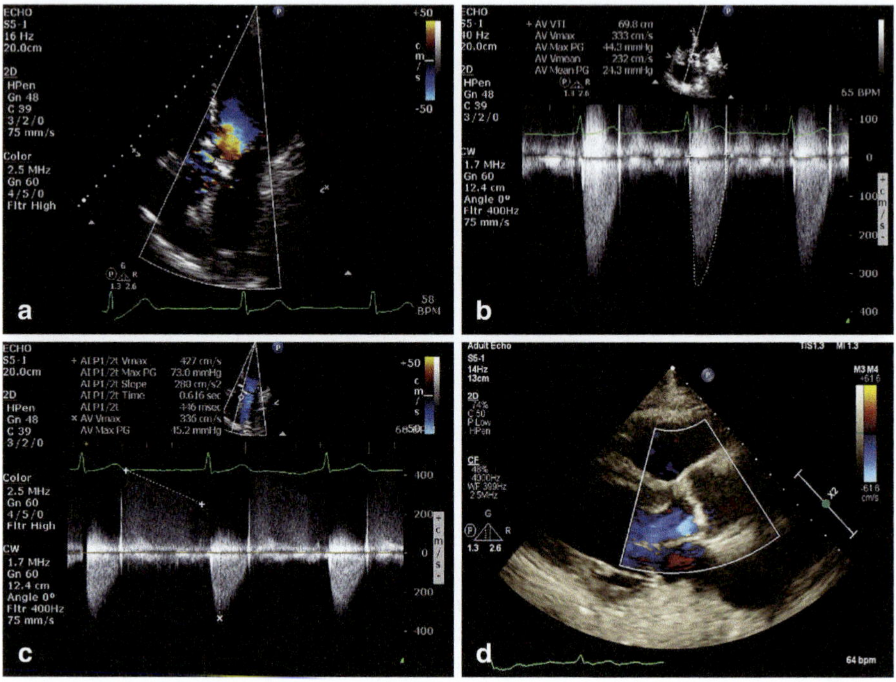

Fig. 1 TTE images of a combined aortic stenosis (**a**, **b**) and regurgitation (**c**, **d**)

reconstructed CT indicated the following mean diameters: 34.9 mm at the sinus of Valsalva and 30.95 mm at the sinotubular junction. Additionally, there was noted tortuosity of the right and left iliac arteries and descending aorta. The minimal dimensions of the left femoral and right external iliac arteries were measured as 9.1 × 9.8 and 8.9 × 10.1 mm, respectively.

3 Preprocedural Considerations, Dilemmas, and Challenges

The patient was evaluated by cardiothoracic surgery and deemed at least moderate surgical risk. Considering the patient's baseline functional capacity, he seemed more suitable for transcatheter aortic valve replacement (TAVR). We decided to use the Sapien Ultra bioprosthesis via the transfemoral route.

4 Procedure, Outcome, and Follow-Up

The patient was admitted for a coronary angiogram followed by TAVR. The coronary angiogram showed nonobstructive coronary artery disease. A repeat coronary angiogram did not reveal significant lesions (Fig. 2a, b, Video 1). However, upon

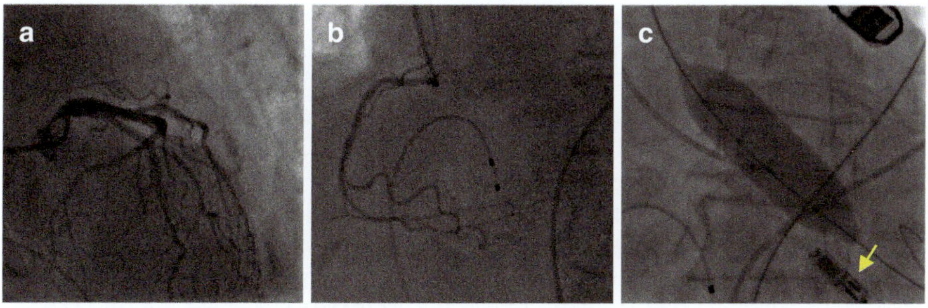

Fig. 2 Urgent coronary angiography and leadless pacemaker implantation (yellow arrow, **c**) following cardiac arrest during TAVR procedure. Figures (**a**) and (**b**) indicate patent left and right coronary arteries. After hemodynamic stabilization, a successful balloon valvuloplasty was performed (**c**)

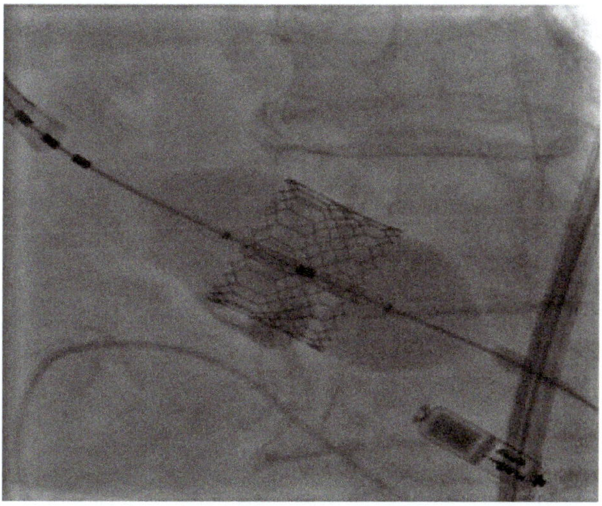

Fig. 3 Successful TAVR procedure performed in standard fashion with balloon-expanding valve

induction of anesthesia, the patient went into ventricular tachycardia followed by transient asystole which required brief cardiopulmonary resuscitation and insertion of emergent leadless permanent pacemaker. In place of TAVR, he underwent balloon aortic valvuloplasty (Fig. 2c, Video 2). During the post-procedure period, he was noted to have a sharp decrease in blood pressure, so midodrine was initiated. He received multiple pure red blood cell transfusions for acute anemia likely secondary to bone marrow suppression, given a history of myelodysplastic syndrome. He was discharged in stable condition.

The patient returned three months later to attempt the TAVR procedure once more. Although his symptoms improved in the short period after the valvuloplasty, he still complains of fatigue, dyspnea on exertion, shortness of breath, and chest pain. After obtaining femoral access, TAVR was successfully performed (Fig. 3). A post-procedure TEE revealed trace central and paravalvular aortic regurgitation. At the end of the case, following the initiation of protamine sulfate and prior to extubation, the patient developed hypotension and bradycardia, requiring intravenous pushes of epinephrine. TTE showed stable valve function, trivial pericardial effusion, and no evidence of aortic root injury. Left ventricular function was preserved. The patient remained stable and was extubated in the catheterization laboratory with grossly intact neurologic function and required one day of ionotropic support before de-escalation. He was discharged in stable condition.

At his 30-day follow-up, the patient complained of severe fatigue, weakness, dyspnea on exertion, supplemental oxygen use throughout the day with activity, and intermittent dizziness. He initially felt well post-TAVR but noted a declined most recently. He denied chest pain, chest pressure, orthopnea, paroxysmal nocturnal dyspnea, fevers, chills, recent infections, palpitations, stroke-like symptoms, and GI bleed. The patient has not required a blood transfusion since the TAVR procedure.

5 Follow-Up

The patient died 6-months following an initial valvuloplasty procedure from sepsis.

6 Discussion

Peri-procedural bradycardia and hypotension during TAVR may challenge the clinician due to a wide differential of potential causes. Underlying conduction disorders, sinus node dysfunction and atrioventricular block (AVB), and vasovagal mediated AVB due to increased parasympathetic tone may contribute to bradycardic events [1].

Conduction disturbances are one of the most common complications of TAVR that may result in marked bradycardia, as seen in some cases of new-onset left bundle branch block (LBBB) and advanced AVB requiring a permanent pacemaker [2, 3]. Prosthesis expansion during TAVR may result in direct injury, hematoma formation, and ischemia of conduction pathways as a result of the close proximity of the bundle of His and left bundle branch to the base of the aortic valve leaflets [3–5]. Therefore, patients with prior conduction disturbances, especially right bundle branch block (RBBB), are at risk of developing complete AVB after TAVR [6, 7]. Specific guidelines regarding indications for pacemaker implantation following TAVR are not well defined and are left for the clinician's judgment [5, 7]. The American College of Cardiology (ACC) recommends adequate risk assessment for conduction disturbances prior to TAVR implantation by standard electrocardiographic techniques [5]. The difference between membranous septum length and implantation depth measured by computed tomography and fluoroscopy was a significant predictor for complete AVB and pacemaker implantation [5, 8]. Peri-procedural pacing for at least 24 hours with continuous cardiac monitoring is indicated for special cases, especially in patients with prior RBBB, new-onset LBBB, or transient high-grade AVB following TAVR [5].

Our patient developed bradycardia and hypotension following the administration of protamine sulfate. Protamine, a reversal agent for heparin, may cause hypotension due to the release of endothelium-derived relaxing factor (EDRF), causing systemic vasodilation, and myocardial depression [9, 10]. Other mechanisms of protamine shock may be related to histamine release, and acute pulmonary hypertension acute pulmonary hypertension causing right ventricular failure and reduced cardiac output [11–13]. Risk factors related to protamine shock include previous pulmonary hypertension, prior protamine exposure, specific fish allergy, rate of infusion, and insulin-dependent diabetes [12, 14]. Kataoka et al. described the case of a TAVR patient who developed protamine shock due to pulmonary hypertension. The patient in this case recovered after catecholamine administration [12]. Another case of protamine shock following cardiopulmonary bypass and coronary artery bypass grafting (CABG) in a patient who was resistant to hemodynamic supportive therapy demonstrated successful treatment with inhaled prostacyclin [11].

Key Points

- Peri-procedural bradycardia and hypotension during TAVR are not uncommon and may challenge the physician due to a broad range of potential causes.
- Conduction disturbance during TAVR may be partially preventable by carefully reviewing the preprocedural electrocardiogram and computed tomography.
- When bradycardia and hypotension occur during the TAVR procedure, extensive searching for the possible causes should be performed, and one of the etiologies may be the common drugs like protamine.

References

1. Kusumoto FM, Schoenfeld MH, Barrett C, Edgerton JR, Ellenbogen KA, Gold MR, Goldschlager NF, Hamilton RM, Joglar JA, Kim RJ, Lee R. 2018 ACC/AHA/HRS guideline on the evaluation and management of patients with bradycardia and cardiac conduction delay: executive summary: a report of the American College of Cardiology/American Heart Association Task Force on Clinical Practice Guidelines, and the Heart Rhythm Society. J Am Coll Cardiol. 2019;74(7):932–87.
2. Miura M, Shirai S, Uemura Y, Hayashi M, Takiguchi H, Ito S, Yano M, Kawaguchi T, Morinaga T, Isotani A, Kakumoto S. Clinical impact of intraventricular conduction abnormalities after transcatheter aortic valve implantation with balloon-expandable valves. Am J Cardiol. 2019;123(2):297–305.
3. Auffret V, Puri R, Urena M, Chamandi C, Rodriguez-Gabella T, Philippon F, Rodés-Cabau J. Conduction disturbances after transcatheter aortic valve replacement: current status and future perspectives. Circulation. 2017;136(11):1049–69.
4. Moreno R, Dobarro D, López de Sá E, Prieto M, Morales C, Calvo Orbe L, Moreno-Gomez I, Filgueiras D, Sanchez-Recalde A, Galeote G, Jiménez-Valero S. Cause of complete atrioventricular block after percutaneous aortic valve implantation: insights from a necropsy study. Circulation. 2009;120(5):e29–30.

5. Lilly SM, Deshmukh AJ, Epstein AE, Ricciardi MJ, Shreenivas S, Velagapudi P, Wyman JF. 2020 ACC expert consensus decision pathway on management of conduction disturbances in patients undergoing transcatheter aortic valve replacement: a report of the American College of Cardiology Solution Set Oversight Committee. J Am Coll Cardiol. 2020;76(20):2391–411.
6. Tovia-Brodie O, Letourneau-Shesaf S, Hochstadt A, Steinvil A, Rosso R, Finkelstein A, Michowitz Y. The utility of prophylactic pacemaker implantation in right bundle branch block patients pre-transcatheter aortic valve implantation. Isr Med Assoc J. 2019;12(21):790–5.
7. Bob-Manuel T, Nanda A, Latham S, Pour-Ghaz I, Skelton WP IV, Khouzam RN. Permanent pacemaker insertion in patients with conduction abnormalities post transcatheter aortic valve replacement: a review and proposed guidelines. Ann Transl Med. 2018;6(1):11.
8. Hamdan A, Guetta V, Klempfner R, Konen E, Raanani E, Glikson M, Goitein O, Segev A, Barbash I, Fefer P, Spiegelstein D. Inverse relationship between membranous septal length and the risk of atrioventricular block in patients undergoing transcatheter aortic valve implantation. J Am Coll Cardiol Interv. 2015;8(9):1218–28.
9. Smith SC, Blair SN, Criqui MH, Fletcher GF, Fuster V, Gersh BJ, Gotto AM, Gould KL, Greenland P, Grundy SM, Hill MN. Preventing heart attack and death in patients with coronary disease. J Am Coll Cardiol. 1995;26(1):292.
10. Shapira N, Schaff HV, Piehler JM, White RD, Sill JC, Pluth JR. Cardiovascular effects of protamine sulfate in man. J Thorac Cardiovasc Surg. 1982;84(4):505–14.
11. Jerath A, Srinivas C, Vegas A, Brister S. The successful management of severe protamine-induced pulmonary hypertension using inhaled prostacyclin. Anesth Analg. 2010;110(2):365–9.
12. Kataoka A, Watanabe Y, Seki S, Takamura S, Hioki H, Kyono H, Sawamura S, Kozuma K. Efficacy of intraoperative transesophageal echocardiography in a case of protamine shock during transcatheter aortic valve implantation. JA Clin Rep. 2016;2(1):1–4.
13. Horrow JC. Protamine: a review of its toxicity. Anesth Analg. 1985;64(3):348–61.
14. Weiss ME, Adkinson NF. Allergy to protamine. Clin Rev Allergy. 1991;9(3–4):339–55.

Left Ventricular Outflow Obstruction Following TAVR

Vivek Patel, Robert Naami, and Mohamed Hassanein

1 Clinical Background

The patient is a 91-year-old female with a past medical history of non-Hodgkin's lymphoma diagnosed 20 years ago, dyslipidemia, benign lung tumor status post-resection, and recent gastrointestinal (GI) bleeding with multiple syncopal events.

Following her last syncopal episode, she was admitted to our center and was found to have an additional lower GI bleed. The patient endorsed symptoms of fatigue and shortness of breath with normal daily activities. She underwent a cauterization procedure and received six units of packed red blood cells. Per her care providers, she had required approximately 12 U of blood transfusion over the last three months due to lower gastrointestinal bleeding. Further coronary angiography work demonstrated non-obstructive coronary disease and moderated severe aortic valve calcification. The patient, therefore, was referred for further evaluation for a valvular intervention.

Supplementary Information The online version contains supplementary material available at [https://doi.org/10.1007/978-3-031-05965-0_17].

V. Patel (✉)
Smidt Heart Institute, Cedars-Sinai Medical Center, Los Angeles, CA, USA
e-mail: vivek.patel@cshs.org

R. Naami
University Hospitals Cleveland Medical Center, Cleveland, OH, USA

M. Hassanein
Cedars Sinai Medical Center, Los Angeles, CA, USA

O. Koren et al. (eds.), *Complex Cases in Structural Heart Intervention*,
https://doi.org/10.1007/978-3-031-05965-0_17

2 Imaging

Pre-procedural TTE demonstrated severe aortic valve stenosis with mean and peak valve gradients of 36 and 51 mmHg, respectively (Fig. 1a, c, Videos 1 and 2). Doppler waveform illustrated a pressure gradient of 103 mmHg at the left ventricular outflow tract (LVOT) with Valsalva. The mitral valve showed moderate stenosis with mean valve gradient of 6 mmHg (Fig. 1b, d, Videos 3, 4 and 5). Left ventricular systolic function was preserved (ejection fraction of 70%). Cardiac reconstructed CT indicated an annular mean internal diameter of 18.8 mm, area of 274.6 mm^2, and perimeter of 59.8 mm. The following mean diameters were measured: 31.9 mm at the Sinus of Valsalva, 29.8 mm at the sinotubular junction, 17.2 mm at the LVOT. The right and left coronary ostia originated at 13.7 and 9.7 mm, respectively, from the native aortic annulus (Fig. 2a–f). Volume rendered image of the aortic valve demonstrated a valve area of 0.94 cm^2 and a membranous structure partially obstructing the LVOT (Figs. 2g, h and 3a, Video 6). Pre-procedural CT also demonstrated mid-right and left femoral arteries with 6.4 × 7.4 and 5.4 × 6.9 mm, respectively. Pre-procedural coronary angiography demonstrated non-obstructive coronary artery disease.

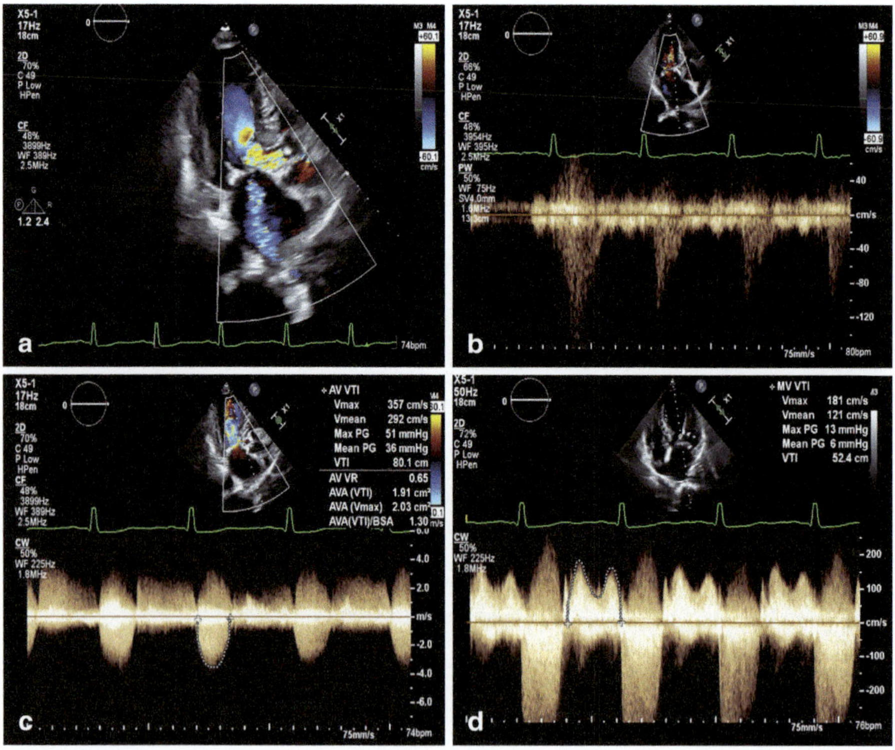

Fig. 1 Preprocedural TTE showed accelerated flow across the aortic valve compatible with severe aortic stenosis in the parasternal long-axis (**a**) and short-axis (**b**) views. Note the flow across the LVOT (**c**) and the mitral valve (**d**). *TTE* transthoracic echocardiography

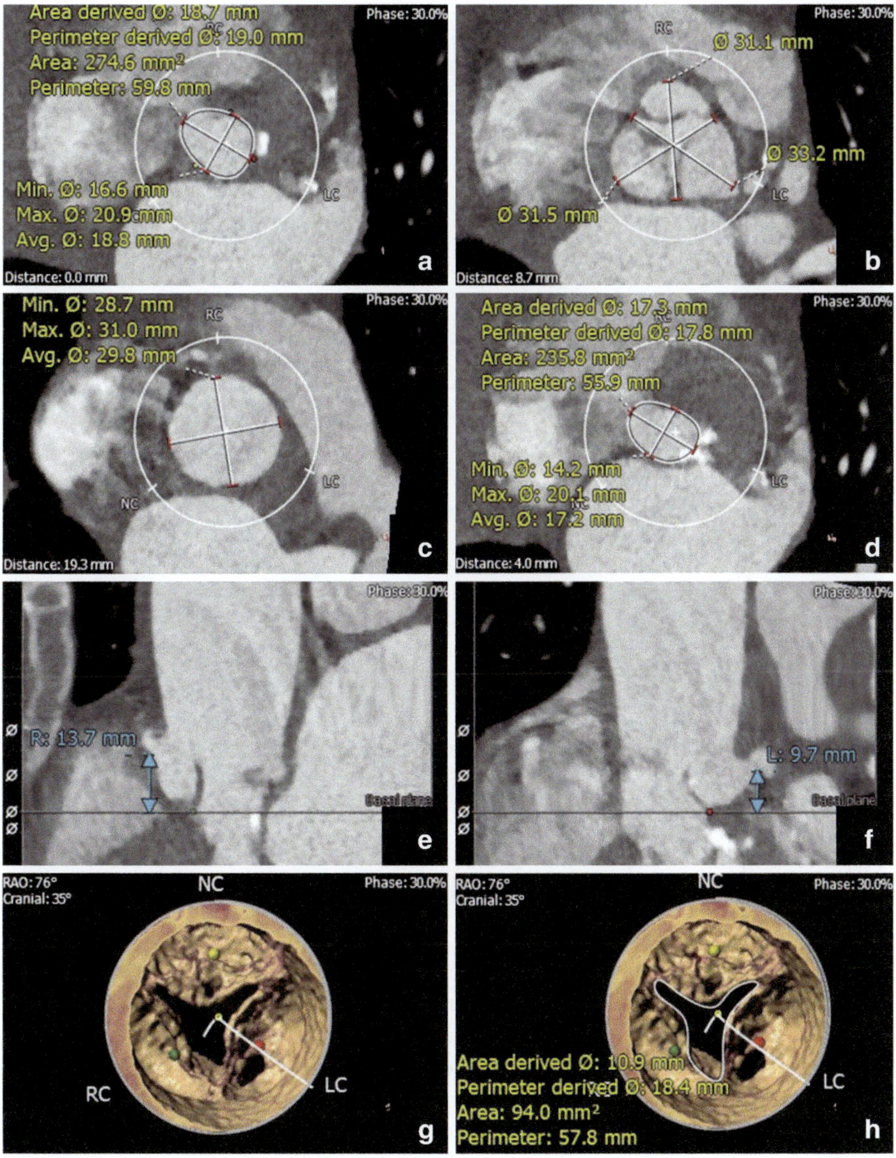

Fig. 2 Pre-procedural CT analysis. Figures (**a**)–(**d**) indicate the dimension of the annulus, the SOV, the sinotubular junction, and the LVOT. Figures (**e**) and (**f**) show the coronary height from the annular plane. Figures (**g**) and (**h**) indicate a volume render image of an aortic valve with planimetry valve area assessment

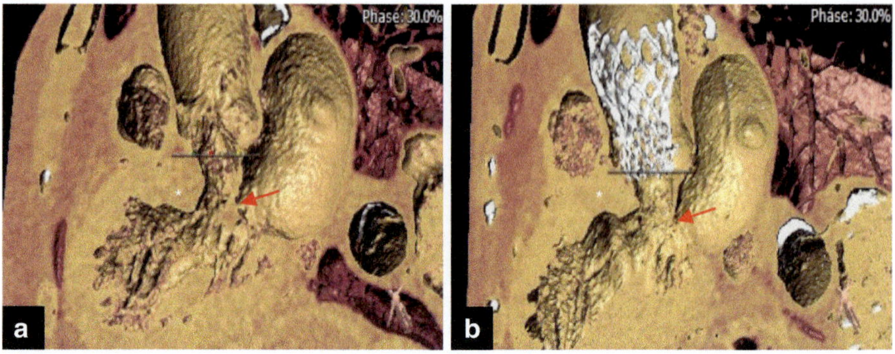

Fig. 3 Volume rendered images of the three-chamber view before (**a**) and after (**b**) TAVR and alcohol ablation. Note the thickness of the interventricular septum (white asterisk) and the position of the anterior mitral leaflet (red arrow)

3 Pre-Procedural Considerations, Dilemmas, and Challenges

The heart team evaluated the patient and decided that TAVR is a suitable alternative to surgical aortic valve replacement due to an STS score of 5.4%. Given LVOT narrowing, the decision was made to use a 23-mm self-expandable bioprosthetic Evolut R valve rather than a balloon-expandable valve. In addition, the patient would be evaluated intraoperatively, using TEE, for alcohol ablative therapy. The left coronary ostium was also of relatively low height and required wiring before valvular deployment.

4 Procedure, Outcome, and Follow-Up

A transesophageal echocardiographic probe was advanced into the mid-esophagus with basline images, including aortic annulus measurement and aortic valve gradients obtained and recorded. Aortic annulus measurement was consistent with previous CT angiographic studies. TEE demonstrated severe aortic valve stenosis, a subaortic membrane measuring 2 cm, and an LVOT diameter of 0.529 cm (Fig. 4).

A 6F XBLAD 3.5 guide catheter and a 0.014 Balance coronary guidewire were used to engage the left coronary artery and wire the LAD for left main protection for low coronary height (Fig. 5b). The 23-mm self-expandable bioprosthetic Evolut R valve was advanced and positioned across the stenotic aortic valve. The valve was deployed in the standard technique with pacing at a lower rate (120 bpm) (Fig. 5a). There was no evidence of left system obstruction (Video 7). Next, the aortic valve gradient was measured. There was a residual LVOT gradient due to a subvalvular tunnel on TTE and simultaneous LV-Ao hemodynamic tracings. The former revealed a severe gradient across the LVOT with a velocity of 486 cm/s (Fig. 6a, b, Video 8). The decision made was to proceed with septal ablation.

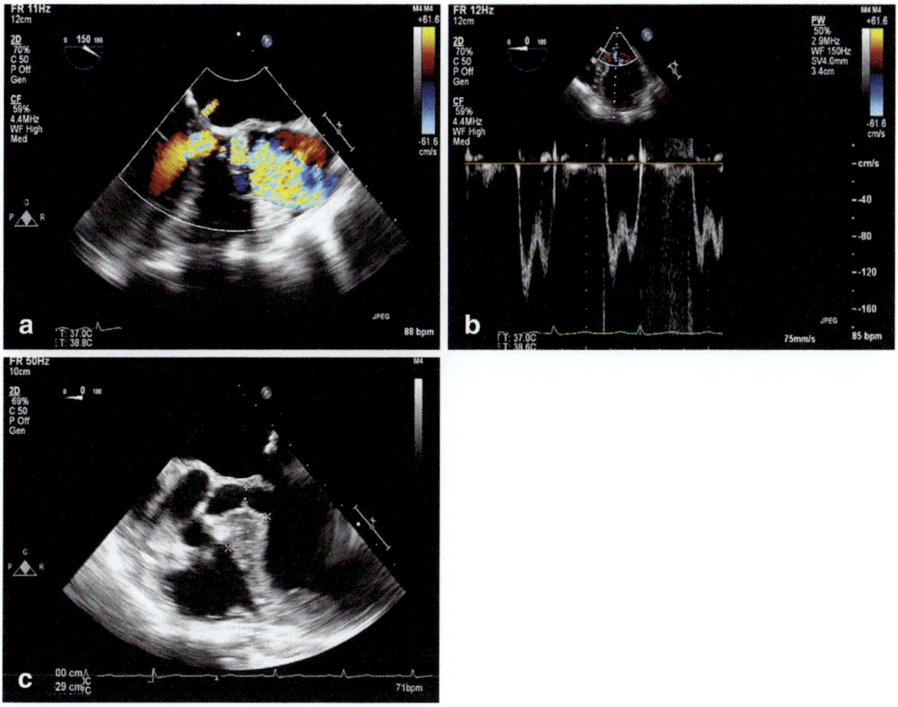

Fig. 4 Procedural TEE views: parasternal long axis view shows severe aortic valve stenosis (**a**) and flow across the LVOT (**b**). Figure (**c**) shows the dimension of the sub aortic membrane and the LVOT at 2 and 0.5 cm respectively

Through the 6F XBLAD 3.5 guide catheter, we advanced a second 0.014 Balance coronary guidewire into the first septal. A 2.0 × 6 mm OTW Medtronic Sprinter balloon was placed in the first septal and inflated to 4 cc. Selective first septal angiogram was performed, which showed no reflux into the LAD. Contrast location was confirmed on TEE in the septal bulge. 2 cc of ethanol was injected (Videos 9 and 10) slowly with a steady decrease in LVOT gradient, a reduction in velocity (121 cm/s), an improvement of mitral systolic anterior motion, and regurgitation (Figs. 5c, d and 6c, d, Videos 6 and 7). However, the patient developed a complete heart block requiring VVI backup pacing. The balloon was deflated and removed with the coronary guidewire. The final angiogram showed obliteration of the first septal and intact TIMI 3 flow down the LAD (Fig. 5e, f, Video 11). The guide catheter and LAD coronary guidewire were removed. A post-procedure TEE revealed no central aortic regurgitation and mild perivalvular regurgitation (Video 12).

At a 30-day follow-up, the patient was doing well and no longer felt fatigued. She could do all normal daily activities without shortness of breath or palpitations. Post-procedural TTE revealed normal LV systolic function, proper bioprosthetic valve positioning with mild aortic stenosis, and a mean valvular gradient of

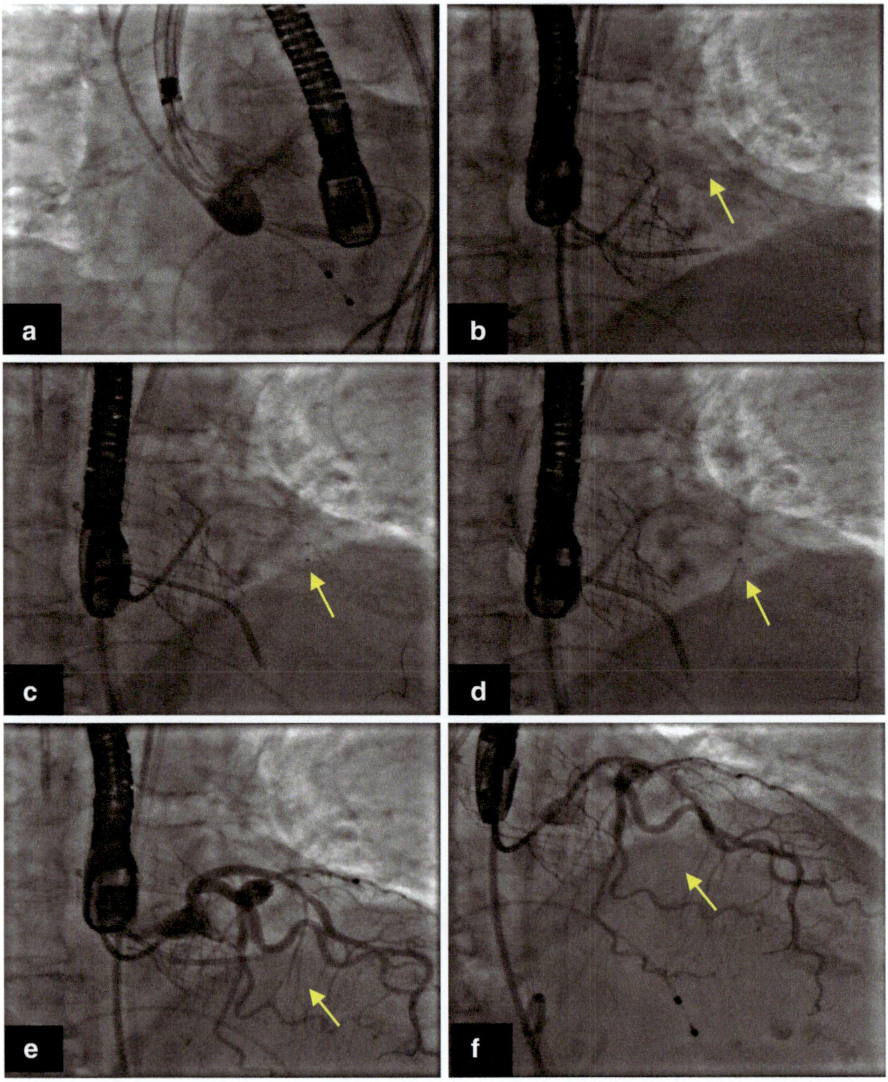

Fig. 5 Fluoroscopic imaging of the TAVR procedure. (**a**) Deployment of self-expanding Evolut R with a coronary guidewire advanced to the left coronary artery. (**b**) Low coronary height (yellow arrow) in respect to the THV. (**c**) Alcohol ablation using a guidewire in the first septal branch (yellow arrow). (**d**) Injection of 2 cc of ethanol in the first septal branch (yellow arrow). (**e**) Flow in the septal branches before the injection of alcohol. (**f**) Lack of flow to the septal branch following alcohol injection

13 mmHg (Fig. 7a–c, Videos 13 and 14). The mitral valve and LVOT gradient was measured to be 7 and 4 mmHg, respectively (Fig. 7d). Volume rendered illustration showed no LVOT obstruction following the TAVR-ablation procedure (Fig. 3b, Video 15).

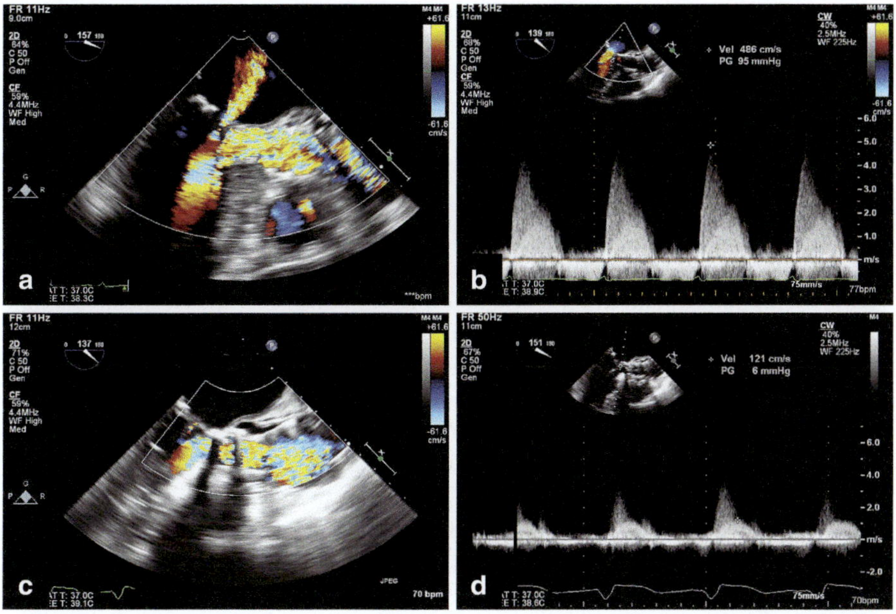

Fig. 6 TEE imaging during TAVR procedure. Figure (**a**) shows color Doppler at LVOT level with severe obstruction and high gradient (**b**) across the LVOT following the THV deployment. Following alcohol ablation, a reduction in gradient across the LVOT was noted (**c**, **d**)

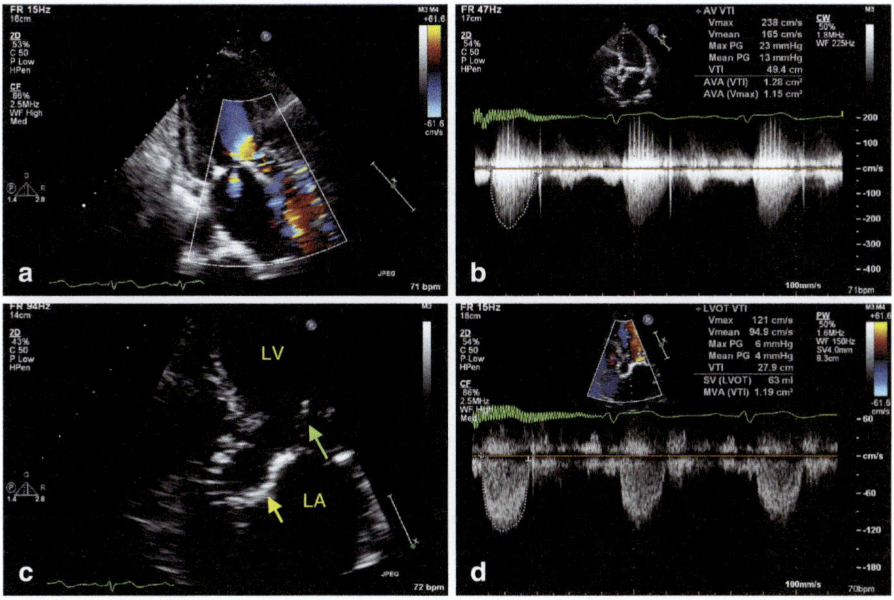

Fig. 7 A 30 days TTE follow-up shows mild aortic stenosis (short axis, **a**), and AV mean gradient of 13 mmHg (**b**). The THV is well seated in aortic position (yellow arrow, Figure **c**) without systolic anterior motion of the anterior mitral leaflets (green arrow, Figure **c**) and normal left ventricular wall thickness. The LVOT gradient remains low with 4 mmHg (**d**)

Unfortunately, the patient died four months following her procedures with a COVID-19 infection.

5 Discussion

A small aortic annulus (SAA) can largely affect the pre- and intraoperative planning of a patient's TAVR procedure in the setting of aortic stenosis. SAA is defined as an annulus with a mean and minimal diameter of <23 and ≤21 mm, respectively, and has historically been associated with poor outcomes in surgical aortic valve replacement (SAVR) [1–3]. While annular root enlargement is an option for SAA patients receiving SAVR, studies have demonstrated higher rates of intraoperative myocardial infarction, stroke, and overall mortality [4–6]. TAVR, conversely, has been shown to be particularly beneficial in patients with SAA, producing larger aortic valves areas associated with lower trans-prosthetic gradients and reduced rates of patient-prosthetic mismatch [7, 8]. In part, this benefit of a transcatheter approach stems from the intentional valve oversizing and the absence of a sewing ring.

Among TAVR valves, self-expanding valves have a better hemodynamic profile in SAA than balloon-expanding valves. This stems from the supra-annular position of the self-expanding valve leaflets which creates a larger orifice area [9, 10]. In one retrospective analysis of SAA patients, the CoreValve was associated with lower peak velocity and lower mean transaortic gradients than the Sapien valve. However, no differences in prosthesis-patient mismatch were observed, and paravalvular aortic regurgitation was more frequent in patients who received the CoreValve system [11].

An additional consideration that can affect post-operative hemodynamics is the formation of a left ventricular outflow obstruction (LVOTO) following TAVR. In patients with aortic stenosis, hypertrophy of the left ventricular myocardium develops due to the increased myocardial load imposed by the valvular obstruction. It can lead to obstructive pathology at the left ventricle's midventricular portion or outflow tract. Importantly, patients may demonstrate hypertrophy without evidence of obstruction on hemodynamic preoperative testing. Rather, upon implantation of the transcatheter prosthesis, the patient may develop acute obstruction upon implantation of the transcatheter prosthesis. It is likely the result of several physiological and anatomic changes, namely the rapid decrease in afterload. In one multivariate analysis, the LVOT diameter, transvalvular velocity, and the presence of accelerated intraventricular flow at baseline were associated with the occurrence of LVOTO with valve deployment [12]. In patients with both dynamic LVO obstruction and aortic stenosis, surgical myectomy and subsequent SAVR is the optimal treatment strategy. Alternatively, combined alcohol septal ablation and transcatheter aortic valve replacement should only be considered for very high surgical risk patients [13]. Namely, alcohol septal ablation should be performed first to avoid the dramatic decompensation following TAVR deployment, given the vulnerable left ventricle [14]. Furthermore, limited studies suggest that a pre-existing dual-chamber ICD may be protective given the increased likelihood of conduction damage from the ablative therapy or subsequent de-novo valve. In the absence of a pacemaker, the patient may require a longer monitoring period with a temporary pacing wire.

Key Points

- LVOT obstruction is a rare complication with a catastrophic consequence after TAVR procedure.
- Patients with hypertrophic cardiomyopathy at baseline may be at particular risk.
- The combined minimal invasive approach, which has proggresively become popular for high-risk surgical patients, is alcohol septal ablation followed by TAVR.
- Operators should be familiar with the technique and patient selection.

References

1. Bahlmann E, Cramariuc D, Minners J, Lønnebakken MT, Ray S, Gohlke-Baerwolf C, Nienaber CA, Jander N, Seifert R, Chambers JB, Kuck KH, Gerdts E. Small aortic root in aortic valve stenosis: clinical characteristics and prognostic implications. Eur Heart J Cardiovasc Imaging. 2017;18:404–12.
2. Dumont E, Xu K, Hahn RT, Leon MB. Impact of aortic annulus size on valve hemodynamics and clinical outcomes after transcatheter and surgical aortic valve replacement: insights from the PARTNER Trial. Circ Cardiovasc Interv. 2014;7:701–11.
3. Kalavrouziotis D, Rodés-Cabau J, Bagur R, Doyle D, De Larochellière R, Pibarot P, Dumont E. Transcatheter aortic valve implantation in patients with severe aortic stenosis and small aortic annulus. J Am Coll Cardiol. 2011;58:1016–24.
4. Repossini A, Di Bacco L, Passaretti B, Grubitzsch H, Schäfer C, Claus B, Giroletti L, Folliguet T, Bisleri G, Fischlein T, Santarpino G, Di Bartolomeo R, Laborde F, Muneretto C. Early hemodynamics and clinical outcomes of isolated aortic valve replacement with stentless or transcatheter valve in intermediate-risk patients. J Thorac Cardiovasc Surg. 2017;153:549–558.e3.
5. Rodés-Cabau J, Pibarot P, Suri RM, Kodali S, Thourani VH, Szeto WY, Svensson LG, Kapetanakis EI, Athanasiou T, Mestres CA, Nashef SA, Aagaard J, Moritz A, Van Ingen G, Chronidou F, Palatianos G, Alivizatos PA, Stavridis GT. Aortic valve replacement: is there an implant size variation across Europe. J Heart Valve Dis. 2008;17:200–5.
6. Wilbring M, Alexiou K, Schumann E, Matschke K, Tugtekin SM. Isolated aortic valve replacement in patients with small aortic annulus-a high-risk group on long-term follow-up. Thorac Cardiovasc Surg. 2013;61:379–85.
7. Baumgartner H, Stefenelli T, Niederberger J, Schima H, Maurer G. "Overestimation" of catheter gradients by Doppler ultrasound in patients with aortic stenosis: a predictable manifestation of pressure recovery. J Am Coll Cardiol. 1999;33:1655–61.
8. Dayan V, Vignolo G, Soca G, Paganini JJ, Brusich D, Pibarot P. Predictors and outcomes of prosthesis-patient mismatch after aortic valve replacement. JACC Cardiovasc Imaging. 2016;9:924–33.
9. Mauri V, Kim WK, Abumayyaleh M, Walther T, Moellmann H, Schaefer U, Conradi L, Hengstenberg C, Hilker M, Wahlers T, Baldus S, Rudolph V, Madershahian N, Rudolph TK. Short-term outcome and hemodynamic performance of next-generation self-expanding versus balloon-expandable transcatheter aortic valves in patients with small aortic annulus: a multicenter propensity-matched comparison. Circ Cardiovasc Interv. 2017;10:e005013.
10. Rogers T, Steinvil A, Gai J, Torguson R, Koifman E, Kiramijyan S, Negi S, Lee Y, Okubagzi P, Satler LF, Ben-Dor I, Pichard AD, Waksman R. Choice of balloon-expandable versus self-

expanding transcatheter aortic valve impacts hemodynamics differently according to aortic annular size. Am J Cardiol. 2017;119:900–4.
11. Smith CR, Leon MB, Mack MJ, Miller DC, Moses JW, Svensson LG, Tuzcu EM, Webb JG, Fontana GP, Makkar RR, Williams M, Dewey T, Kapadia S, Babaliaros V, Thourani VH, Corso P, Pichard AD, Bavaria JE, Herrmann HC, Akin JJ, Anderson WN, Wang D, Pocock SJ, PARTNER Trial Investigators. Transcatheter versus surgical aortic-valve replacement in high-risk patients. N Engl J Med. 2011;364:2187–98.
12. Tsuruta H, Hayashida K, Yashima F, Yanagisawa R, Tanaka M, Arai T, Minakata Y, Itabashi Y, Murata M, Kohsaka S, Maekawa Y, Takahashi T, Yoshitake A, Shimizu H, Fukuda K. Incidence, predictors, and midterm clinical outcomes of left ventricular obstruction after transcatheter aortic valve implantation. Catheter Cardiovasc Interv. 2018;92(4):E288–98. Epub 2018 Jan 23. PMID: 29359402. https://doi.org/10.1002/ccd.27508.
13. Krishnaswamy A, Tuzcu EM, Svensson LG, Kapadia SR. Combined transcatheter aortic valve replacement and emergent alcohol septal ablation. Circulation. 2013;128(18):e366–8.
14. Rowin EJ, Kimmelstiel C. Combined alcohol septal ablation and transcatheter aortic valve replacement: drunk and playing with fire. Catheter Cardiovasc Interv. 2020;95(4):838–9. PMID: 32159290. https://doi.org/10.1002/ccd.28795.

TAVR in Previous Two TAVRs in SAVR

Vivek Patel, Robert Naami, and Arvind Reddy Devanabanda

1 Clinical Background

The patient presented for outpatient evaluation and surgical risk assessment for mitral and aortic valve replacement. The patient is a 67-year-old male with a severe and symptomatic aortic paravalvular leak. Past medical history is remarkable for a Bentall procedure with #27 Freestyle porcine aortic valve replacement for type 1A aortic dissection (with residual enlarging of the distal aortic arch and proximal descending aorta) (Fig. 1) and two TAVR-in-Valve (with two separate 29-mm Evolut valves) interventions for bioprosthetic aortic valve insufficiency, severe mitral regurgitation, non-ischemic cardiomyopathy secondary to valvular heart disease (EF 30%, NYHA IV, stage C), atrial flutter status post radiofrequency ablation and subsequent atrial fibrillation, sick sinus syndrome status post atrioventricular node ablation, toxin-induced liver cancer status post orthotopic liver transplant, and end-stage renal disease status post kidney transplant and now awaiting a second orthotopic kidney transplant. Over the past several months, the patient endorsed progressive fatigue, shortness of breath with minimal exertion, two pillow orthopnea, paroxysmal nocturnal dyspnea, and significant anxiety. He denied chest palpitations, lower extremity edema, or syncope.

V. Patel (✉)
Smidt Heart Institute, Cedars-Sinai Medical Center, Los Angeles, CA, USA
e-mail: vivek.patel@cshs.org

R. Naami
University Hospitals Cleveland Medical Center, Cleveland, OH, USA

A. R. Devanabanda
Cedars Sinai Medical Center, Los Angeles, CA, USA

O. Koren et al. (eds.), *Complex Cases in Structural Heart Intervention*,
https://doi.org/10.1007/978-3-031-05965-0_18

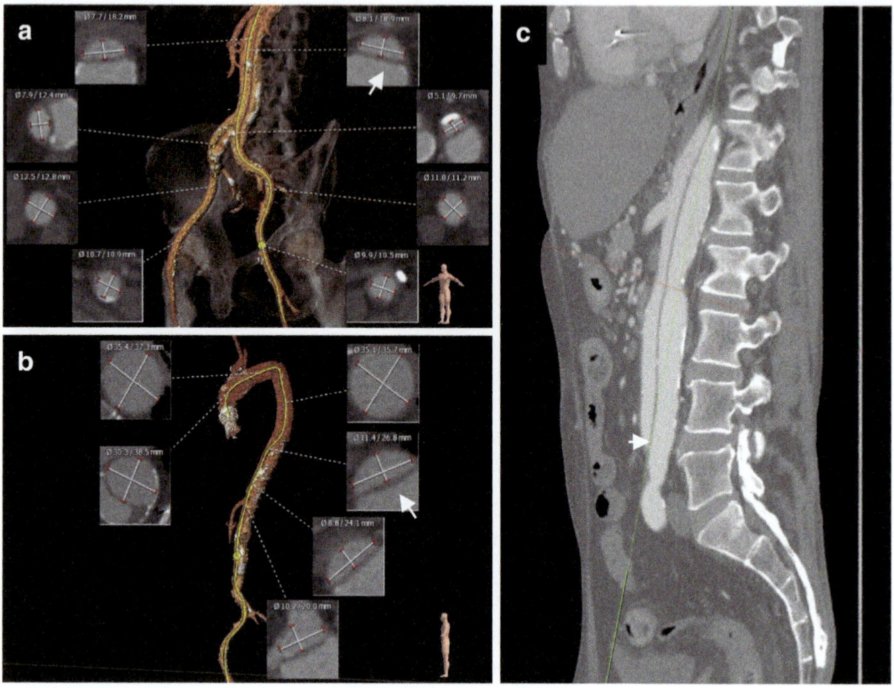

Fig. 1 Abdominal aorta and bilateral iliofemoral dimension measurements (**a**, **b**). Note the abdominal aorta dissection (white arrow) (**c**) extending towards the common iliac arteries

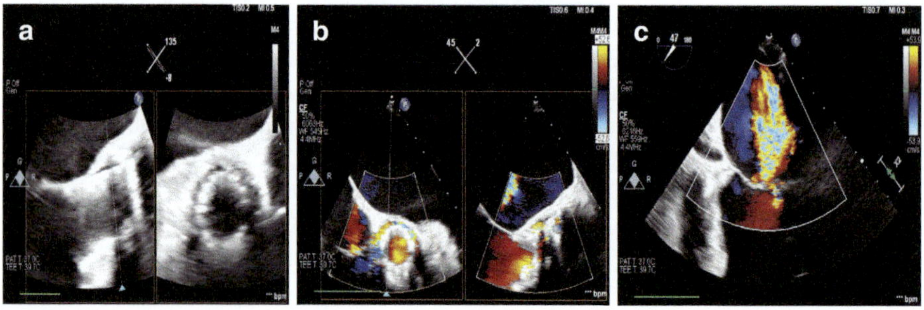

Fig. 2 Self-expanding transcatheter valve (Evolut R) in short axis TEE view (**a**) indicating circumferential paravalvular leak (short axis TEE view, **b**) and an increase in the regurgitation flow jet over the mitral annulus (two-chambers TEE view, **c**)

2 Imaging

Pre-procedural TEE revealed normal left ventricular chamber size with moderately reduced systolic function (LVEF of 30–35%) and severe mitral regurgitation. A self-expanding Medtronic Evolut TAV (×2) was found within a surgical bioprosthetic valve with very severe paravalvular regurgitation involving ~45% of the sewing ring circumference and mild transvalvular aortic regurgitation (Fig. 2).

TTE showed a transaortic peak gradient of 45 mm Hg and mean gradient of 25 mmHg. Cardiac reconstructed CT indicated an annular mean internal diameter of 22.9 mm, area of 337.5 mm², and perimeter of 65.2 mm. The following mean diameters were measured: 19.8 mm at the Sinus of Valsalva and 20.3 mm at the LVOT. The right coronary ostia originated at 15.1 and 35.0 mm from the native annulus and previously implanted self-expanding valve. The left coronary ostia originated at 19.0 and 36.9 mm from the native annulus and previously implanted self-expanding valve (Fig. 3).

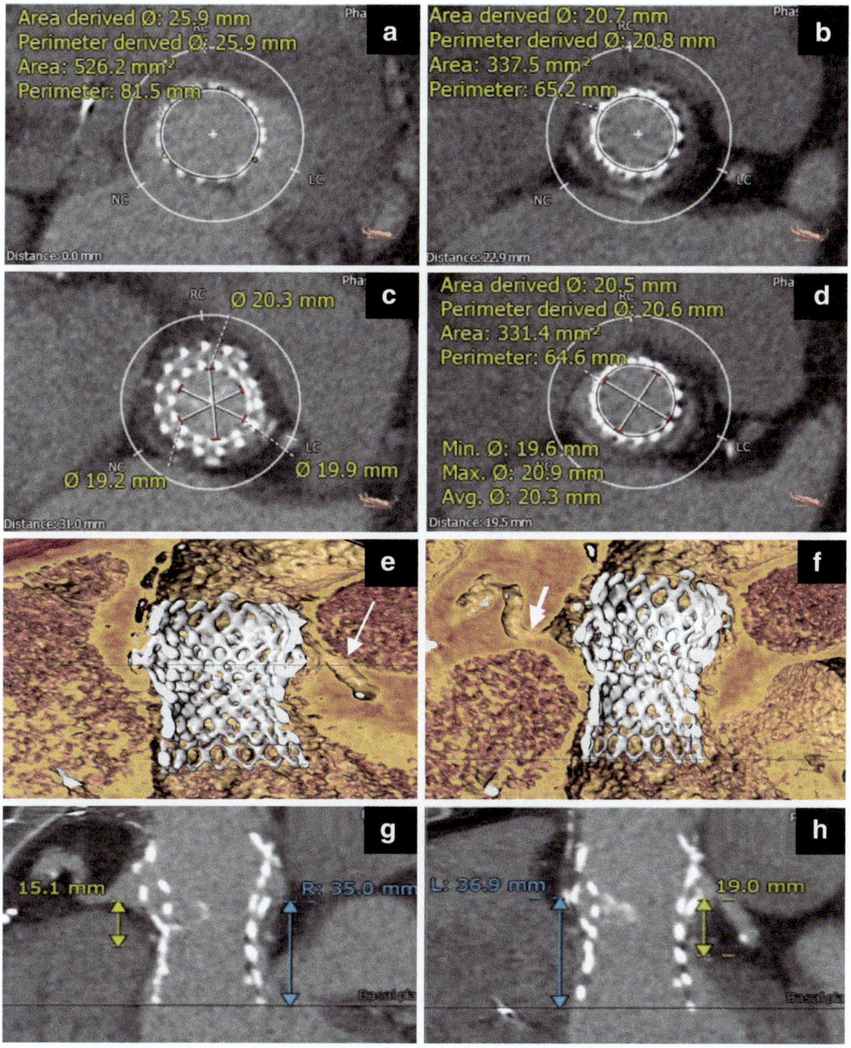

Fig. 3 Pre-TAVR cardiac CT image analysis. THV dimensions at the inflow of transcatheter aortic valve (**a**), THV dimensions at the native annulus level (**b**). The diameter of the SOV (**c**) and the LVOT (at 4 mm below the native annulus, **d**) and the left (**e**) and the right (**f**) coronary arteries (white arrow) in respect to the THV and to the annulus level (**g**, **h**). *THV* transcutaneous heart valve, *SOV* sinus of Valsalva, *LVOT* left ventricle outflow tract

3 Pre-Procedural Considerations, Dilemmas, and Challenges

Given our patient's severely depressed left ventricular ejection fraction, he has been deemed a poor surgical candidate (Society of Thoracic Surgery Score of 20%) for re-do sternotomy, re-do aortic valve replacement, and mitral valve repair or replacement. Interventional cardiology was consulted, and the patient was found to be an appropriate candidate for subclavian access transcatheter aortic valve replacement (TAVR) using a 26-mm Edwards Sapien Ultra valve given the extensive residual aortic dissection. The subclavian approach was chosen for THV placement to avoid the small false lumen in the residual aortic dissection and allow direct entry into the true lumen of the aortic arch (Fig. 4). The extent of paravalvular leak precludes transcatheter plugging options.

4 Procedure and Outcome

The delivery system and 26 mm Sapien-3 THV were advanced using subclavian access and positioned across the regurgitant aortic valve using the standard technique. With rapid pacing, the valve was successfully deployed (Fig. 5). A post-procedure TEE revealed trace central aortic regurgitation such that post-dilation was performed with an additional 2 mL. Subsequent TEE showed no paravalvular leak (Fig. 6). The valve delivery system and sheath were subsequently removed, with an angiography of the subclavian artery performed upon withdrawal, demonstrating no vessel injury or flow limitation.

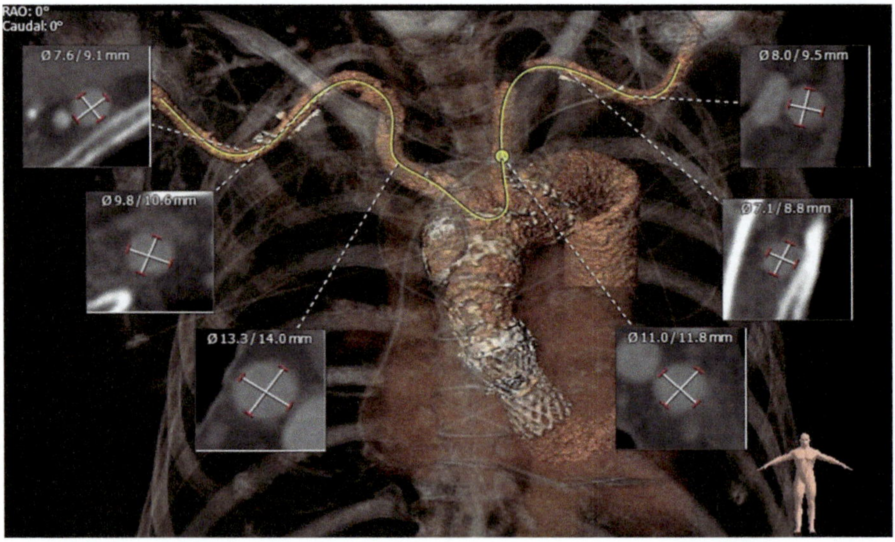

Fig. 4 Reconstructed CT analysis of the luminal diameter of the subclavian arteries

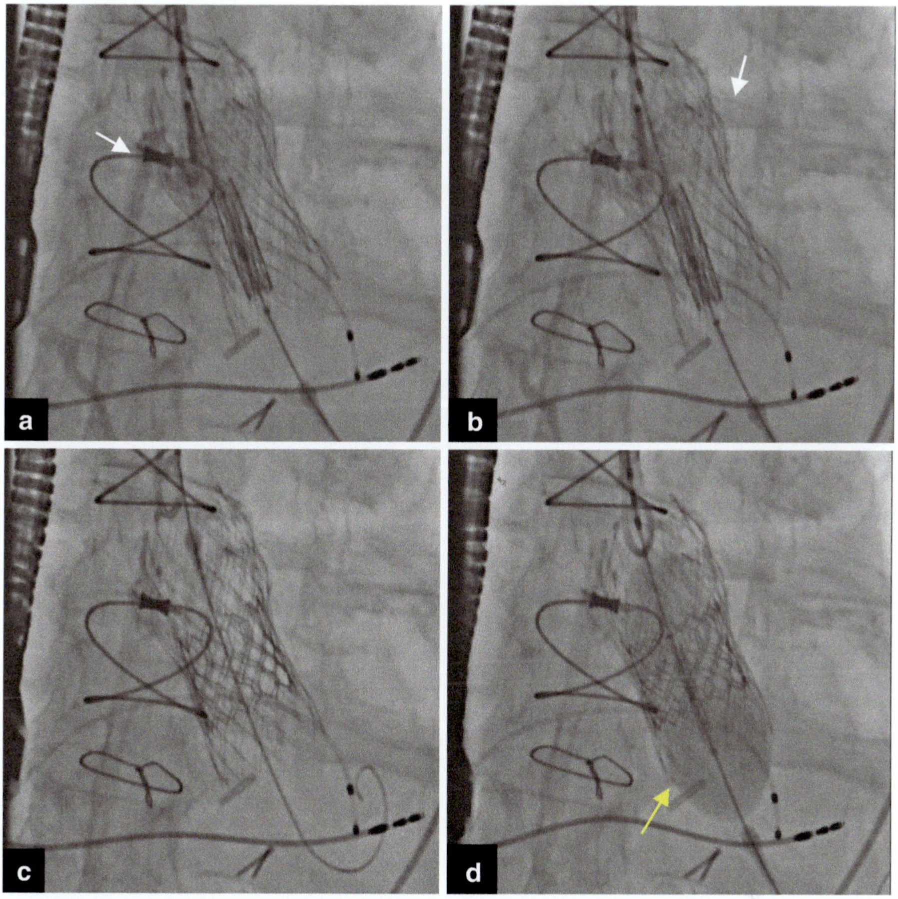

Fig. 5 Fluoroscopic view of TAVR procedure. Note the trace amount of contrast in the right (white arrow, **a**) and the left coronary arteries (white arrow, **b**), the deployment of a balloon-expandable valve (Sapien-3) on prior self-expanding valve (**c**), and the post-deployment balloon dilatation (white arrow, **d**)

5 Follow-Up

On a 30-day follow-up, the patient showed an improvement in his symptoms. He denied chest pressures, fatigue, shortness of breath, and orthopnea. TTE demonstrated unchanged left ventricular systolic function (EF 35%), bioprosthetic stented-valve in the aortic position without evidence of a paravalvular leak, aortic valve area of 1.8 cm^2, peak transaortic gradient of 22 mmHg, and a mean transaortic gradient of 12 mmHg. Mitral regurgitation severity improved from moderate to mild (Fig. 7).

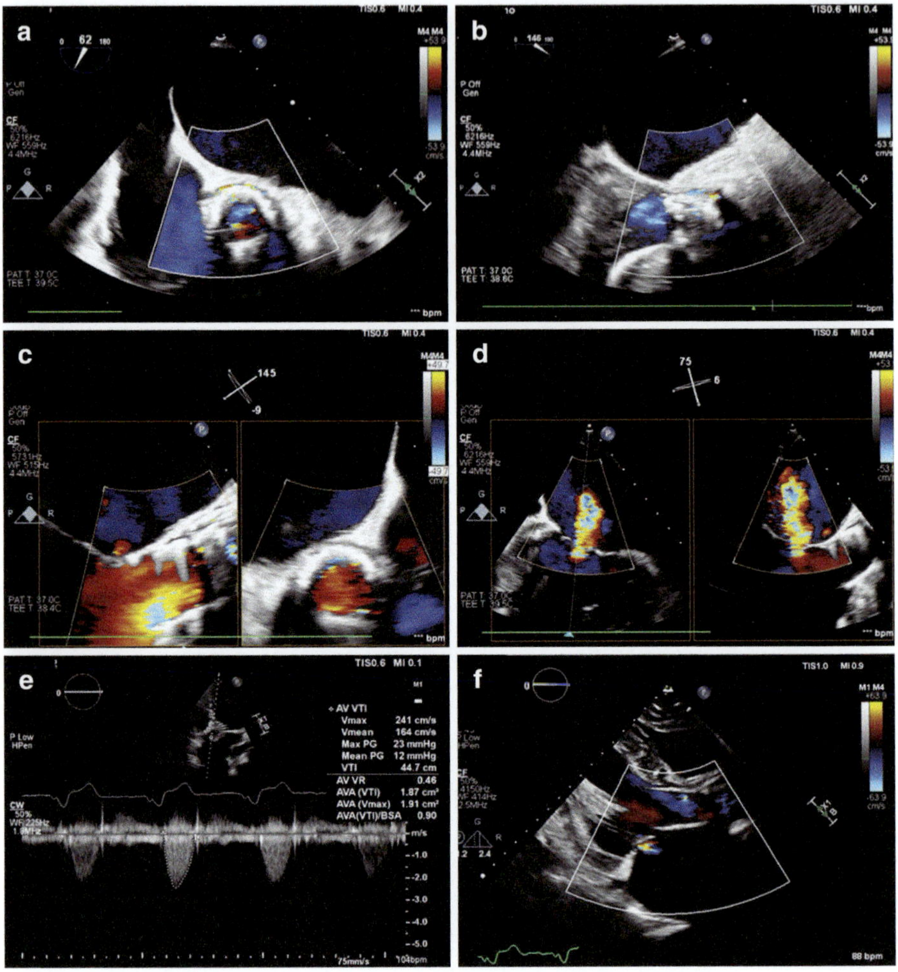

Fig. 6 Procedural TEE images: mild circumferential paravalvular leak (PVL) and mild aortic regurgitation (AR) after deployment of a balloon-expandable valve (RV inflow outflow view (**a**) and long axis view (**b**)). Figure **c** shows an improvement of the PVL and the AR following post-procedure Balloon inflation (**c**) and a reduction in regurgitation flow over the mitral valve (**d**). TTE at 30-day follow-up shows mild aortic stenosis (**e**), no aortic regurgitation and mild mitral regurgitation (**f**)

6 Discussion

Redo TAVR for treating the postprocedural, late occurrence of paravalvular regurgitation and transcatheter aortic valve prosthesis failure is safe and associated with favorable clinical and echocardiographic outcomes [1].

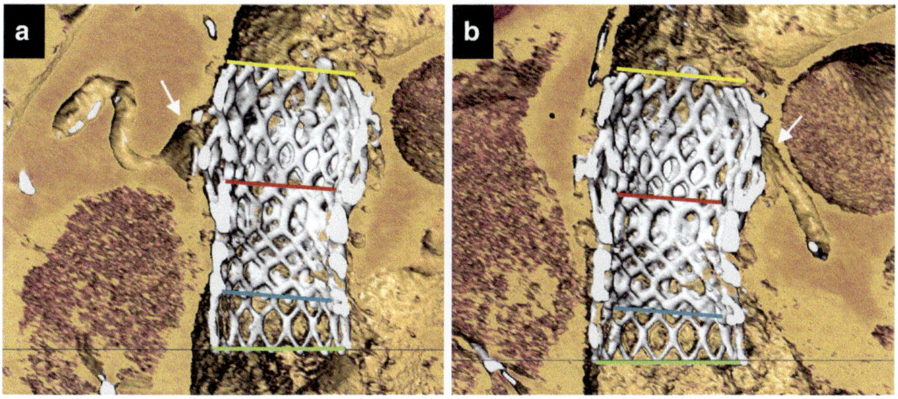

Fig. 7 To avoid obstruction of the coronary arteries (white arrows, Right coronary artery (**a**), Left coronary Artery (**b**)), the balloon-expandable valve Sapien 3 was deployed relatively lower with respect to the annular level. Green and blue lines show the inflow of a self-expanding and a balloon-expanding valve, respectively, and the red and yellow lines indicate THVs outflow

The subclavian approach for TAVR is a safe and feasible option compared to the femoral approach in type B aortic dissections [2]. It should be taken under consideration when the latter is not optimal.

A post-dilation approach in TAVR for selected patients significantly minimized the rates of paravalvular regurgitation without increasing 30-day and 1-year mortality [3, 4]. This technique enables us to adjust and perform fine-tuning after valve positioning and assist in controlling the extent of subvalvular leaks, a matter of great importance in high-risk patients.

This case accentuates the need for a thorough evaluation and assessment of all methods at hand, along with the importance of clinical judgment. Furthermore, it shows the utility of subclavian access for TAVR, especially in the cases of residual aortic dissections.

Key Points

- As TAVR extends to low-risk and younger patients, the valve-in-valve procedure will become more common.
- Transfemoral access is the most common and widely used approach.
- Alternative access, as the subclavian, should be more explored in the context of aortic dissections.

References

1. Barbanti M, Webb JG, Tamburino C, Van Mieghem NM, Makkar RR, Piazza N, Latib A, Sinning JM, Won-Keun K, Bleiziffer S, Bedogni F. Outcomes of redoing transcatheter aortic valve replacement for the treatment of the postprocedural and late occurrence of paravalvular regurgitation and transcatheter valve failure. Circ Cardiovasc Interv. 2016;9(9):e003930.
2. Petronio AS, De Carlo M, Bedogni F, Maisano F, Ettori F, Klugmann S, Poli A, Marzocchi A, Santoro G, Napodano M, Ussia GP. 2-Year results of CoreValve implantation through the sub-

clavian access: a propensity-matched comparison with the femoral access. J Am Coll Cardiol. 2012;60(6):502–7.
3. Harrison JK, Hughes GC, Reardon MJ, Stoler R, Grayburn P, Hebeler R, Liu D, Chang Y, Popma JJ, CoreValve US Clinical Investigators. Balloon post-dilation following implantation of a self-expanding transcatheter aortic valve bioprosthesis. J Am Coll Cardiol Interv. 2017;10(2):168–75.
4. Wang N, Lal S. Post-dilation in transcatheter aortic valve replacement: a systematic review and meta-analysis. J Interv Cardiol. 2017;30(3):204–11.

TAVR in Pseudoaneurysm of Sinus of Valsalva

Vivek Patel, Robert Naami, and Sabah Skaf

1 Clinical Background

The patient is a 72-year-old female with a past medical history of hypertension, hyperlipidemia, subacute lacunar cerebral vascular accident, cavernous cerebral malformations secondary to cerebral amyloid angiopathy, iron deficiency anemia, pulmonary hypertension, arteriovenous malformations, intestinal bleeding, and severe aortic stenosis (Heyde's syndrome). The patient began to experience unusual fatigue and weight loss in the past year and was subsequently found to have severe aortic stenosis. In the interim months, the patient was hospitalized for agitation, confusion, and altered mental status and was found to have aortic valve endocarditis. During her hospital stay, she underwent a transesophageal echocardiogram, which was concerning for severe aortic regurgitation due to flail of the non-coronary cusp and pseudoaneurysm due to a contained rupture in the Sinus of Valsalva. The patient completed a 6-week course of antibiotics and is here for continued evaluation of her severe, symptomatic aortic stenosis. The patient denied chest pain, cough, syncope, seizures, asthma, COPD, fever, and hospitalization due to congestive heart failure exacerbation.

Supplementary Information The online version contains supplementary material available at [https://doi.org/10.1007/978-3-031-05965-0_19].

V. Patel (✉)
Smidt Heart Institute, Cedars-Sinai Medical Center, Los Angeles, CA, USA
e-mail: vivek.patel@cshs.org

R. Naami
University Hospitals Cleveland Medical Center, Cleveland, OH, USA

S. Skaf
Cedars Sinai Medical Center, Los Angeles, CA, USA

O. Koren et al. (eds.), *Complex Cases in Structural Heart Intervention*,
https://doi.org/10.1007/978-3-031-05965-0_19

2 Imaging

TTE showed normal LV systolic function (EF 72%) and severe calcific aortic valve with AV area 0.6 cm^2, mean transaortic gradient of 44 mmHg, and peak transaortic gradient of 82 mmHg. Coronary angiogram revealed nonobstructive coronary disease. Cardiac reconstructed CT indicated an annular mean internal diameter of 19.1 mm, area of 259.8 mm^2, and a perimeter of 58.5 mm. The following mean diameters were measured: 22.9 mm at the Sinus of Valsalva, 21.4 mm at the STJ, and 16.2 mm at the LVOT. The coronary ostia originated at 12.1 and 12.8 mm (for the RCA and LCA) above the annular plane (Fig. 1). The pseudoaneurysm was measured to have 8.9 mm mean height from the aortic annular plane and 5.0 mm diameter (Fig. 2). CT data was used to construct volume rendered images of the pseudoaneurysm (Fig. 3). Pre-procedural TEE revealed severe aortic insufficiency (Fig. 4, Video 1).

3 Pre-Procedural Considerations, Dilemmas, and Challenges

Following evaluation by the multidisciplinary heart team, the patient was determined to be inappropriate for conventional surgery due to history of cerebral amyloid angiopathy and associated increased risk of intracranial hemorrhage in the setting of full anticoagulation. Instead, patient opted for transfemoral TAVR using 23-mm self-expandable bioprosthetic Evolut valve with closure of the pseudoaneurysm.

4 Procedure, Outcome, and Follow-Up

Attention was first directed to the pseudoaneurysm. After root angiography confirmed large aortic pseudoaneurysm (PSA) with a neck measuring roughly 1 × 1.5 cm, a 6F Hockey stick via radial sheath was used to engage, and scion wire was passed into PSA. A Lantern microcatheter was inserted after Trapper was used to secure. Ruby coils measuring 6 × 20 mm were inserted but were pulled out of PSA likely due to severe aortic insufficiency. These were then removed. A Pod 14 × 60 cm coil was also attempted but appeared insecure again due to aortic insufficiency. At this point, it was felt that without securing the aortic insufficiency, stable coil placement was unlikely. Therefore, attention was turned to completing TAVR. A 23-mm self-expandable bioprosthetic Evolut was advanced and positioned across the stenotic aortic valve. With pacing at lower rate, the valve was deployed in the standard technique (Fig. 5). A post-procedure TEE revealed improved aortic opening, reduced flow to the PSA, central aortic regurgitation and trace perivalvular regurgitation (Fig. 6, Video 2). It was confirmed with aortic root angiography.

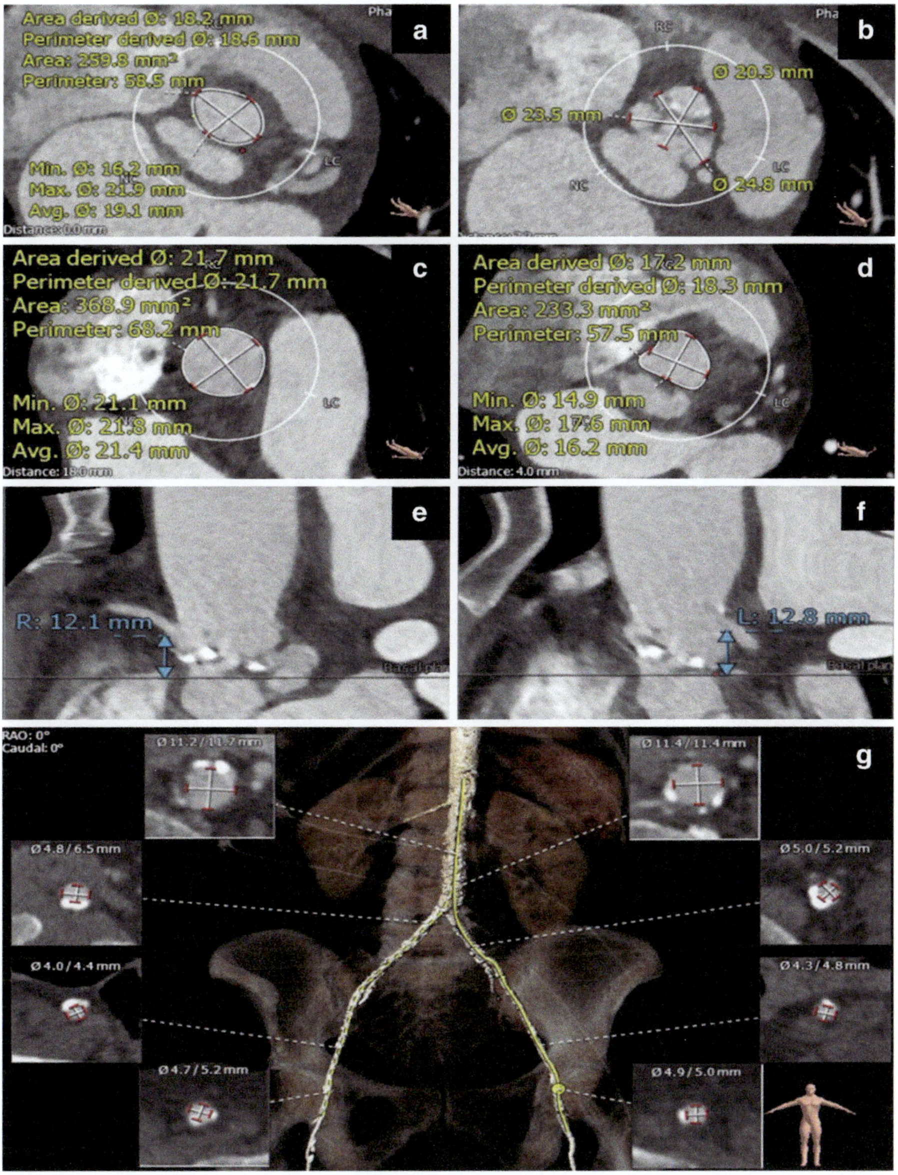

Fig. 1 Pre-TAVR reconstructed CT Analysis showing the dimension of the annulus (**a**), sinus of valsalva (**b**), sinotubular junction (**c**) and the left ventricular outflow track (**d**). The right coronary (**e**) and the left (**f**) coronary height and the minimal luminal diameter across the abdominal aorta and the iliofemoral arteries (**g**)

We removed the valve delivery system; however, hemostasis was not achieved at the left femoral access site. Selective iliofemoral angiography revealed a spiral dissection with a possible tear at the CFA site. After discussion with the vascular

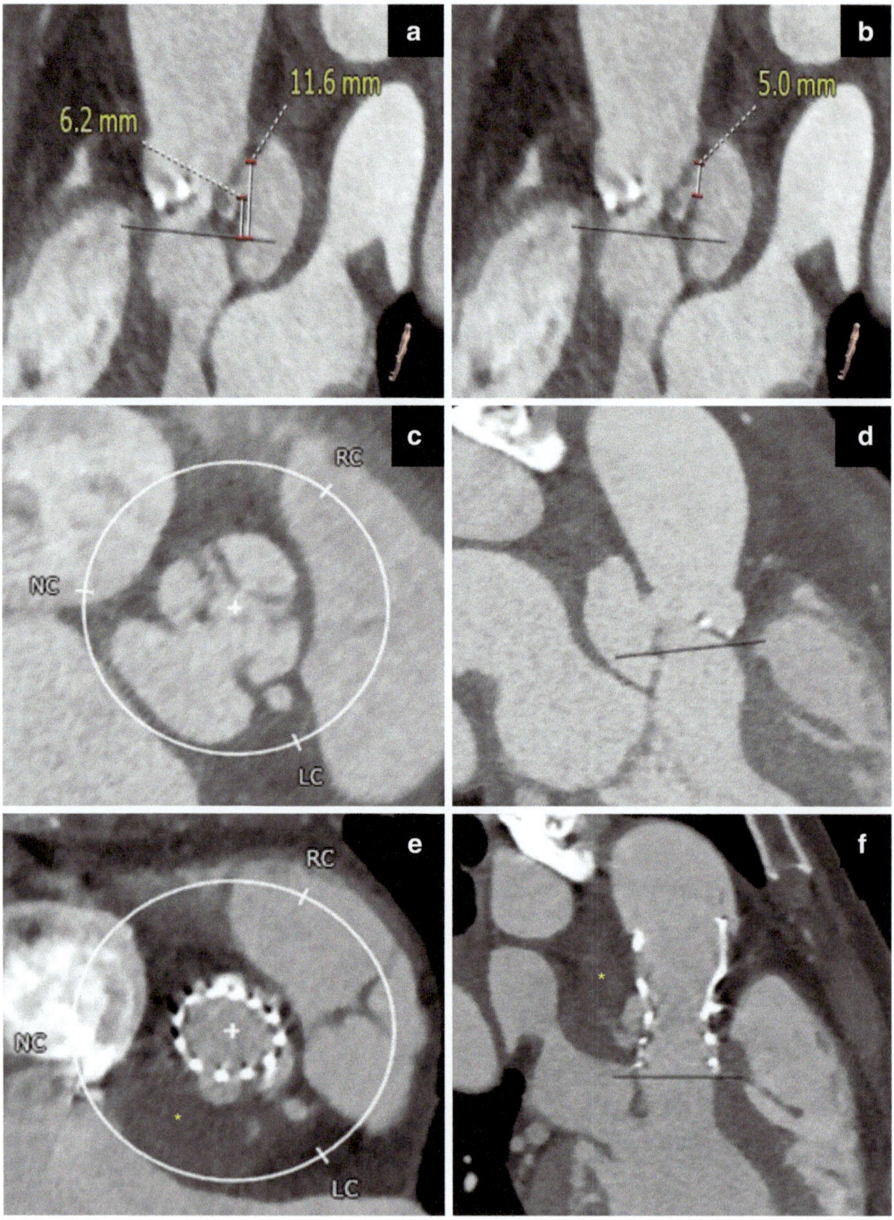

Fig. 2 Reconstructed CT images of the SOV pseudoaneurysm before (**a–d**) and after (**e**, **f**) the TAVR procedure. Note the neck height (**a**) and its diameter (**b**), and its dimension in the short (**c**, **e**) and long (**d**, **f**) axis. Note the clot (yellow asterisk) in the pseudoaneurysm following the THV deployment

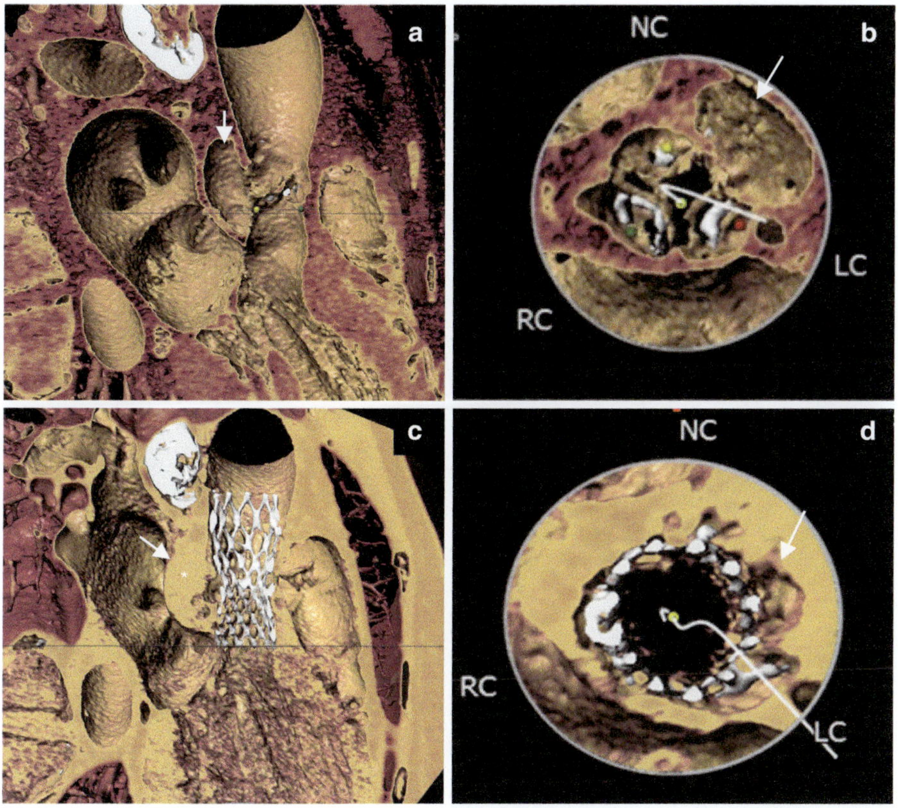

Fig. 3 Volume render images showing a SOV pseudoaneurysm (White arrow) before (**a**, **b**) and after (**c**, **d**) the TAVR procedure. Note the clot in the pseudoaneurysm following THV deployment (white asterisk, **c**)

surgery team, we thought that landing a covered stent may jeopardize the SFA bifurcation; therefore, we decided to proceed with surgical repair. The patient remained hemodynamically stable throughout the procedure. The remaining hospital course was uneventful, and the patient was discharged home.

On a 30-day and 3-month follow-ups, the patient reported feeling well with a noticeable improvement in symptoms. TTE on 30-day follow-up shows a well-placed bioprosthetic valve with no significant aortic regurgitation. The aortic valve mean pressure gradient was 17.0 mmHg (Video 3). A post-TAVR CT angiogram revealed intact aortic valve bioprosthesis without change to PSA size. However, the pseudoaneurysm did contain clots and had less contrast, which caused mild left atrial compression (Figs. 2 and 3).

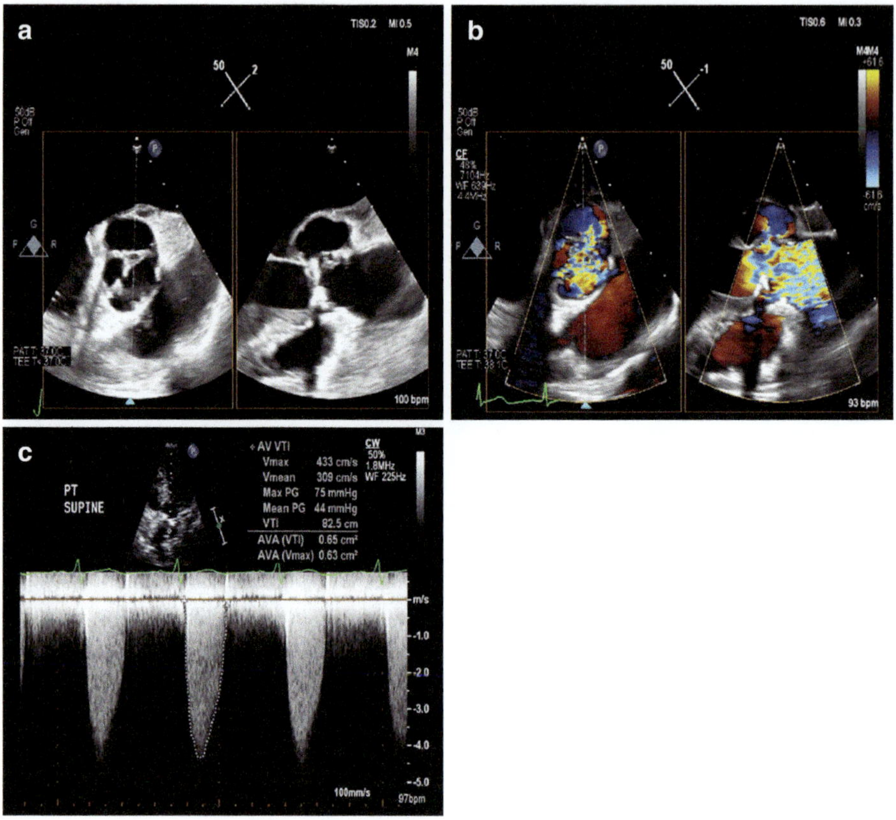

Fig. 4 Pre-procedural TEE indicating a significant aortic insufficiency before the procedure. Note AV anatomy (long axis AV view, **a**), color Doppler flow across the LVOT (**b**) and the gradient over aortic valve (Apical view, **c**). *LVOT* left ventricle outflow tract

5 Discussion

The sinuses of Valsalva (SOV) are a collection of pockets within the aortic root, between the aortic annulus and sinotubular junction. The sinuses prevent blockage of the coronary artery ostia by opening the aortic valve during systole. In a healthy state, each sinus measures a diameter, on average, of less than 4.0 cm in men and 3.6 cm in women. However, weakening at the level of the elastic lamina of one or multiple sinuses predisposes the spaces to pathological dilations or aneurysms, which are most seen in the right coronary sinus. SOV aneurysms (or SOVA) affect nearly 0.1% of the population, making up nearly 4% of all congenital heart diseases and affect men more commonly than women. The median age was 45 years old in one retrospective study of nearly 100 patients undergoing SOVA repair [1, 2].

SOV aneurysms (or SOVA) have been linked to congenital and acquired processes. These include genetic connective tissue disorders such as Ehlers–Danlos

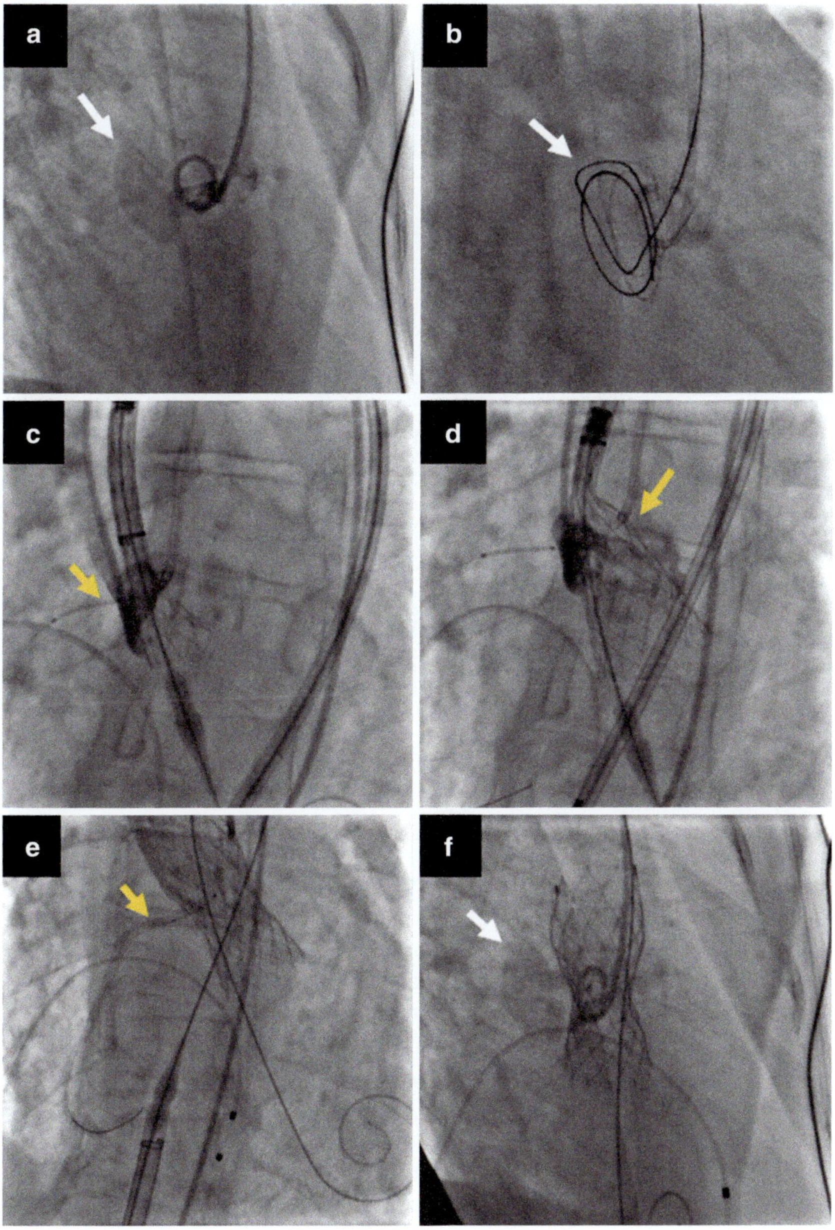

Fig. 5 Fluoroscopic view of the TAVR procedure. Note the full dimension of the pseudoaneurysm (white arrow, **a**) while trying to close it with a penumbra peripheral occlusion (POD) 14 × 60 cm coil (white arrow, **b**). Following unsuccessful closure of the pseudoaneurysm with a coil, a self-expanding THV was positioned lower to avoid RCA occlusion (yellow arrow, **c**) and then was partially deployed (yellow arrow, **d**). Once RCA patency was confirmed (yellow arrow, **e**) the THV was fully opened. Following the THV deployment, the flow to the pseudoaneurysm was reduced (white arrow, **f**)

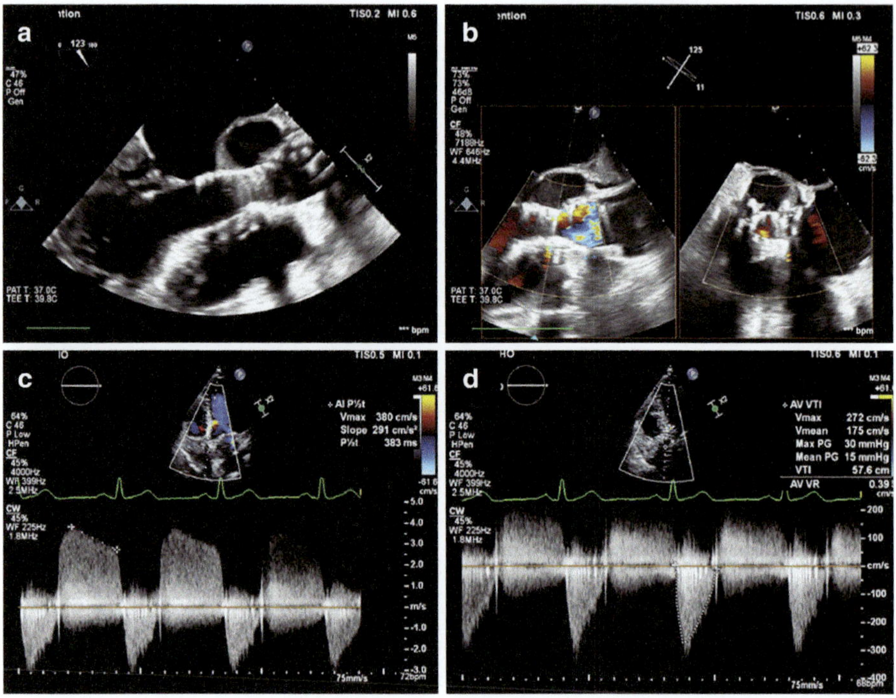

Fig. 6 Post-procedural TTE showing a well seated bioprosthetic THV in aortic position (**a**), a reduction in the flow across the valve and toward pseudoaneurysm's neck (**b**), a diastolic eccentric regurgitation jet (**c**), mean aortic valve gradient of 15 mmHg (**d**)

and Marfan's syndrome. Conversely, acquired etiologies include infections (e.g., syphilis, endocarditis), inflammatory states (e.g., atherosclerosis, vasculitis), and chest trauma [3]. SOVA sequela depends on which sinus is affected. However, complications often include rupture. For example, a SOVA and subsequent rupture of the right coronary sinus may extend and cause shunting to the right ventricle or right atrium and lead to right ventricular dysfunction [4, 5].

The imaging modality of choice when diagnosing SOVA is 2D transesophageal echocardiography. Echo often demonstrates an abnormal enclosed space bulging into the right or left ventricular cavity [6, 7]. An alternative diagnostic tool is cardiac catheterization; however, it is reserved to interogate coronary anatomy in patients requiring surgical repair. Additionally, cardiac computed tomography aids in quantifying the SOVA size and morphology. Moreover, color flow Doppler helps assess hemodynamic changes in the setting of complications such as rupture [8, 9].

Indications and methods of SOVA repair depend on the aneurysm's size, the patient's comorbidities, and associated cardiac symptoms. Non-ruptured sinus of Valsalva aneurysm should be surgically repaired if associated with significant symptoms or is rapidly enlarging as delineated by the 2010 American Guidelines for Thoracic Aortic Disease [10, 11]. Alternatively, a ruptured SOVA can be repaired using surgical or transcatheter methods. Surgical repair is more conventional, particularly when rupture is associated with regurgitation or septal defect. Alternatively, transcatheter repair using closure devices has demonstrated favorable outcomes. In a retrospective study of 33 patients with ruptured SOVA, transcatheter closure was successfully achieved using occluder devices in all but one patient. Moreover, there were no adverse outcomes (i.e., infective endocarditis, device displacement, arrhythmias, or death) in a median follow-up of 6 years [12, 13].

Key Points

- SOV aneurysm/pseudoaneurysm is rare.
- Among known risk factors are congenital connective tissue diseases, infection, inflammation, and mechanical trauma.
- Surgical correction is the therapy of choice.
- Operators should be familiar with the minimally invasive techniques for selected high surgical risk patients.

References

1. Galeczka M, Glowacki J, Yashchuk N, Ditkivskyy I, Rojczyk D, Knop M, Smerdzinski S, Cherpak B, Szkutnik M, Bialkowski J, Fiszer R, Lazoryshynets V. Medium- and long-term follow-up of transcatheter closure of ruptured sinus of Valsalva aneurysm in Central Europe population. J Cardiol. 2019;74(4):381–7.
2. Mustafa S, Mookadam F, Cooper L, Adam G, Zehr K, Stulak J, Holmes D. Sinus of Valsalva aneurysms—47 years of a single center experience and systematic overview of published reports. Am J Cardiol. 2007;99(8):1159–64.
3. Stöger G, Borger MA, Misfeld M. A giant aneurysm of the left sinus of Valsalva. Eur J Cardiothorac Surg. 2019;56(3):627.
4. Ohno N, Watanabe K, Maeda T, Kato O, Ueno G, Yoshizawa K, Fujiwara K. A rare case of unruptured extracardiac multiple sinus of Valsalva aneurysms originating from the orifices with partial aortic wall defects. Surg Case Rep. 2019;5(1):47.
5. Seo KW, Park JS. Sinus of Valsalva aneurysm and multiple aortic aneurysms provoked by viral myocarditis. Korean Circ J. 2019;49(2):194–6.
6. Diwakar A, Patnaik SS, Hiremath CS, Chalam KS, Dash P. Rupture of sinus of valsalva—a 15 years single institutional retrospective review: preoperative heart failure has an impact on postoperative outcome? Ann Card Anaesth. 2019;22(1):24–9.
7. Serban AM, Bătrâna N, Cocoi M, Ianoş R, Moţ S, Kovacs E, Axente DD, Man C, Molnar A. The role of echocardiography in the diagnosis and management of a giant unruptured sinus of Valsalva aneurysm. Med Ultrason. 2019;21(2):194–6.
8. Terdjman M, Bourdarias JP, Farcot JC, Gueret P, Dubourg O, Ferrier A, Hanania G. Aneurysms of sinus of Valsalva: two-dimensional echocardiographic diagnosis and recognition of rupture into the right heart cavities. J Am Coll Cardiol. 1984;3(5):1227–35.
9. Wierda E, Koolbergen DR, de Mol BAJM, Bouma BJ. Rupture of a giant aneurysm of the sinus of Valsalva leading to acute heart failure: a case report demonstrating the excellence of echocardiography. Eur Heart J Case Rep. 2018;2(3):090.
10. Urbanski PP, Hirao S, Irimie V. Root repair in patient with huge sinus Valsalva aneurysm and severe aortic regurgitation. Gen Thorac Cardiovasc Surg. 2020;68(5):530–3.
11. Wingo M, de Angelis P, Worku BM, Leonard JR, Khan FM, Hameed I, Lau C, Gaudino M, Girardi LN. Sinus of Valsalva aneurysm repairs: operative technique and lessons learned. J Card Surg. 2019;34(6):400–3.

12. Hajizeinali A, Hosseinsabet A. Percutaneous device closure of a ruptured aortic sinus of Valsalva aneurysm in a patient with a mechanical bileaflet aortic valve. Turk Kardiyol Dern Ars. 2019;47(3):243.
13. Xiao JW, Niu MN, Wang QG, Zhang DZ, Han XM, Zhang P, Cui CS, Zhu XY. Safety and efficacy of transcatheter closure of ruptured sinus of Valsalva aneurysm. Zhonghua Xin Xue Guan Bing Za Zhi. 2018;46(10):799–803. Chinese.

TAVR Valve Dislodgement Due to Retrieval of Coronary Stent and Guidewire

Vivek Patel, Nathan Drillings, and Sabah Skaf

1 Clinical Presentation

A 51-year-old male with a history of SAVR with Medtronic Freestyle complete sub-coronary valve presented to emergency care in our hospital. He was found to be septic and in acute hypoxemic respiratory failure.

2 Images and Supported Data

TTE and TEE reveal new severe bioprosthetic aortic insufficiency with evidence of flow reversal in the abdominal aorta and severe diastolic dysfunction. Cardiac reconstructed CT indicates an annular mean internal diameter of 28.2 mm, area of 602.4 mm^2, and perimeter of 87.9 mm. The following mean diameters were measured: 43.0 mm at the Sinus of Valsalva, 29.1 mm at the STJ, and 737.7 mm^2 at LVOT (Fig. 1). The coronary ostia originated at an optimal height. The right coronary artery was 20.1 mm above the annular plane, and the left coronary artery

Supplementary Information The online version contains supplementary material available at [https://doi.org/10.1007/978-3-031-05965-0_20].

V. Patel (✉)
Smidt Heart Institute, Cedars-Sinai Medical Center, Los Angeles, CA, USA
e-mail: vivek.patel@cshs.org

N. Drillings
Psychobiology, University of California (UCLA), Los Angeles, CA, USA

S. Skaf
Cedars Sinai Medical Center, Los Angeles, CA, USA

O. Koren et al. (eds.), *Complex Cases in Structural Heart Intervention*,
https://doi.org/10.1007/978-3-031-05965-0_20

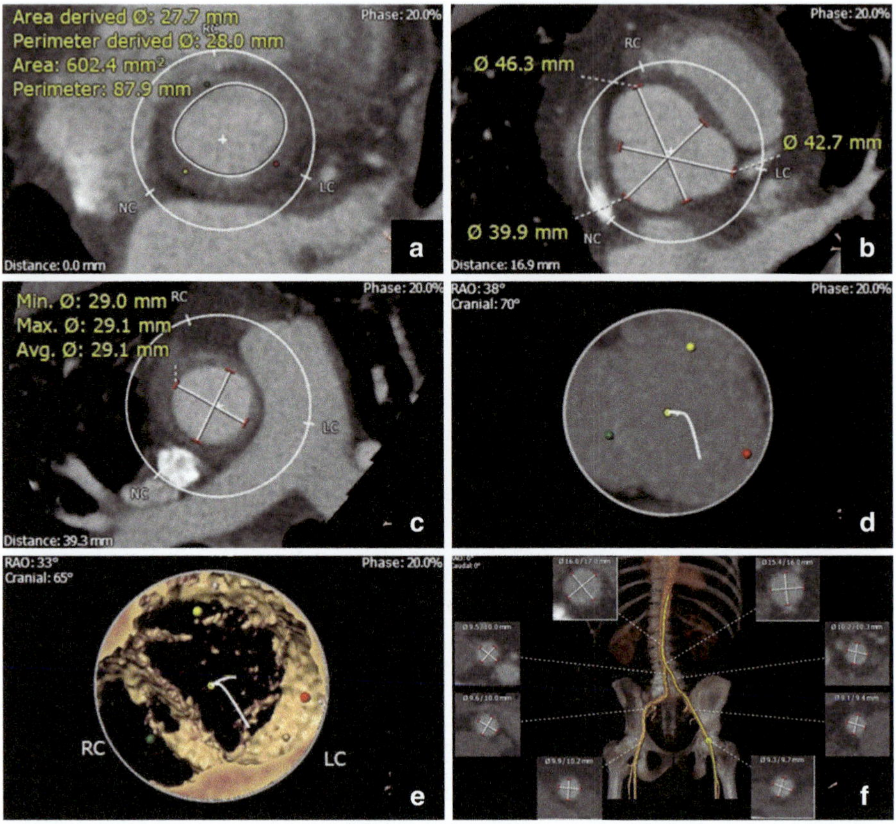

Fig. 1 Reconstructed pre TAVR CT analysis. (**a**) Annulus dimensions. (**b**) Sinus of Valsalva dimension. (**c**) Sinotubular junction dimension. (**d**) Aortic valve calcification score in Hounsfield unit. (**e**) Volume rendered image of aortic valve. (**f**) Abdominal aorta and bilateral iliofemoral arteries measurements

ostium was estimated to be 25.7 mm above the annular plane (Fig. 2). The right femoral artery approach was feasible with a minimal lumen diameter of 9.5 × 10.0 mm measured at the right common iliac artery.

3 Pre-Procedural Consideration: Pitfalls, Dilemmas and Challenges, Technique

Pre-procedure dilemmas were focused on choosing the largest THV possible without compromising future coronary access or risking immediate coronary obstruction. We decided to proceed with the highest diameter possible and use a protecting device for coronary access. The actual diameter of the freestyle valve was 25 mm, which allowed us to use a 29-mm balloon-expandable Sapien-3. CT analysis of the distance between a virtual 29-mm Sapien-3 THV and the coronary ostia was

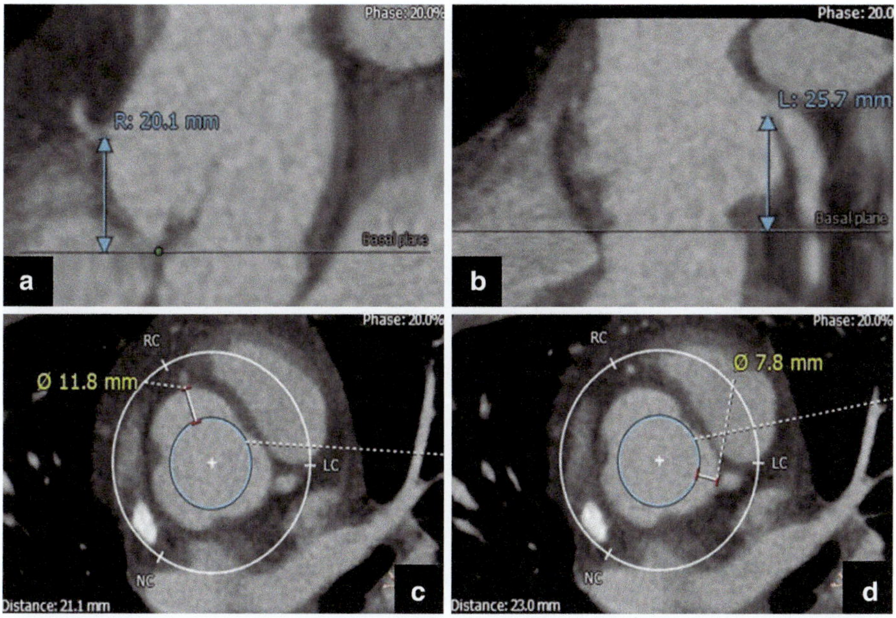

Fig. 2 Coronary heights from the annular plane on CT pre-TAVR analysis: right coronary artery height (**a**); left coronary artery height (**b**), the distance from virtual THVs to the coronary ostium, the distance from 29-mm virtual THV to RCA ostium (**c**); the distance between 29-mm THV and LCA ostium (**d**)

11.8 mm for the RCA and 7.8 mm for LCA (Fig. 2). Pre-procedural coronary angiogram revealed no significant lesions (Fig. 2).

A 29-mm Edwards Sapien S3 valve delivery system was positioned across the aortic valve. With rapid pacing at 180 beats per minute, the valve was deployed in the standard technique with an extra inflation volume of 3 mL. A post-procedure TEE revealed no central aortic regurgitation and no perivalvular regurgitation (Fig. 3e, f). However, during the deployment, the Sion guidewire was looped in the left ventricle (Video 1). After the valve deployment, the Xience stent was stuck between the previous surgical bioprosthesis and the TAVR stent frame (Fig. 4b, Videos 2 and 3). Multiple attempts to remove the Xience stent and the Sion guidewire were made. Unfortunately, this resulted in the migration of the TAVR bioprosthesis in the aortic root (Fig. 4c, Videos 4 and 5). Hemodynamically, the patient remained stable. The guide catheter and the Xience stent were then removed. Another 6F EBU guide catheter was used to engage the left coronary artery, and an angiogram showed preserved flow in the left main coronary artery (Fig. 4d, Video 6). We anticipated that an attempt at pulling the TAVR valve within the ascending aorta using a snaring device might cause aortic dissection. Therefore, we decided to deploy the second TAVR valve within the first TAVR valve to secure it and treat the original aortic regurgitation (Videos 7 and 8). Angiographically, the TAVR valve was tilted free in the aortic root. A reliant stent graft balloon was advanced, crossed the Sapien valve, and subsequently inflated to correct the valve angle.

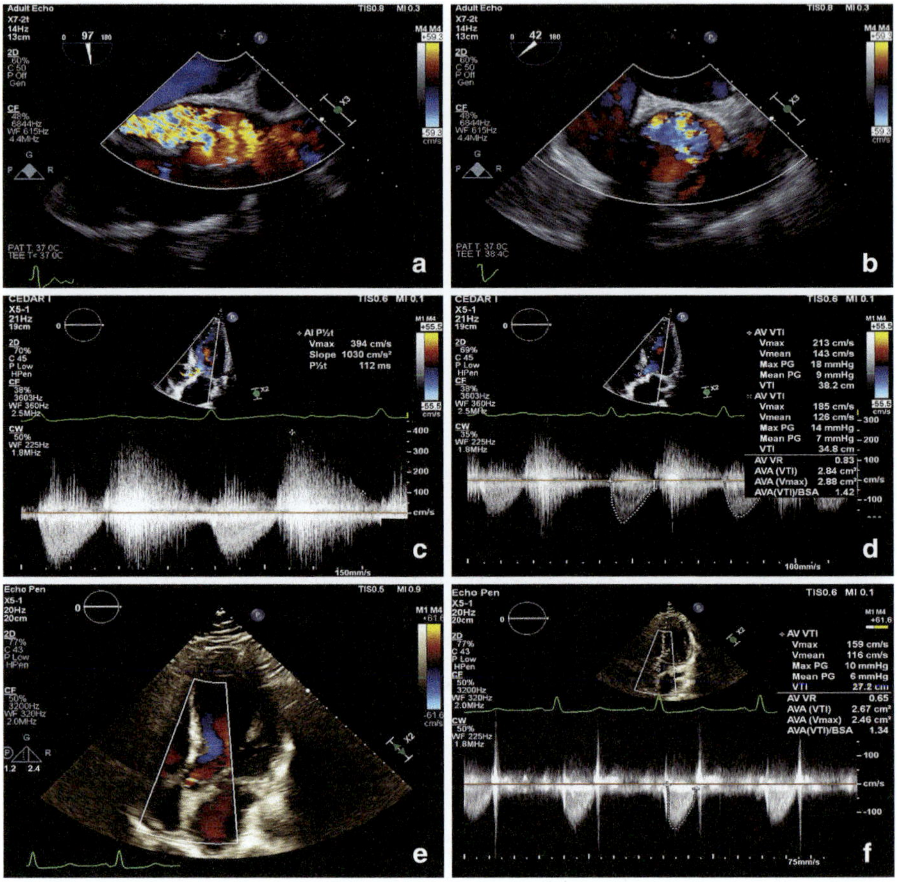

Fig. 3 TEE significant aortic insufficiency is seen on the mid-esophageal TEE view (**a**), short axis view (**b**), diastolic eccentric regurgitation jet seen on an apical long-axis view (**c**), pre-procedural AV gradient is measured in an apical long axis view (**d**), post-procedural 5 chamber view of aortic valve (**e**), post-procedural AV gradient is measured in an apical long axis view (**f**)

A 29-mm Edwards Sapien S3 valve delivery system was positioned across the native aortic valve while overlapping with the first Sapien valve. With rapid pacing at 180 beats per minute, the valve was deployed in the standard technique with an extra inflation volume of 5 mL. A post-procedure TEE revealed no central aortic regurgitation and no perivalvular regurgitation.

4 Outcome and Follow-Up

A post-procedural next-day TTE revealed no central aortic regurgitation and mild perivalvular regurgitation. The THV was well situated in the aortic position with normal leaflet motion.

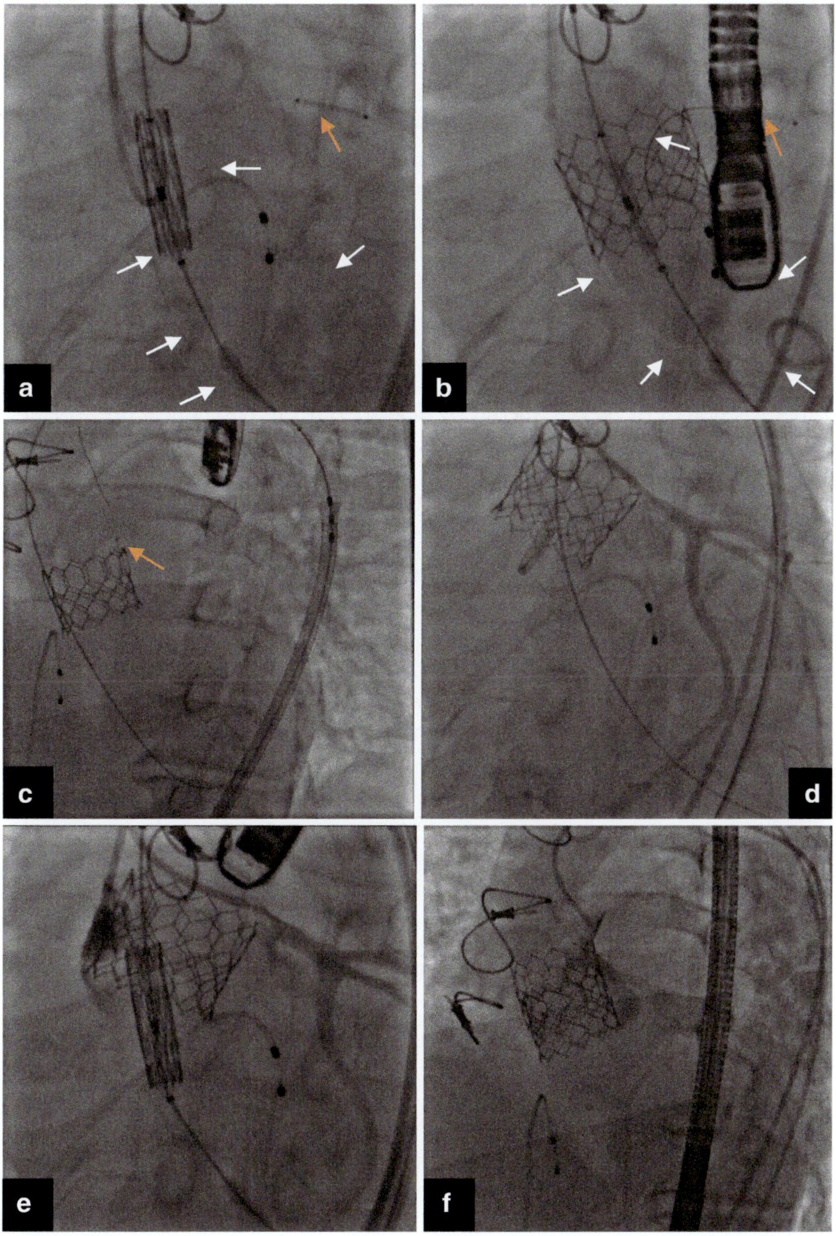

Fig. 4 Fluoroscopic view of TAVR procedure: position of Xience stent (orange arrow) and Sion guidewire (white arrows) before the TAVR valve deployment (**a**), Position of Xience stent (orange arrow) and Sion guidewire (white arrows) after the TAVR valve deployment (**b**), Xience stent can be seen stuck between TAVR and previous freestyle valve (**c**), valve dislodgment after the attempt of removing guide wire and stent (**d**), second TAVR valve deployment and contrast can be seen in the left coronary artery (**e**), balloon-expandable Sapien-3 deployment over previous TAVR valve and good flow in left coronary artery (**f**)

5 Discussion

Entrapped wire over a THV is a rare but potentially serious complication. Unlike known PCI techniques (GC wire, balloon inflation, snaring, microcatheter), entrapped wire in THV during TAVR seems to be more challenging [1]. A literature review on similar cases yields little information on how to bail out from this situation. Our experience focuses on using a wire manipulation technique by positioning the wire to the side of the wire entrapment and slowly applying rotational movement to loosen the firm contact between the wire and the THV strut. Once the contact is loosened, we could then apply gentle pressure to pull it back. This maneuver should be repeated until the entire wire is pulled backed completely. Of note, this technique was not used in this case.

Embolization of the percutaneous device is a rare but potentially life-threatening complication [2]. Management strategies depend on the type, size, and location of the embolized device, timing of diagnosis, and clinical presentation of the patient. The potential for aortic dissection because of manipulation of a THV in the aorta is an obvious concern [3]. In this case, the THV valve was not repositioned due to a high risk of aortic dissection. However, if feasible, one option could be to position the dislodged valve in the descending aorta using a snare catheter, paying close attention to not obstruct flow to any important branches of the aorta. An alternative option is to decide if it is possible to overlap a new prosthesis within the embolized TAVR valve. Several criteria need to be considered, such as the coronary height, coronary engagement after the deployment, and the location of the embolized TAVR valve. Increased awareness of predisposing factors, preventive measures, and appropriate bail-out options and techniques are strongly advisable.

Key Points

- Embolization of the percutaneous device is a rare but potentially life-threatening complication.
- The operator should be familiar with known risk factors.
- Entrapped wire in THV during TAVR seems to be a more challenging case, especially in the case of valve-in-valve.
- Appropriate bail-out options and techniques are strongly advisable.

References

1. Al-Moghairi AM, Al-Amri HS. Management of retained intervention guide-wire: a literature review. Curr Cardiol Rev. 2013;9(3):260–6. PMID: 23116055; PMCID: PMC3780351. https://doi.org/10.2174/1573403x11309030010.
2. Stolcova M, Ciatti F, Cardaioli F, Demola P, Nai Fovino L, Fabris T, Mattesini A, Matsuda Y, Ristalli F, Di Mario C, Tarantini G, Meucci F, Fraccaro C. Embolizzazione di protesi durante impianto transcatetere di valvola aortica [Prosthesis embolization during transcatheter aortic valve implantation]. G Ital Cardiol (Rome). 2020;21(11):35–44. Italian. PMID: 33295333. https://doi.org/10.1714/3487.34671.

3. Tay EL, Gurvitch R, Wijeysinghe N, Nietlispach F, Leipsic J, Wood DA, Yong G, Cheung A, Ye J, Lichtenstein SV, Carere R, Thompson C, Webb JG. Outcome of patients after transcatheter aortic valve embolization. JACC Cardiovasc Interv. 2011;4(2):228–34. PMID: 21349463. https://doi.org/10.1016/j.jcin.2010.10.010.

TAVR in Aortic Root Homograft and Challenging Access

Vivek Patel, Quentin Wise, and Ahmed Al Badri

1 Clinical Background

A 57-year-old male patient presented to our clinic with dyspnea on moderate exertion and fatigue. The surgeon evaluated the patient and found him to be of high surgical risk for re-do sternotomy and surgical aortic valve replacement. The patient was selected for transcatheter heart valve repair. This patient had a history of a type A aortic dissection status post-David procedure (valve-sparing aortic root replacement) and type B aortic dissection with an enlarging descending thoracic aortic aneurysm. This patient also had a history of the right to left carotid-carotid bypass, left carotid-left subclavian artery bypass, thoracic endovascular aortic repair using a Gore thoracic branch device (TBE) for the innominate artery, left subclavian artery coil embolization, followed by left renal artery angioplasty with stent placement.

Supplementary Information The online version contains supplementary material available at [https://doi.org/10.1007/978-3-031-05965-0_21].

V. Patel (✉)
Smidt Heart Institute, Cedars-Sinai Medical Center, Los Angeles, CA, USA
e-mail: vivek.patel@cshs.org

Q. Wise
Interventional Cardiology, Cedars-Sinai Medical Center, Los Angeles, CA, USA

A. Al Badri
Cedars Sinai Medical Center, Los Angeles, CA, USA

O. Koren et al. (eds.), *Complex Cases in Structural Heart Intervention*,
https://doi.org/10.1007/978-3-031-05965-0_21

2 Imaging

TTE and TEE revealed severe aortic valve regurgitation with holo-diastolic flow reversal in the descending aorta and mild aortic stenosis with a mean gradient of 14 mmHg (Fig. 1, Video 1). Echocardiography also showed severe aortic valve regurgitation with normal left ventricular function. Cardiac reconstructed CT indicated an annular mean internal diameter of 26.8 mm, area of 587.0 mm^2, and perimeter of 86.7 mm. The following mean diameters were measured: 34.4 mm at the

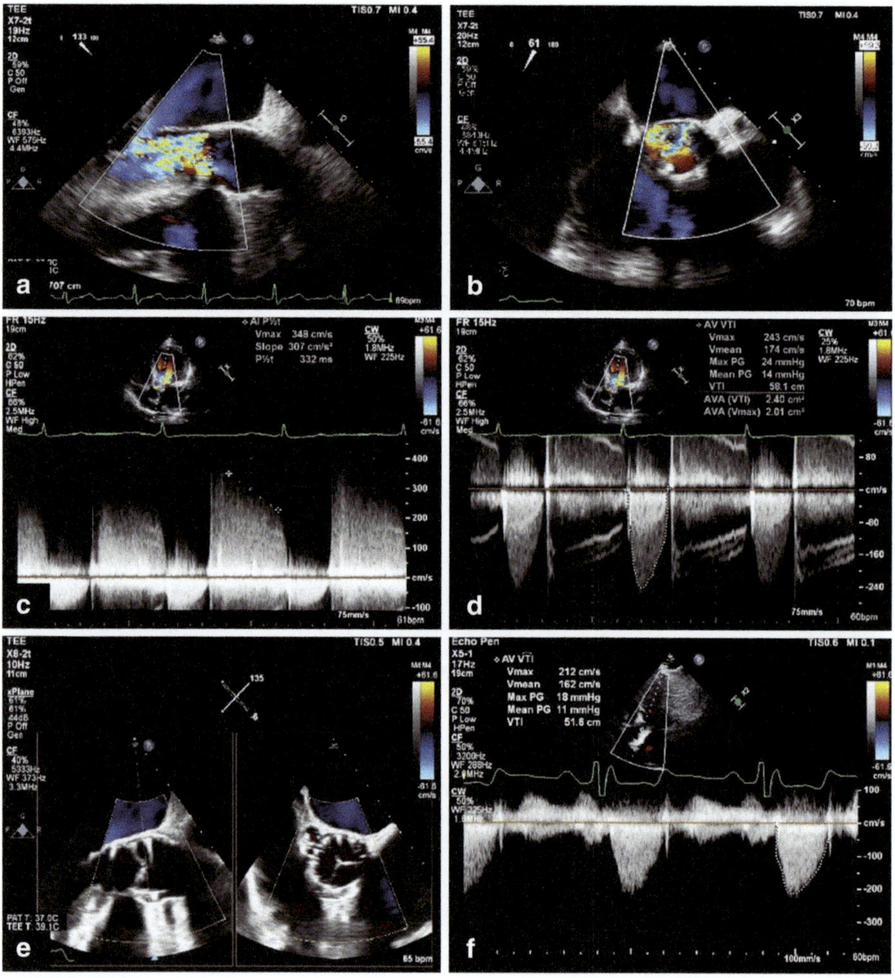

Fig. 1 TEE significant aortic insufficiency is seen on the mid-esophageal TEE view (**a**), short axis view (**b**), diastolic eccentric regurgitation jet seen on an apical long-axis view (**c**), pre-procedural AV gradient is measured in an apical long axis view (**d**), post-procedural long axis and short axis view of the aortic valve (**e**), post-procedural AV gradient is measured in an apical long axis view (**f**)

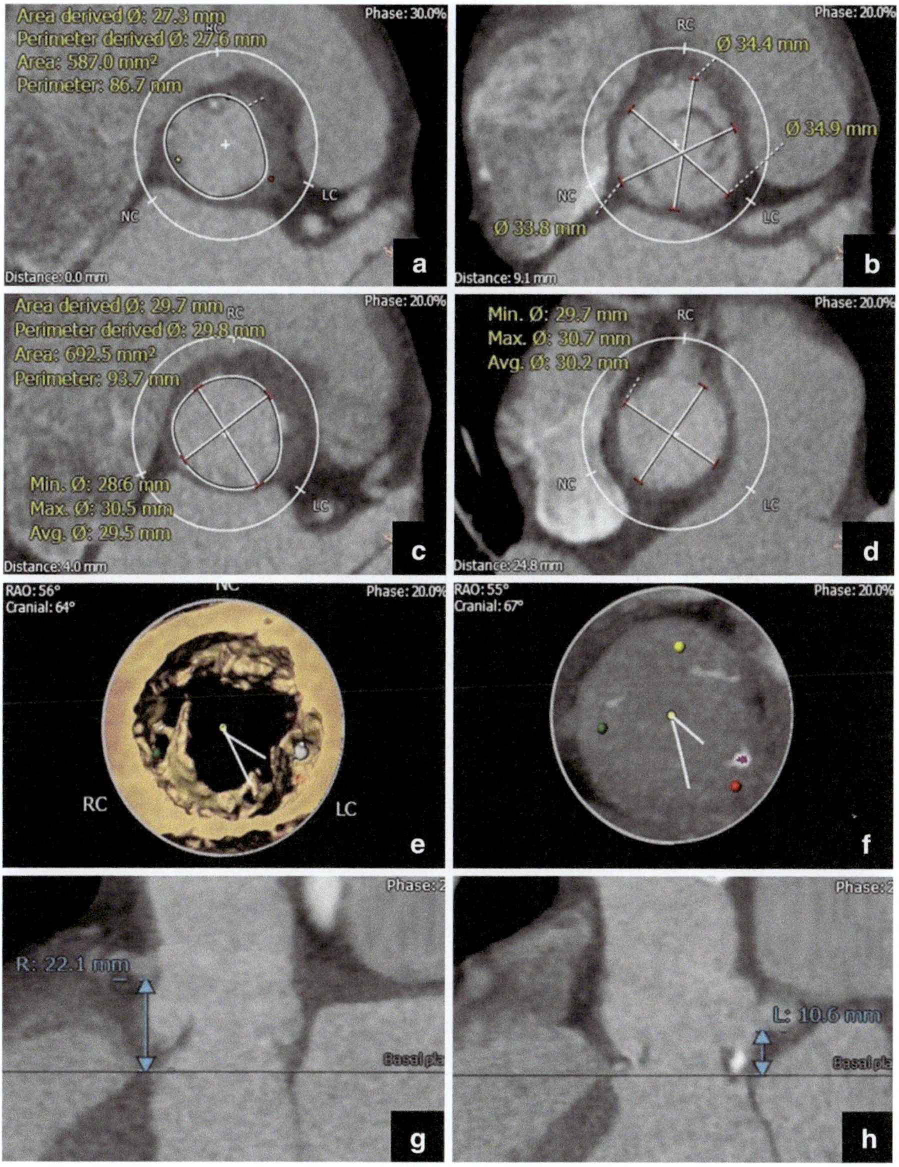

Fig. 2 CT pre-TAVR analysis. Annulus dimensions (**a**), sinus of Valsalva dimension (**b**), left ventricular outflow track dimensions (**c**), sinotubular junction dimension (**d**), volume rendered image of the aortic valve (**e**), calcium score (**f**), right coronary height (**g**), left coronary height (**h**)

Sinus of Valsalva, 30.2 mm at the STJ, and 692.5 mm² at LVOT. The right and left coronary heights measured respectively 22.1 and 10.6 mm. The left coronary height was borderline (Fig. 2). CT showed the presence of graft in the descending aorta and graft between the brachiocephalic artery and the aortic arch. A dissection was present from the abdominal aorta to the left femoral artery (Fig. 3).

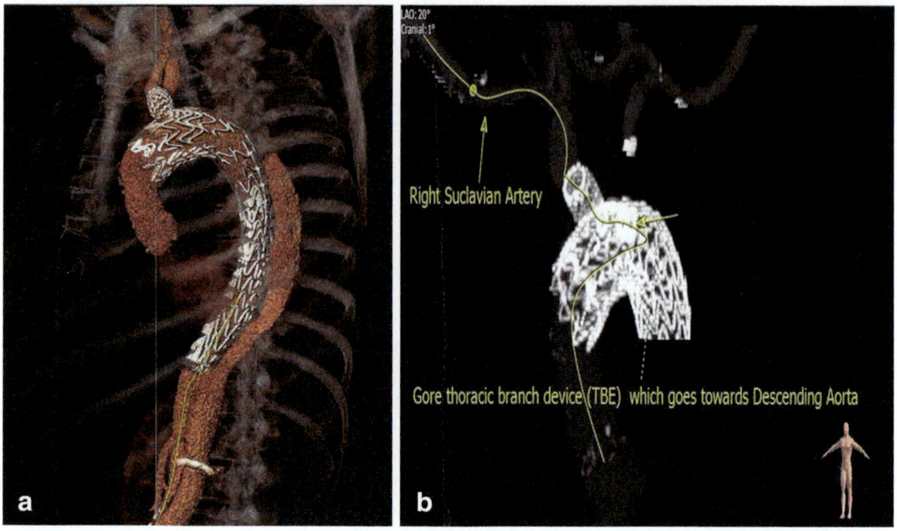

Fig. 3 Endovascular graft in descending aorta (**a**), Gore thoracic branch device in brachiocephalic artery (arrow showing the graft distal part position in the aortic arch) (**b**)

3 Pre-Procedural Considerations, Dilemmas, and Challenges

There were multiple challenges present in this case. The first dilemma was choosing a balloon-expandable or self-expanding valve and what size to use considering the homograft, mild aortic valve calcification, dissection, and repair in aortic vessels. The second dilemma was choosing a safe access site considering known dissection in the abdominal aorta and left femoral artery. The subclavian and carotid arteries were turned down as preferred accesses due to prior aortic arch branching, multiple bypasses, and the abdominal aorta's true lumen diameter being 4.4 × 12.0 mm (Fig. 2b).

Considering the presence of homograft, mild calcium on the aortic valve, vascular anatomy, and relatively borderline left coronary height, we chose a 29-mm Sapien-3 valve with extra volume if needed, because of the flexibility of the delivery system and low-profile characteristics. We decided to attempt a left femoral access approach.

4 Procedure, Outcome, and Follow-Up

IVUS catheter was used to confirm the true lumen in the iliac arteries and abdominal aorta (Video 2). The delivery system was advanced from the AA using the IVUS catheter to the annulus. The annulus was measured at 636 mm^2 during the procedure with TEE to confirm the suitability of the 29-mm S3 Valve. A 29-mm Edwards

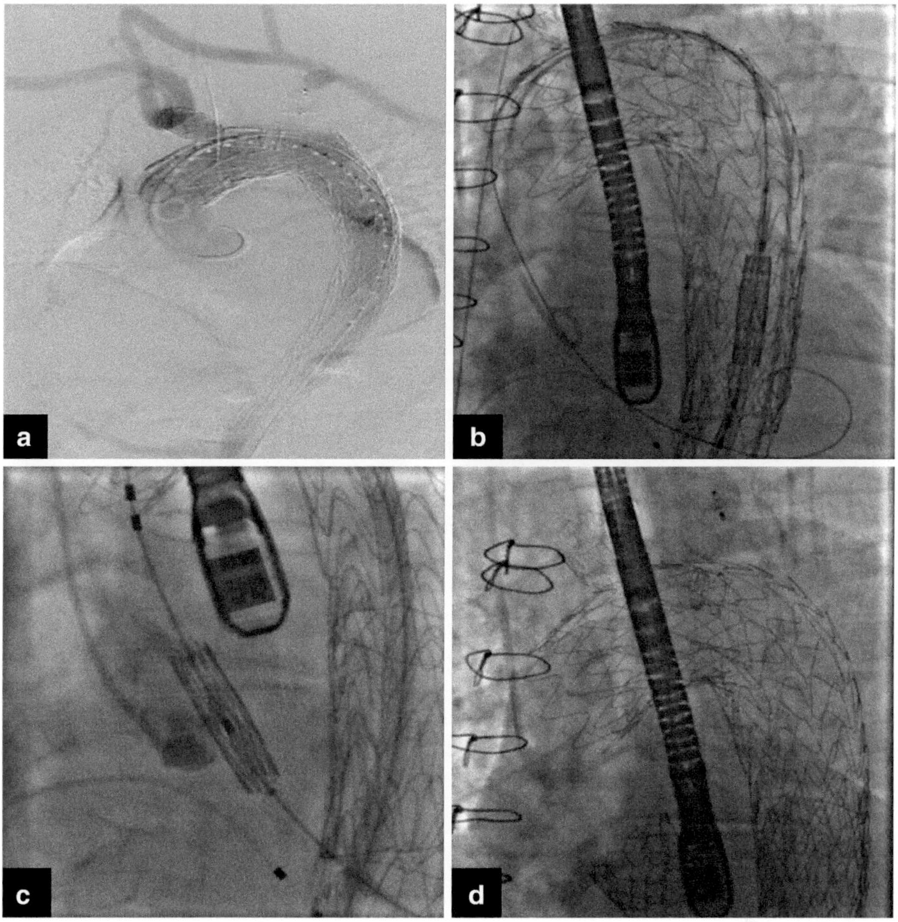

Fig. 4 Fluoroscopic view of TAVR procedure: endovascular graft in aortic arch, and branching graft in right subclavian artery (**a**), TAVR delivery system in endovascular graft (**b**), balloon-expandable Sapien-3 valve across homograft before deployment (**c**), balloon-expandable Sapien-3 deployment over homograft (**d**)

Sapien S3, with an extra 5 mL volume, was positioned across the stenotic aortic valve and deployed with rapid pacing at 180 beats per minute (Fig. 4, Videos 3 and 4).

A post-procedure TEE revealed no significant aortic regurgitation and trivial paravalvular regurgitation. The THV was well seated in the aortic position with normal leaflet motion. At the 30-day follow-up, the patient felt significantly better, with no shortness of breath and less fatigue (Fig. 3b).

5 Discussion

Repeat surgical valve replacement after a failed homograft can be challenging and high risk. TAVR has recently emerged as an alternative procedure for patients. There is limited data available for TAVR in failed homograft in big registries such as PARTNER 2 Valve-in-Valve Registry and CoreValve US Expanded Use Study [1, 2]. Selection and sizing of TAVR prostheses in AR patients are crucial for procedural success. Different criteria need to be considered, such as aortic valve calcification, LVOT area, annulus area, and coronary height [3]. TAVR for failing aortic homograft may be feasible and safe when the patient has a high surgical risk. This case shows the feasibility and safety of the TAVR procedure in the presence of type B dissection and previous endovascular graft. As TAVR is becoming more acceptable for younger patients, we will see more complex cases with such a combination [4]. Pre-procedural planning is crucial for such cases.

Key Points

- Selection of the TAVR prosthesis in AR patients is crucial for procedural success.
- It is important to choose the proper valve size taking into consideration the low degree of calcification and consequent less secure anchoring of the TAVR valve.
- Pre-procedural imaging is crucial for safety and better outcomes for TAVR in failed homograft and history of type B dissection.
- TAVR can be successfully performed in patients with aortic dissection treated with endovascular stent grafts. However, care should be exercised and adjunctive medical devices, such as the IVUS Catheter, can be used to ensure true lumen positioning of the catheters.
- Oversizing is important when treating aortic regurgitation.

References

1. Mangieri A, Giannini F, Laricchia A, Romano V, Lanzillo G, Pagnesi M, Ponticelli F, Ancona M, Latib A, Colombo A. Transcatheter treatment of pure aortic regurgitation in a horizontal aorta complicated by valve embolization and aortic dissection. Cardiovasc Revasc Med. 2019;20(6):535–6. https://doi.org/10.1016/j.carrev.2018.12.013.
2. Hollander KN, Montealegre-Gallegos M, Mahmood F. Valve-in-valve-in homograft: a case of a repeat transcatheter aortic valve replacement in a patient with an aortic homograft. Ann Card Anaesth. 2016;19(4):737–9. https://doi.org/10.4103/0971-9784.191575.
3. Saji M, Hoyt WJ Jr, Ailawadi G, Mulloy DP, Ghanta RK, Ragosta M, Scott LD. Transcatheter aortic valve replacement in a young adult patient with a failed homograft. Pediatr Cardiol. 2016;37(5):986–8. https://doi.org/10.1007/s00246-016-1399-2.
4. Kilic A, Siki MA, Szeto WY, Bavaria JE, Anwaruddin S, Desai ND. Concomitant endografting of a type B aortic dissection during transfemoral aortic valve replacement. Ann Thorac Surg. 2017;103(3):e223–4. https://doi.org/10.1016/j.athoracsur.2016.08.070.

Aortic Root Rupture Following TAVR Procedure

Ofir Koren, Vivek Patel, Siamak Kohan, and Hezzy Shmueli

1 Clinical Presentation

A 78-year-old female with a history of severe aortic stenosis, hypothyroidism, and degenerative joint disease presented with NYHA III congestive heart failure (CHF). Given her critically narrow aortic valve and her high NT-pro B type-natriuretic peptide (BNP) blood levels, the patient was considered for a transcatheter aortic valve replacement (TAVR). She was considered an intermediate-risk patient during her preoperative visit using the investigational Sapien 3 valve as part of the PARTNER 2 registry.

2 Images and Supported Data

A preoperative transthoracic echocardiogram (TTE) revealed normal left ventricular ejection fraction, severe diastolic dysfunction, severe aortic valve stenosis, and mild to

Supplementary Information The online version contains supplementary material available at [https://doi.org/10.1007/978-3-031-05965-0_22].

O. Koren
Smidt Heart Institute, Cedars-Sinai Medical Center, Los Angeles, CA, USA

Faculty of Medicine, Technion, Israel Institute of Technology, Haifa, Israel
e-mail: Ofir.Koren@cshs.org

V. Patel (✉)
Smidt Heart Institute, Cedars-Sinai Medical Center, Los Angeles, CA, USA
e-mail: vivek.patel@cshs.org

S. Kohan
Kaiser Permanente Los Angeles Medical Center, Los Angeles, CA, USA

H. Shmueli
Cardiology Department, Soroka University Medical Center, Beer Sheva, Israel

O. Koren et al. (eds.), *Complex Cases in Structural Heart Intervention*,
https://doi.org/10.1007/978-3-031-05965-0_22

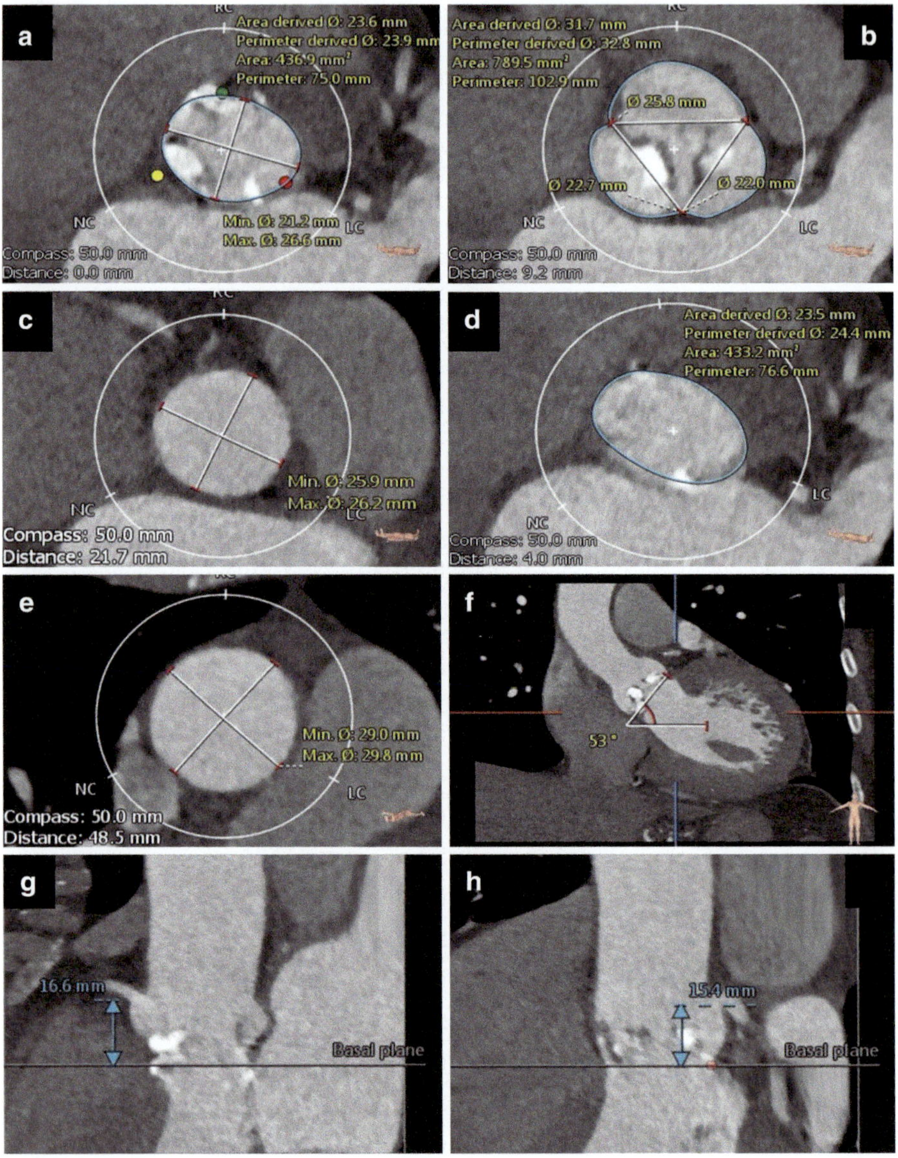

Fig. 1 Reconstructed CT analysis before the procedure. Note the annulus (**a**) and the SOV (**b**) dimensions, the STJ (**c**) and LVOT height and diameter (**d**) and the maximal luminal diameter of ascending aorta (**e**). The aortic angulation is 53°(**f**), and the Ostia of the coronary arteries are high enough above the annular plane indicating low risk for coronary obstruction (**g, h**)

moderate mitral regurgitation. The mean transaortic gradient was 55 mmHg, and the aortic valve area was 0.5 cm^2. Subsequent coronary angiograms showed no obstructive coronary artery disease. Preoperative CT measuring the aorta landmarks revealed low-risk features for coronary obstruction (Fig. 1) and calcifications throughout the aorta (Fig. 2). A baseline transesophageal echocardiogram (TEE) evaluated the aortic annulus and aortic valve gradients, consistent with previous CT angiograms.

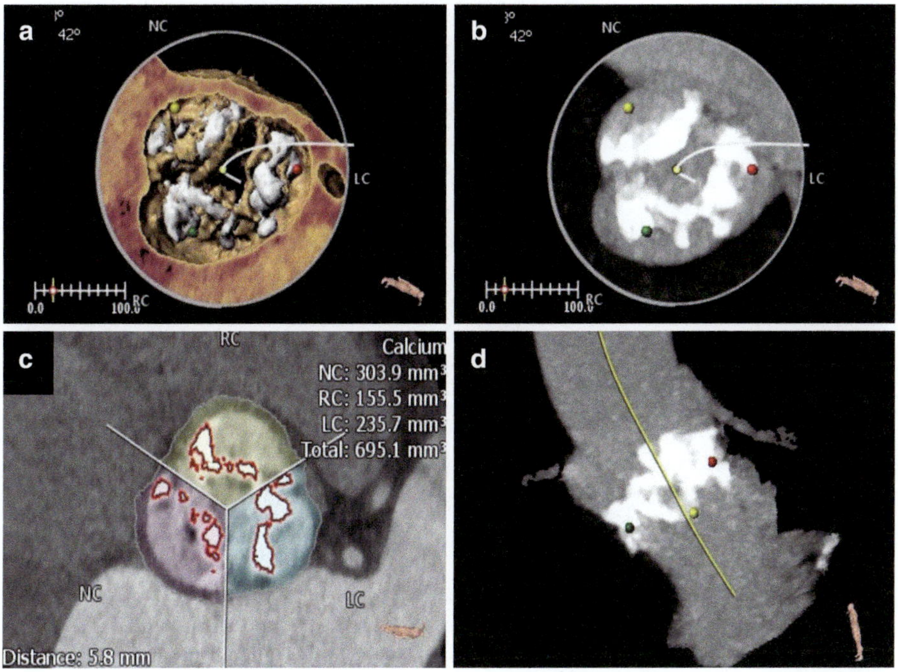

Fig. 2 Reconstructed CT analysis before the procedure. Note the extent of calcification (**a**, **b**) and its distribution in respect to the coronary cusps (**c**) and the aortic root (**d**)

3 Pre-Procedural Consideration: Pitfalls, Dilemmas, and Challenges

Prevention of an aortic rupture depends on the balance between the sizing of the new valve to prevent paravalvular leak (PVL) and the diameter of the native aortic annulus [1]. Thus, preliminary assessment of patients should include accurate assessment of the "device landing zone," which includes the aortic root and left ventricular outflow tract [1, 2]. In case of discrepancies between the measurements from TTE, TEE, and CT, we repeat the measurements to choose a valve size accurately [1]. Another consideration includes the calcifications in this zone as seen on preoperative CT.

4 Technique

The patient underwent a transfemoral TAVR using a 26-Sapien 3 Valve. We used the 5 French micropuncture kit to access femoral arteries and veins, confirmed by femoral angiography. A 6 French dilator was introduced into the right femoral artery to deploy Perclose suture, followed by an 11 French Terumo sheath. A 6 French Terumo sheath was introduced into the left femoral artery, and a 5 French long

Terumo sheath was introduced into the left femoral vein. The pacing was achieved through a 5 French balloon-tipped temporary transvenous pacemaker at the RV apex through the femoral venous sheath.

A multipurpose catheter was advanced over a J-tipped wire into the ascending aorta. This multipurpose catheter was exchanged for a Lunderquist wire, and the 11 French Terumo sheath was exchanged for a 14 French Sapien 3 sheath. Then, an 11 French sheath was placed within this.

A pigtail catheter was advanced through the 6 French sheaths in the left femoral artery to get a baseline aortic root angiogram. Then, an AL-1 catheter and straight wire were advanced through the large sheath to cross the stenotic aortic valve. An Amplatz extra-stiff wire (0.025 × 260 cm) was advanced into the LV cavity. At this point, the wire was removed, and transaortic valvular gradients were obtained. The 26-mm Sapien 3 Commander valve delivery system was exchanged for the AL-1 catheter.

We could not cross the calcified aortic valve with the Sapien 3 system. Thus, we removed the sheath and the delivery system over an Amplatz stiff wire and inserted another 14 French sheath into the right femoral artery. We dilated the aortic valve using balloon valvuloplasty with a Z-Med II balloon (20 mm × 4 cm) and inflated it two times with rapid pacing (Videos 1 and 2, Fig. 3). The valvuloplasty balloon was exchanged for the 26-mm Sapien 3 Commander valve delivery system, positioned across the valve, and then deployed in the standard technique with rapid pacing at 180 beats per minute (Video 3, Fig. 3). The delivery system was exchanged for a 6 French multipurpose catheter into the LV for hemodynamic monitoring.

The blood pressure immediately dropped, and chest compressions were initiated. Simultaneously, a TEE probe was inserted. An ascending aortogram confirmed a pericardial effusion (Video 4) with an aortic root rupture and frank bleeding near the left coronary artery (Videos 5, 6 and 7, Figs. 3 and 4). Subsequently, a micropuncture needle performed a pericardiocentesis into the pericardial space, and a pericardial drain was placed. The patient was put on cardiopulmonary bypass, and a sternotomy was performed with the assistance of cardiovascular surgery. We proceeded with aorto-mitral curtain repair and a surgical aortic valve replacement with a 19 mm Sorin Mitroflow surgical bioprosthesis. The surgery was successful without any noticeable events. Postprocedural TEE showed a well-seated bioprosthetic valve, moderate to severe mitral regurgitation, no valvular or paravalvular leak, and normal biventricular systolic function (Videos 8 and 9, Fig. 5). The current peak transaortic pressure gradient was 21 mmHg, and the mean transaortic pressure gradient was 10 mmHg.

At the end of the procedure, the patient was weaned off bypass, the heparin was reversed, the 14 French sheath was removed, and perclose sutures were deployed for hemostasis. No femoral arterial dissection was seen on ultrasound. Chest tubes were placed in the mediastinum and both pleural. During the procedure, there was a total of 70 cc of Visipaque contrast used, and there was a total of 17.8 min of fluoroscopic time.

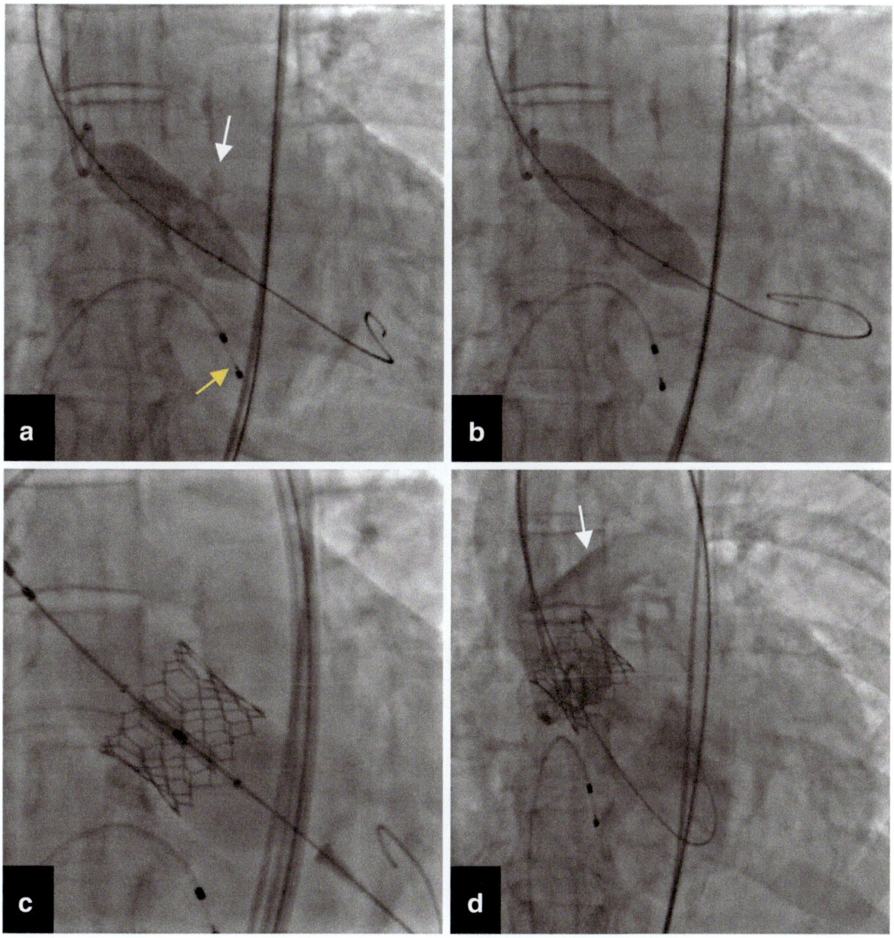

Fig. 3 Fluoroscopic view of the procedure. Two rounds of Balloon dilatation (**a**, **b**) performed due to an inability in crossing the aortic valve. Note the significant calcification over the AV (white arrow) and the temporary pacing lead in the RC (orange arrow). Deployment of a 26 mm balloon expendable valve over the calcified AV (**c**) leads to aortic root rupture near the LCA and immediate pericardial effusion (**d**, white arrow)

5 Outcome and Follow-Up

The patient was transferred to the cardiac ICU in stable condition while intubated. Three days postoperatively, the patient's course was complicated by sinus arrest with junctional escape rhythm (requiring epinephrine) and atrial fibrillation with the rapid ventricular response given a left bundle branch block with sinus node dysfunction requiring a permanent pacemaker. The patient was discharged after two weeks in stable condition. The patient was alive six years following the procedure.

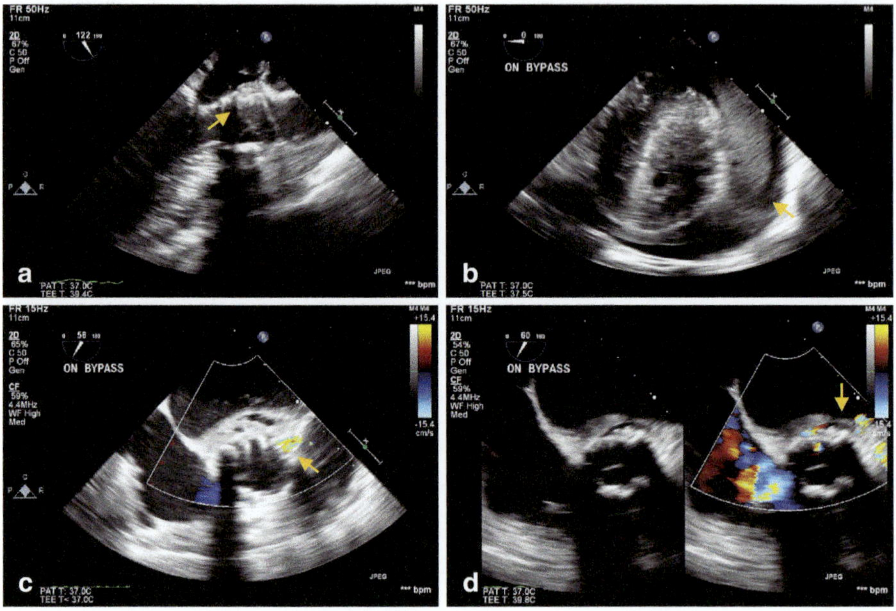

Fig. 4 Transesophageal echocardiography following valve deployment (**a**, orange arrow) indicating severe pericardial effusion (**b**, orange arrow). During vascular bypass, a Doppler flow over the aortic valve in short axis view indicated abnormal flow near the LCA (**c**, orange arrow) and aortic-mitral continuity (**d**, orange arrow)

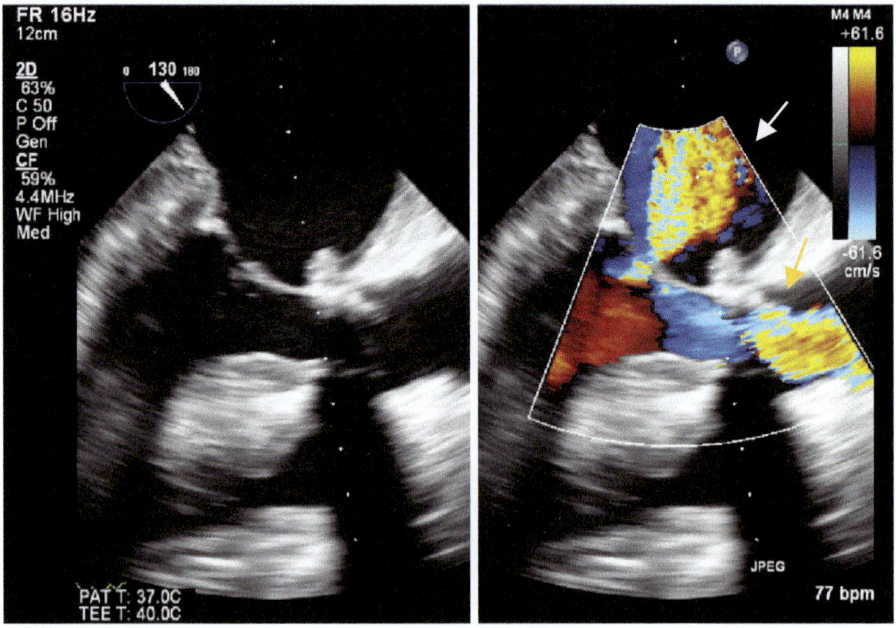

Fig. 5 Transesophageal echocardiography following open heart valve surgery, a Sorin Mitroflow bioprosthesis 19 mm valve (orange arrow) shows a well-positioned and functioning prosthesis and a hyperdynamic LV with moderate to severe mitral regurgitation with an eccentric jet. (white arrow)

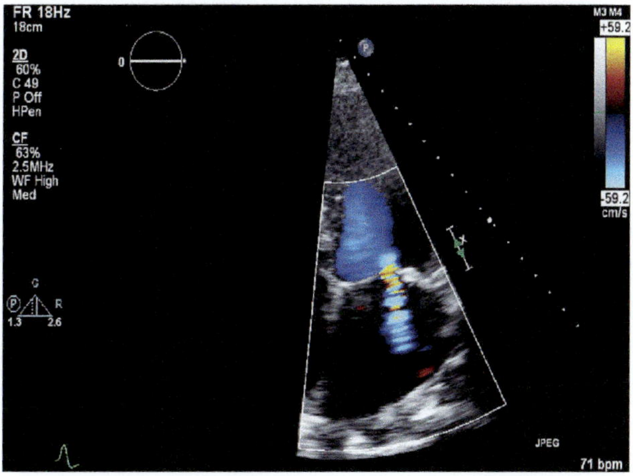

Fig. 6 Transthoracic echocardiography for the 1-year follow up after the surgery indicated a well-positioned bioprosthetic valve, good LV function and mixed mitral regurgitation and stenosis with only moderate severity

Repeat TEE at 1-year follow-up indicated a well-positioned bioprosthetic valve with mixed mitral regurgitation and stenosis with moderate severity (Fig. 6, Video 10).

6 Discussion

TAVR is a treatment for symptomatic severe aortic stenosis patients who are not appropriate or at high risk for surgical aortic valve replacement. A rare but life-threatening complication is an aortic root rupture. The prevalence of aortic root rupture in patients that underwent TAVR was reported between 0.4% and 1%; however, the prevalence has been decreasing given increasing expertise and the use of pre-procedural multislice CT [1, 3–5].

The risk factors associated with aortic root rupture can be split into anatomical and procedural risk factors. Anatomical risk factors include significant calcification, small aortic valve annulus (<20 mm), narrow aortic root, short distance from the coronary ostia to annulus, severe asymmetric sub-aortic LV hypertrophy, global LVH, smaller body surface area, female gender, and nodules (>4 mm) [1–3]. This patient had several risk factors for an aortic rupture, including significant calcification of aortic valve and root, female gender, and dilation of the native valve before valve deployment. Calcification of any of these areas such as aortic root leaflet, annulus, left ventricular outflow tract (LVOT), walls of sinus of Valsalva, or bicuspid valve increases the risk [2]. Procedural risk factors include overdilation of the prosthesis, oversizing the valve, and balloon-expandable valves [1, 6]. Overdilation of the prosthesis may occur in the setting of dilation of the stenotic native aortic valve before valve deployment or additional ballooning to address paravalvular leak after the valve deployment [1–3, 6, 7]. Oversizing of the valve (≥20%) is a significant risk factor in the setting of calcification or other factors [2, 3, 6, 7]. In balloon-expandable valve, oversizing ≥20% predicted an eightfold increased risk in contained rupture [8]. Barbanti et al. compared patients with TAVR with balloon-expandable prostheses complicated by rupture versus those without rupture and revealed these risk factors: LVOT/sub-annular calcification (odds ratio 10.9) and prosthesis oversizing (odds ratio 8.4) [7].

In addition to an accurate assessment of the anatomy of the patient, other preventative considerations include assessing the patient for high-risk factors, choosing a smaller valve, incomplete inflation of the balloon during deployment, higher valve positioning to prevent deployment in the LVOT, avoiding re-ballooning to prevent PVL in those with significant calcifications, considering conventional surgery instead of TAVR, and even avoiding the procedure or transferring to a center with more experience in TAVR [2, 7, 9]. In patients with significant calcifications, it may be safer to do the procedure with self-expanding or inflatable valves instead of balloon-expandable, which are rarely associated with rupture when post-dilation is not performed [3, 9].

Aortic valve rupture is a life-threatening complication of TAVR and can be successfully treated with appropriate recognition and management. Diagnosis depends on the patient's stability and requires echocardiography, aortography, or direct exploration with surgery [2]. Patients with acute hemodynamic instability or those with symptoms and unclear hemodynamics should be considered for an immediate cardiopulmonary bypass to maintain stability [1, 2]. If feasable, a reversal of the anticoagulation should be initiated as early as possible, followed by percutaneous pericardial drainage [3].

Some patients may require immediate surgery with aortic valve replacement, even those initially considered inoperable [1]. The mortality of surgically treated patients is estimated to be 50–75% [2, 3, 7]. Any LVOT and myocardial rupture should be managed with a reconstruction of the LVOT to avoid damaging the coronary arteries [1]. A second TAVR can theoretically be performed if the rupture is identified and treated on time. This will mainly depend on if the rupture site is cranial or caudal to the skirt of the THV [3].

Key Points

- Patients considered for TAVR should have accurate and reliable preoperative measurements of the aortic root and surrounding structures.
- Any discrepancies between aortic root measurements should be assessed before the procedure.
- The benefits of pre-dilation of the stenotic valve or additional ballooning to prevent PVL should be balanced with the risk of aortic root rupture, especially those with existing calcifications.
- Aortic root rupture should be immediately suspected in any patient with hemodynamic instability after a TAVR.

References

1. Pasic M, Unbehaun A, Dreysse S, Buz S, Drews T, Kukucka M, D'Ancona G, Seifert B, Hetzer R. Rupture of the device landing zone during transcatheter aortic valve implantation: a life-threatening but treatable complication. Circ Cardiovasc Interv. 2012;5(3):424–32.
2. Pasic M, Unbehaun A, Buz S, Drews T, Hetzer R. Annular rupture during transcatheter aortic valve replacement: classification, pathophysiology, diagnostics, treatment approaches, and prevention. JACC Cardiovasc Interv. 2015;8(1 Part A):1–9.
3. Coughlan JJ, Kiernan T, Mylotte D, Arnous S. Annular rupture during transcatheter aortic valve implantation: predictors, management and outcomes. Interv Cardiol Rev. 2018;13(3):140.
4. Généreux P, Head SJ, Van Mieghem NM, Kodali S, Kirtane AJ, Xu K, Smith C, Serruys PW, Kappetein AP, Leon MB. Clinical outcomes after transcatheter aortic valve replacement using valve academic research consortium definitions: a weighted meta-analysis of 3,519 patients from 16 studies. J Am Coll Cardiol. 2012;59(25):2317–26.
5. Walther T, Hamm CW, Schuler G, Berkowitsch A, Kötting J, Mangner N, Mudra H, Beckmann A, Cremer J, Welz A, Lange R. Perioperative results and complications in 15,964 transcatheter aortic valve replacements: prospective data from the GARY registry. J Am Coll Cardiol. 2015;65(20):2173–80.
6. Tsuda M, Mizote I, Mukai T, Sakata Y. Aortic root rupture during balloon-expandable transcatheter aortic valve replacement in a patient without recognized risk factors for aortic root rupture: a case report. Eur Heart J Case Rep. 2020;4(3):1–4.
7. Barbanti M, Yang TH, Rodès Cabau J, Tamburino C, Wood DA, Jilaihawi H, Blanke P, Makkar RR, Latib A, Colombo A, Tarantini G. Anatomical and procedural features associated with aortic root rupture during balloon-expandable transcatheter aortic valve replacement. Circulation. 2013;128(3):244–53.
8. Blanke P, Reinöhl J, Schlensak C, Siepe M, Pache G, Euringer W, Geibel-Zehender A, Bode C, Langer M, Beyersdorf F, Zehender M. Prosthesis oversizing in balloon-expandable transcatheter aortic valve implantation is associated with contained rupture of the aortic root. Circ Cardiovasc Interv. 2012;5(4):540–8.
9. Barbanti M. Avoiding coronary occlusion and root rupture in TAVI—the role of pre-procedural imaging and prosthesis selection. Interv Cardiol Rev. 2015;10(2):94.

TAVR in Patient with a Large Apical Left Ventricular Thrombus

Ofir Koren, Dhairya Patel, and Hasan Jilaihawi

1 Clinical Presentation

A 72-year-old male with progressive shortness of breath (NYHA class III), severe AS, and left ventricular apical thrombus requested a second opinion after he was deemed to be of prohibitive risk for surgical AVR. His past medical history was remarkable for hypertension, diabetes mellitus, stage IV chronic kidney disease (eGFR = 14), CAD, and ischemic cardiomyopathy. The patient was placed on warfarin.

2 Images and Supported Data

Preliminary echocardiography (TTE and TEE) showed severely depressed LV function (LVEF = 25%) with global hypokinesis, critical AS with mild regurgitation, and a large LV apical thrombus measuring 3 cm in diameter (Fig. 1, Video 1). AV area (using continuity equation) measured 0.54 cm^2 and the peak gradient was 30 mmHg (mean 17 mmHg). RV function was mildly reduced with pulmonary artery pressure of 34 mmHg. Reconstructed cardiac CT indicated an annular mean

Supplementary Information The online version contains supplementary material available at [https://doi.org/10.1007/978-3-031-05965-0_23].

O. Koren (✉)
Smidt Heart Institute, Cedars-Sinai Medical Center, Los Angeles, CA, USA

Faculty of Medicine, Technion, Israel Institute of Technology, Haifa, Israel
e-mail: Ofir.Koren@cshs.org

D. Patel
Smidt Heart Institute, Cedars-Sinai Medical Center, Los Angeles, CA, USA

H. Jilaihawi
Heart Valve Center, NYU Langone Health, New York, NY, USA

O. Koren et al. (eds.), *Complex Cases in Structural Heart Intervention*,
https://doi.org/10.1007/978-3-031-05965-0_23

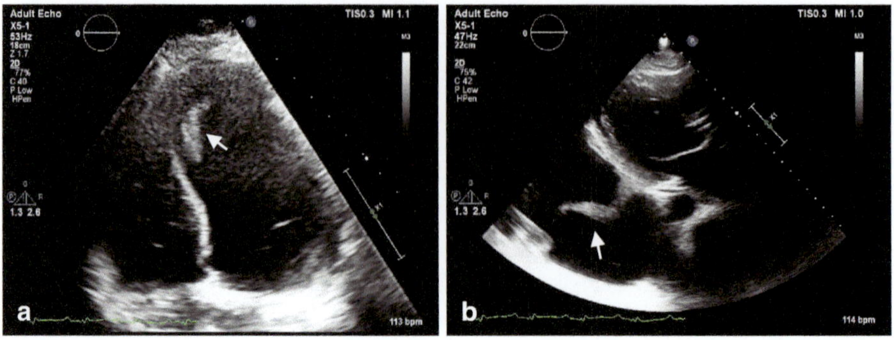

Fig. 1 Pre-procedural echocardiography indicating left ventricle apical thrombus. (**a**) 4C TTE view of an apical left ventricular thrombus (white arrow). (**b**) Inflow-outflow view

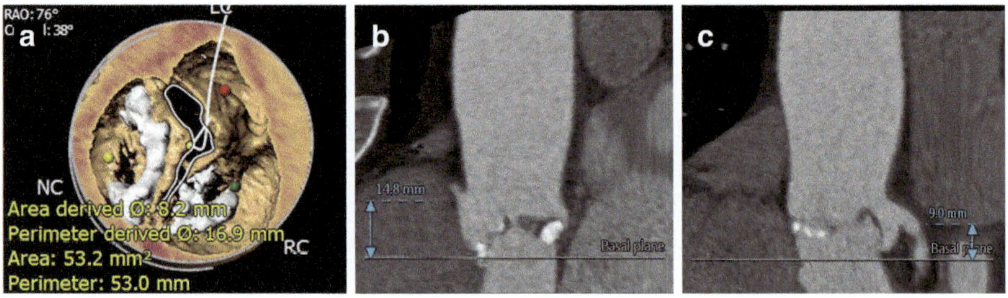

Fig. 2 Pre-procedural reconstructed CT images of the aortic annulus and the coronary arteries. (**a**) AV annular area. (**b**) Right coronary height. (**c**) Left coronary height

Fig. 3 Reconstructed CT images of the left ventricle with a large apical thrombus (yellow arrow)

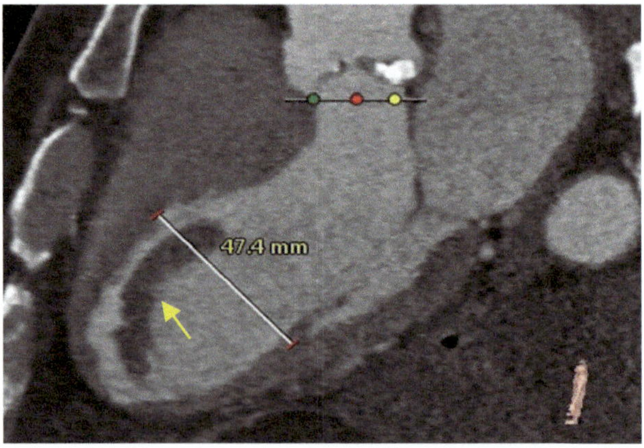

internal diameter of 23.1 mm, area of 414.1 mm^2, and perimeter of 72.6 mm. AV area by CT planimetry was 0.53 cm^2 (Video 2). The following mean diameters were measured: 31.9 mm at the Sinus of Valsalva, 23.8 mm at the STJ, and 29.1 mm at the LVOT. The coronary ostia originated at 14.8 and 9.0 mm (for the RCA and LCA, respectively) above the annular plane (Fig. 2). An elongated mass was confirmed in the LV apical region (Fig. 3). Analysis of the ascending aorta and its branches

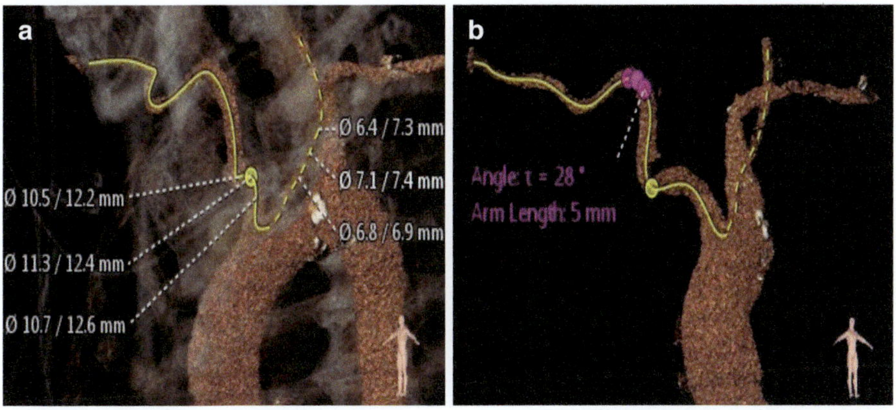

Fig. 4 Reconstructed CT images of aortic arch and it branches. (**a**) Deem view of a sharp angle at the mid brachiocephalic trunk. (**b**) Segmentation only view indicating an angle of 28° over the brachiocephalic trunk (**b**)

indicated a suitable diameter for the cerebral protection device, with a sharp angulation of 28° at the middle part of the right brachiocephalic artery (Fig. 4). Annular analysis was compatible with the 23 Sapien-3 Ultra and the 29 mm Evolut Pro+ THVs.

3 Pre-Procedural Consideration: Pitfalls, Dilemmas, and Challenges

The heart team estimated that the risk for cardiac surgery was prohibitive for this patient due to his existing comorbidities. Considering the surgical risk combined with the patient's preference for a non-invasive approach, we decided to proceed with TAVR using a Sapien-3 ultra THV and a cerebral embolic protection device (Sentinel System, Claret Medical and Boston Scientific, Santa Rosa, CA, USA). The challenge was to avoid the apical thrombus' detachment during LV wire manipulation or RV pacing, leading to an acute embolic event. Furthermore, the preliminary data from the chest CT indicated the presence of coronary artery disease. We deferred the coronary angiogram until the TAVR procedure was completed.

4 Technique

A Claret Sentinel device was guided using fluoroscopy and brief angiography from a pigtail catheter and directed into the ascending aorta with the proximal filter deployed in the right brachiocephalic trunk and the distal filter deployed in the left carotid (Fig. 5). The sharp angle seen on the brachiocephalic artery did not interfere

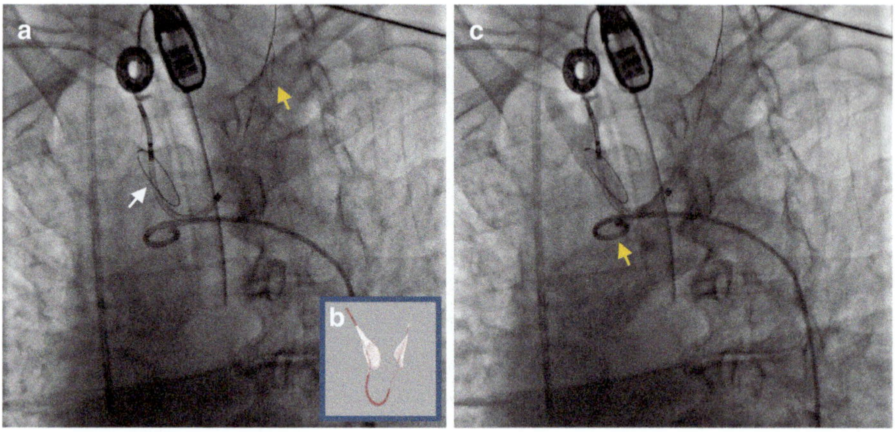

Fig. 5 Fluoroscopy view of a cerebral protection device (CPD) deployed at the branches of the aortic arch. (**a**) A proximal filter located at the brachiocephalic trunk (white arrow) and the distal filter at the left carotid (yellow arrow). (**b**) The Sentinel (Claret Medical and Boston Scientific, Santa Rosa, CA, USA) Cerebral Protection device. (**c**) CPD deployment using fluoroscopy landmarks and brief angiography from a pigtail catheter (yellow arrow)

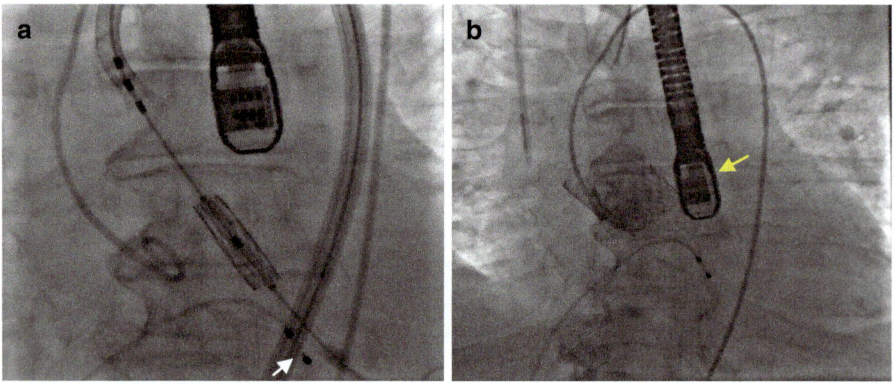

Fig. 6 Fluoroscopy images during the procedure. (**a**) A 23-mm balloon expandable THV positioned over the aortic valve with a pacing lead in the RV (white arrow). (**b**) Bioprosthetic aortic valve deployment guided by TEE (yellow arrow)

with the device insertion. We used an AL-1 catheter together with a straight wire for valve crossing and the pre-shaped Amplatz extra-stiff wire (Cook Medical, Inc., Bloomington, IN) to advance it into the LV cavity while keeping it above the apical region. Sapien-3 ultra THV was deployed using a standard TAVR technique (18 cc in the inflation device) with rapid RV pacing at 180 beats per minute (Fig. 6). The Sentinel device was removed by first recapturing the distal filter, followed by the proximal filter. No macroscopic clots were noted upon extraction of the device. A post-procedure TEE revealed no central aortic regurgitation and only traced perivalvular regurgitation. A mobile thrombus was still noted in the left ventricle.

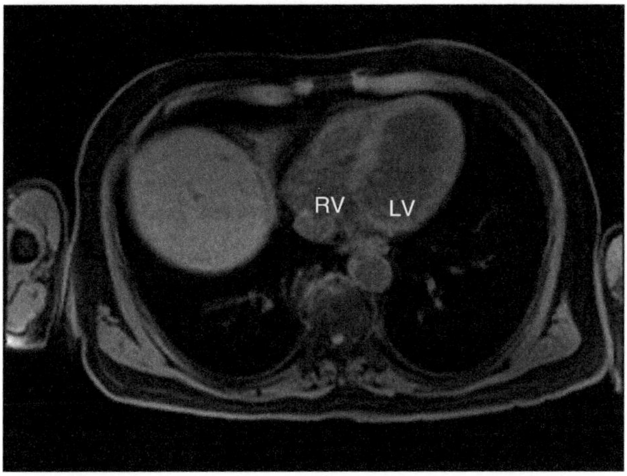

Fig. 7 Cardiac MRI at follow-up indicated the disappearance of the LV thrombus

5 Outcome and Follow-Up

The patient had an uneventful hospital course with no signs of decompensated heart failure. He could walk without shortness of breath and had no evidence of neurological deficit. A total of 80 cc of a third-generation iodine contrast agent (Visipaque, iodixanol) was used without evidence of acute deterioration of renal function. The patient continued treatment with warfarin. Cardiac MRI performed two months later showed thrombus resolution (Fig. 7). During 1-year TTE follow-up, we noted a significant improvement in LV function (LVEF was estimated as 62%) and no evidence of LV thrombus.

6 Discussion

LV apical thrombus is rare but can result in devastating thromboembolism, especially in the context of a TAVR procedure, where thrombus can be detached during the manipulation of LV guidewire/RV pacing [1].

Ischemic cerebrovascular events (ICVE) are among the most severe complications following TAVR, likely secondary to catheter manipulation in the aorta, manipulation of the valve-delivery system, and calcific embolism debris of native aortic valve at the time of deployment [2–4]. The risk of ICVE ranges from 2.7% to 11% at 30 days following TAVR and is associated with a 3.5- to 6-fold increase in mortality at 30 days and 1-year, respectively [5–9]. Most of the ICVE are "silent" (asymptomatic) and can only be detected by specific neuroimaging modalities such as diffusion-weighted magnetic resonance imaging (DW-MRI) or transcranial Doppler [10]. Nevertheless, these silent events may not be benign and may have a long-term impact on a patient's neurocognitive function [11–13].

Cerebral protection devices (CPD) address this issue by protecting the major cerebral arteries from large emboli. CPDs are not recommended for routine use in TAVR but may be utilized in high-risk patients. Recent studies show a significant reduction of ICVE among patients in whom CPD was used, but further randomized control studies are needed to prove clinical benefit [13–17].

Stroke is one of the most devastating complications in patients following TAVR procedures, associated with higher morbidity and mortality rates. All efforts should be made to minimize its occurrence by improving patient selection, avoiding prolonged and unnecessary catheter manipulation while crossing the AV, and using CPDs.

Key Points

- Multimodality imaging is important for understanding the disease and planning the transcatheter procedure to avoid complications in such cases.
- Predictors of ICVE following TAVR include severe AV calcification, prolonged catheter manipulation, and the presence of LV thrombus.
- ICVEs following TAVR are predominantly embolic in origin and are associated with increased morbidity and mortality.
- It is important to minimize LV manipulation while crossing the native aortic valve and implanting the TAVR device.
- Patient selection and risk stratification are key to mitigating embolic complications.
- CPDs are relatively easy to use and are currently the focus of ongoing clinical trials.

References

1. Demirci G, Güner EG, Çörekcioğlu B, et al. Left ventricular apical thrombi: silent but terrifying. J Card Surg. 2020;35(12):3623–5. https://doi.org/10.1111/jocs.15085.
2. Kapadia S, Agarwal S, Miller DC, et al. Insights into timing, risk factors, and outcomes of stroke and transient ischemic attack after transcatheter aortic valve replacement in the PARTNER trial (placement of aortic transcatheter valves). Circ Cardiovasc Interv. 2016;9(9):e002981. https://doi.org/10.1161/CIRCINTERVENTIONS.115.002981.
3. Athappan G, Gajulapalli RD, Sengodan P, et al. Influence of transcatheter aortic valve replacement strategy and valve design on stroke after transcatheter aortic valve replacement: a meta-analysis and systematic review of the literature. J Am Coll Cardiol. 2014;63(20):2101–10. https://doi.org/10.1016/j.jacc.2014.02.540.
4. Vlastra W, Jimenez-Quevedo P, Tchétché D, et al. Predictors, incidence, and outcomes of patients undergoing transfemoral transcatheter aortic valve implantation complicated by stroke. Circ Cardiovasc Interv. 2019;12(3):e007546. https://doi.org/10.1161/CIRCINTERVENTIONS.118.007546.
5. Gasior T, Mangner N, Bijoch J, Wojakowski W. Cerebral embolic protection systems for transcatheter aortic valve replacement. J Interv Cardiol. 2018;31(6):891–8. https://doi.org/10.1111/joic.12573.
6. Teitelbaum M, Kotronias RA, Sposato LA, Bagur R. Cerebral embolic protection in TAVI: friend or foe. Interv Cardiol. 2019;14(1):22–5. https://doi.org/10.15420/icr.2018.32.2.

7. Kroon H, von der Thusen JH, Ziviello F, et al. Heterogeneity of debris captured by cerebral embolic protection filters during TAVI. EuroIntervention. 2021;16(14):1141–7. https://doi.org/10.4244/EIJ-D-20-00744.
8. Mastoris I, Schoos MM, Dangas GD, Mehran R. Stroke after transcatheter aortic valve replacement: incidence, risk factors, prognosis, and preventive strategies. Clin Cardiol. 2014;37(12):756–64. Epub 2014 Nov 17. PMID: 25403514; PMCID: PMC6647626. https://doi.org/10.1002/clc.22328.
9. Eggebrecht H, Schmermund A, Voigtländer T, Kahlert P, Erbel R, Mehta RH. Risk of stroke after transcatheter aortic valve implantation (TAVI): a meta-analysis of 10,037 published patients. EuroIntervention. 2012;8(1):129–38. https://doi.org/10.4244/EIJV8I1A20.
10. Kahlert P, Knipp SC, Schlamann M, et al. Silent and apparent cerebral ischemia after percutaneous transfemoral aortic valve implantation: a diffusion-weighted magnetic resonance imaging study. Circulation. 2010;121(7):870–8. https://doi.org/10.1161/CIRCULATIONAHA.109.855866.
11. Floyd TF, Giovannetti T. Neurocognitive outcomes in older adults after transcatheter aortic valve replacement. J Thorac Cardiovasc Surg. 2012;144(6):1539. https://doi.org/10.1016/j.jtcvs.2012.08.050.
12. Vermeer SE, Prins ND, den Heijer T, Hofman A, Koudstaal PJ, Breteler MM. Silent brain infarcts and the risk of dementia and cognitive decline. N Engl J Med. 2003;348(13):1215–22. PMID: 12660385. https://doi.org/10.1056/NEJMoa022066.
13. Vermeer SE, Longstreth WT Jr, Koudstaal PJ. Silent brain infarcts: a systematic review. Lancet Neurol. 2007;6(7):611–9. https://doi.org/10.1016/S1474-4422(07)70170-9.
14. Kapadia SR, Kodali S, Makkar R, et al. Protection against cerebral embolism during transcatheter aortic valve replacement. J Am Coll Cardiol. 2017;69(4):367–77. https://doi.org/10.1016/j.jacc.2016.10.023.
15. Shah AS, Akhmerov A, Gupta N, Chakravarty T, Makkar RR, Azizzadeh A. Use of a dual-filter cerebral embolic protection device in thoracic endovascular aortic repair. Ann Vasc Surg. 2020;65:54.e1–4. https://doi.org/10.1016/j.avsg.2020.01.077.
16. Cubero-Gallego H, Pascual I, Rozado J, et al. Cerebral protection devices for transcatheter aortic valve replacement. Ann Transl Med. 2019;7(20):584. https://doi.org/10.21037/atm.2019.09.25.
17. Bagur R, Solo K, Alghofaili S, et al. Cerebral embolic protection devices during transcatheter aortic valve implantation: systematic review and meta-analysis. Stroke. 2017;48(5):1306–15. https://doi.org/10.1161/STROKEAHA.116.015915.

TAVR in Patients with Repaired Tetralogy of Fallot

Ofir Koren, Isabel Ben Guy, and Wen Cheng

1 Clinical Presentation

The patient is a 75-year-old male with a tetralogy of Fallot. (TOF) He underwent a "Brock" procedure consisting of right ventricular outflow tract dilation to relieve right ventricular infundibular obstruction at ten years of age. Six years later, the patient was found to have elevated right ventricular pressures and underwent complete repair of TOF, consisting of: patch closure of the ventricular septal defect (VSD), resection of infundibular muscular obstruction, and patch reconstruction of the RVOT. He did well post-surgery and resumed a normal activity level with limited restrictions. At adult age, the patient underwent pacemaker implantation for sick sinus syndrome following failed atrial flutter ablation. He additionally received a PCI at 74 for a severe disease of the proximal LAD.

Supplementary Information The online version contains supplementary material available at [https://doi.org/10.1007/978-3-031-05965-0_24].

O. Koren (✉)
Smidt Heart Institute, Cedars-Sinai Medical Center, Los Angeles, CA, USA

Faculty of Medicine, Technion, Israel Institute of Technology, Haifa, Israel
e-mail: Ofir.Koren@cshs.org

I. Ben Guy
Lithuania University of Health Sciences (LSMU), Kaunas, Lithuania

W. Cheng
Cedars Sinai Medical Center, Los Angeles, CA, USA

O. Koren et al. (eds.), *Complex Cases in Structural Heart Intervention*,
https://doi.org/10.1007/978-3-031-05965-0_24

2 Images and Supported Data

TTE demonstrated severe aortic valve stenosis with peak gradients of 88 and a mean of 58 mmHg. The aortic valve area was 0.5 cm^2 via the continuity equation. Cardiac reconstructed CT demonstrated an aortic annulus area of 768.7 mm^2, a perimeter of 99.4 mm, and a mean diameter of 32.3 mm. The mean SOV area and diameter were 1022.8 mm^2 and 35.2 mm, respectively. Meanwhile, STJ and LVOT areas were 755.6 and 683.6 mm^2, respectively (Fig. 1a–f). The right and left coronary arteries were 17.9 and 14.1 mm above the annulus basal plane (Fig. 2a, b). The aorto-ventricular angulation was measured to be 95° (Fig. 2c). The annulus was highly calcified, particularly at the SOV, with a 775.2 mm^3 column of calcium at the HU850 threshold (Fig. 3a–f). Using volume rendering of the reconstructed CT imaging, the VSD surgical patch appeared to extend from the posterior portion of the LVOT. It

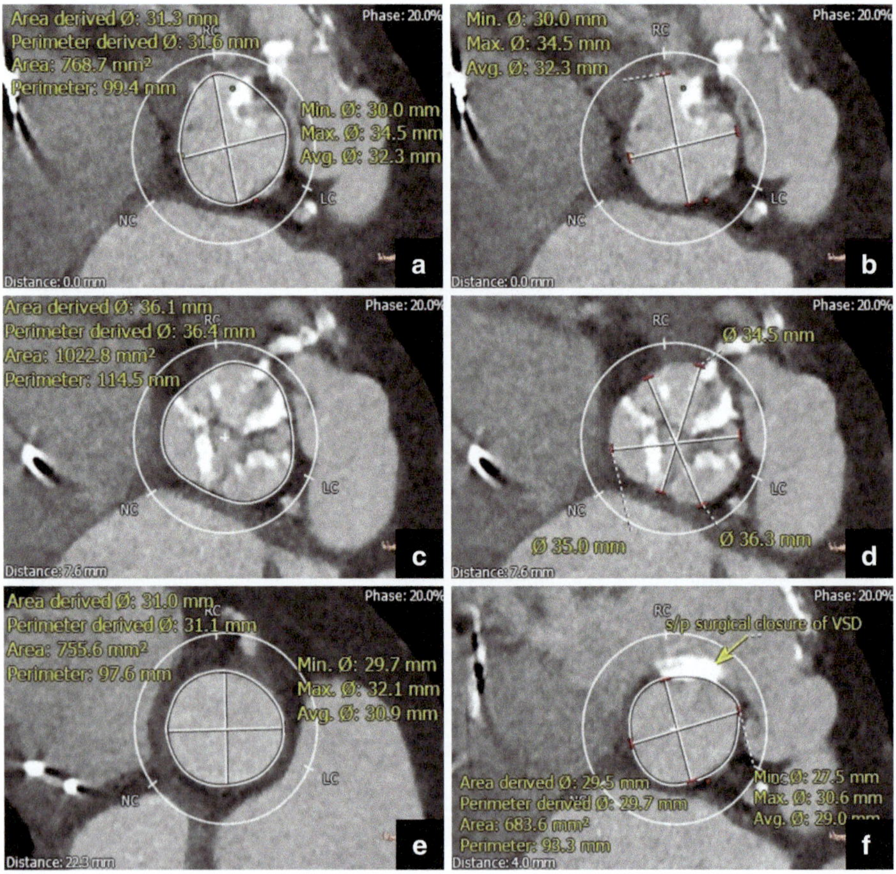

Fig. 1 Reconstructed CT analysis before the procedure. Note the annulus dimensions (**a**, **b**), the SOV area (**c**) and diameter (**d**), the STJ (**e**) and LVOT area (**f**)

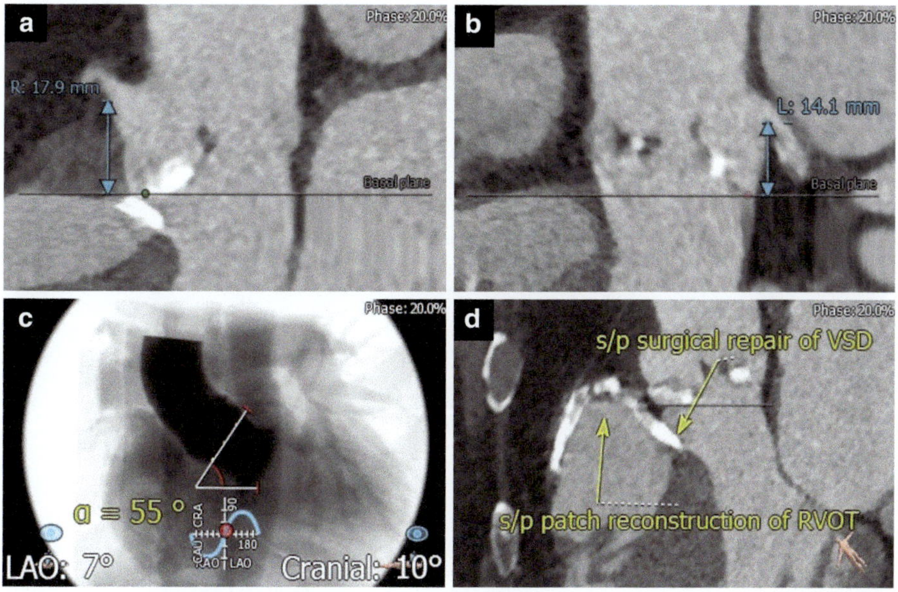

Fig. 2 Reconstructed CT analysis before the procedure. Note the right (**a**) and left (**b**) coronary artery height from the annular basal plane, the aortic angle (**c**) and the RVOT patch extending from the posterior border of the LVOT and through the NCC and RCC (**d**)

bordered with the left and noncoronary cusps (Figs. 2d and 4a, b). Pre-procedural TEE demonstrated severe aortic valve calcification with significant stenosis and mild regurgitation (Fig. 5a–c, Video 1). The right ventricle was severely dilated with intact systolic function and accompanied by mild tricuspid regurgitation and moderate pulmonic regurgitation (Fig. 5d, e, Video 2). The mitral valve was remarkable for mild to moderate regurgitation secondary to mitral valve prolapse (Fig. 5f). Intracardiac echocardiography (ICE) was completed preoperatively to delineate the right-sided disease further. The study demonstrated moderately dilated yet fully functional RV, mild tricuspid regurgitation, and moderate pulmonic valve regurgitation with maximal flow acceleration of 2.15 m/s (Fig. 6).

3 Pre-Procedural Consideration

We present a 75-year-old male patient with a history of corrected TOF who develops severe symptomatic calcific aortic valve stenosis. The patient has chronic diastolic heart failure with NYHA class III–IV symptoms. The patient was evaluated by cardiothoracic surgery and was deemed to be of high surgical risk and appropriate for TAVR. The heart team decided the best therapeutic option was TAVR.

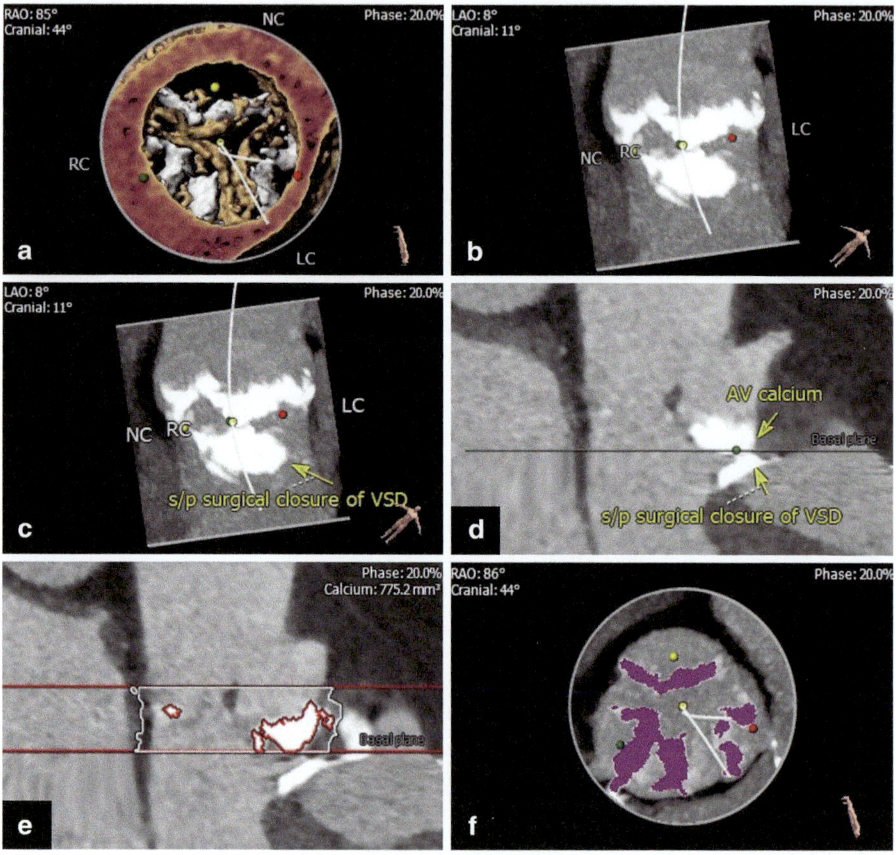

Fig. 3 Reconstructed CT analysis before the procedure. Note the annulus area (**a**) and the distribution of calcification in regard to the coronary cusps (**b**) and the surgical patch (**c**, **d**). The volume of calcification measured using 850 Hounsfield unit as a threshold (**b**) indicated a significant SOV (**e**) and annulus (**f**) calcification

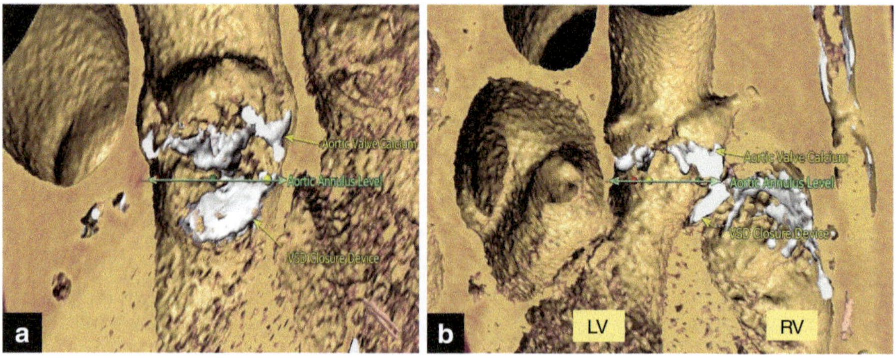

Fig. 4 Volume rendered 3D reconstructed CT image of Aortic Valve (**a**) and surrounding structure (**b**). The VSD patch border with the non-coronary and the right coronary cusps and how it affects the aortic root anatomy

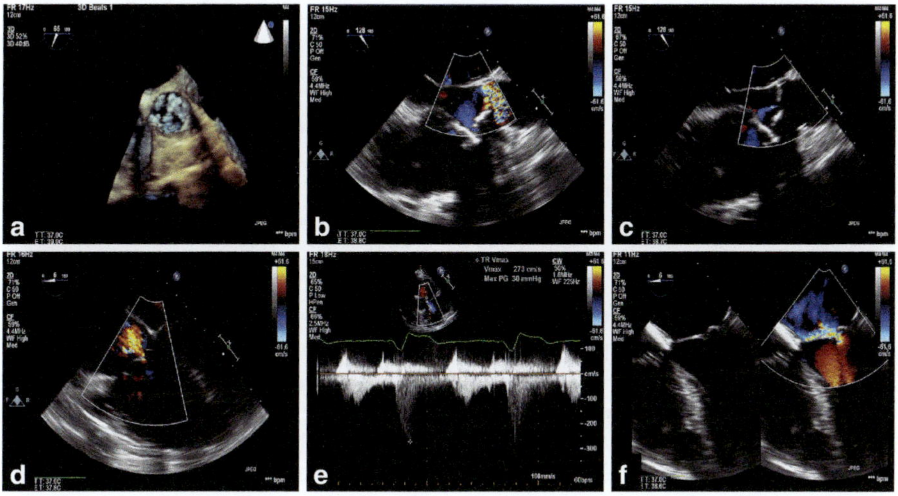

Fig. 5 Transesophageal echocardiography before the procedure indicating severely calcified aortic valve (**a**) with significant stenosis (**b**) and mild regurgitation (**c**), severely dilated right ventricle with mild tricuspid regurgitation (**d**), moderate pulmonic regurgitation (five-chamber TTE view, **e**) and mild to moderate mitral regurgitation with eccentric and anteriorly directed jet because of mitral valve prolapse (**f**)

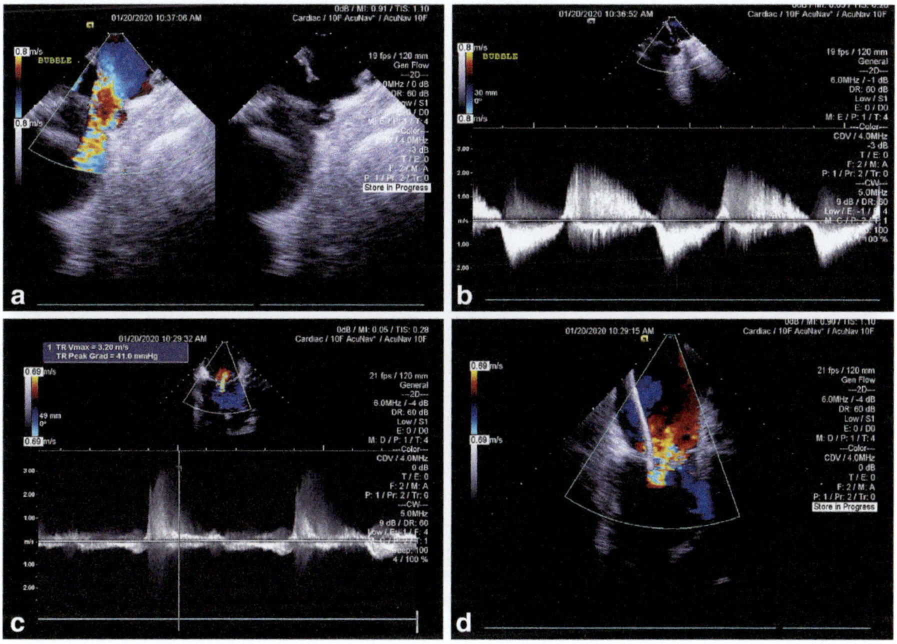

Fig. 6 Intracardiac echocardiography (ICE) before the procedure indicating fully functioning RV with moderate dilatation, a moderate native pulmonic regurgitation (per color and spectral Doppler, **a**) with a maximal flow acceleration of 2.15 m/s across the valve (**b**) and mild tricuspid regurgitation (**c**, **d**)

4 Technique

A 29-mm Edwards Sapien S3 valve delivery system was positioned across the stenotic aortic valve (Fig. 7a). With rapid pacing at 180 beats per minute, the valve was deployed in the standard technique (−2 mL in the inflation device) (Video 3). Additional post balloon dilatation was performed (+2 inflation device) (Video 4) due to a paravalvular leak (Figs. 7b, c and 8a–c). A post-procedure TEE revealed trace central aortic regurgitation and moderate to severe perivalvular regurgitation, mainly from VSD patch (Figs. 7d and 8d, Videos 5, 6 and 7). We decided to perform second valve implantation with lower positioning, anticipating the sealing skirt would reduce the paravalvular leakage. A second 29-mm Edwards Sapien S3 valve was positioned across the stenotic aortic valve. With rapid pacing at 180 beats per minute, the valve was deployed in the standard technique (+2 mL in the inflation device) (Fig. 7e, Video 8). A post-procedure TEE revealed trace central aortic regurgitation and mild perivalvular regurgitation (Figs. 7f and 8e). The valve delivery

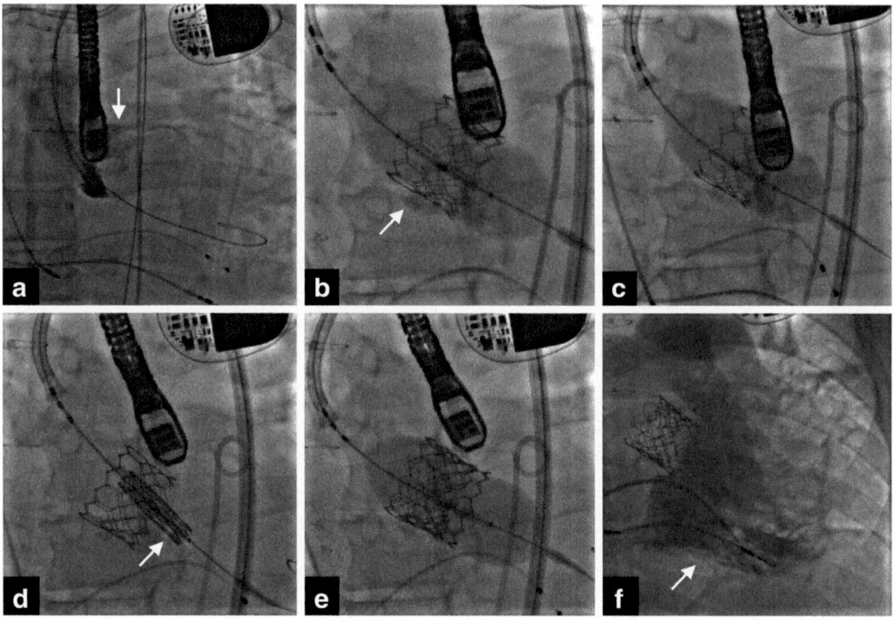

Fig. 7 Fluoroscopy views of the procedure. Positioning of the THV over the AV annulus based on co-planar view landmarks (**a**). Note the flow to the coronary artery (white arrow, **a**). First full deployment of a Sapien-3 bioprosthetic valve, (white arrow, **b**) a moderate paravalvular leak was noticed, which required post-deployment balloon dilatation with an additional 2 cc's of volume in the inflating device (**c**). A post-procedure TEE revealed trace central aortic regurgitation and moderate to severe perivalvular regurgitation, mainly from the VSD patch which required deployment of a second Sapien-3 valve at a lower position (white arrow, **d**). Following full deployment (**e**) only trace AR and mild PVL were noticed. At the end of the procedure, a right ventriculography was performed (white arrow, **f**) to assess the dimension of the ventricle and the severity of the pulmonic regurgitation

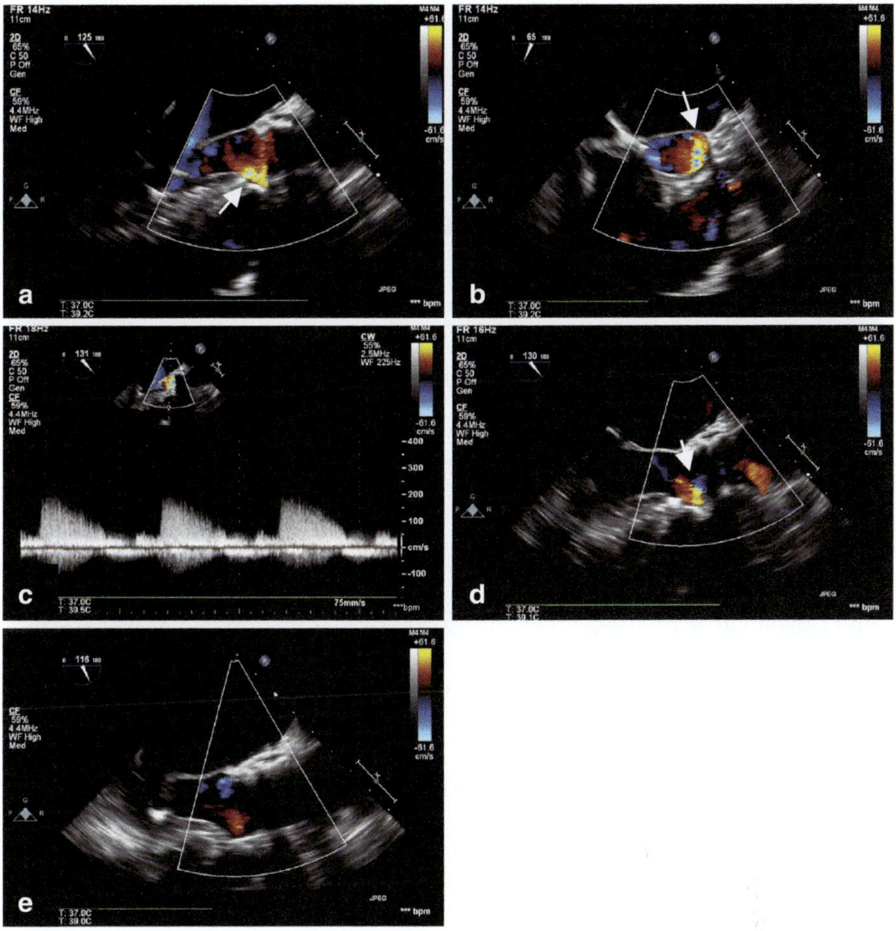

Fig. 8 Transesophageal echocardiography during the procedure. Following the first THV deployment, a moderate paravalvular leak (PVL) was mainly seen on the location of the surgical patch (white arrow, **a–c**). Post-deployment balloon dilatation did not seem to resolve the PVL (white arrow, **d**). A second THV was deployed at a lower position with significant reduction in the regurgitation jet (**e**)

system was then taken out. The Sentinel device was then recaptured and removed. A 6F multipurpose catheter was placed into the LV to measure post-valve deployment hemodynamics and then removed.

5 Outcome and Follow-Up

The remainder of the hospitalization was unremarkable. The patient tolerated the procedure well and had no heart failure symptoms or chest pain. Post-procedural TTE demonstrated improved aortic stenosis without significant aortic regurgitation

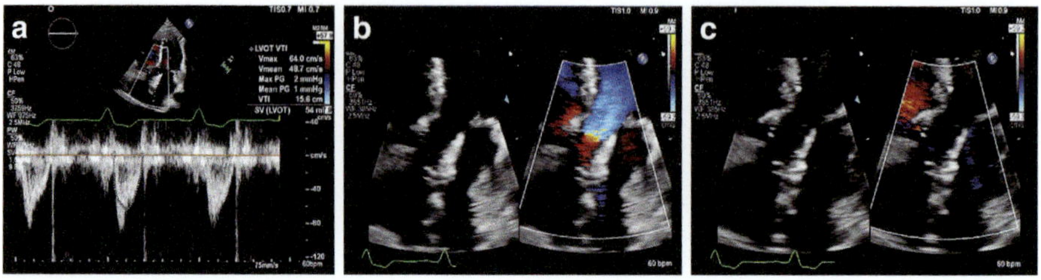

Fig. 9 Transthoracic echocardiography after the procedure. A significant reduction in the AV systolic flow over the AV (**a**, **b**) with only a trace of aortic regurgitation (**b**) and widely open leaflets (**c**)

(Fig. 9, Video 9). On a 30-day follow-up, the patient expressed substantial improvement in his quality of life. He could take short walks without developing shortness of breath or early fatiguability.

6 Discussion

Adult congenital heart disease refers to cardiovascular malformations that are present at birth. Studies estimate a prevalence of 0.6% within the general population [1]. In 2010, it was estimated that 1.4 million adults in the USA lived with congenital heart disease. Recently, with improvements in surgical and medical treatment of congenital heart patients, adult patients now outnumber pediatric patients living with congenital heart disease. Tetralogy of Fallot (TOF) is the most common form of cyanotic adult congenital heart disease. It combines four congenital disabilities: a malaligned ventricular septal defect, right ventricular outflow tract obstruction leading to right ventricular hypertrophy, and anteriorly displaced aortic valve. Surgical repair is generally performed in early childhood and consists of closure of the ventricular septal defect and relief of the right ventricular outflow tract obstruction. Following correction, patients' complications are arrhythmia and pulmonary valve regurgitation leading to right heart failure [2–5]. Additionally, adults with repaired TOF have an increased risk of sudden cardiac death (SCD), with an incidence of around 2% every ten years of follow-up [6–8]. Primary prevention ICD should be considered for these patients who otherwise meet standard qualifying criteria.

While pulmonary valve regurgitation is the most common valvular dysfunction following TOF repair, calcific aortic valve stenosis can develop over the lifespan of corrected TOF patients who reach an older age [9–12]. To the best of our knowledge, this is a unique case of a patient with corrected TOF who developed heart defects at an advanced age. He therefore requires percutaneous techniques such as coronary artery stent grafting and TAVR.

The synthetic patch used to close the VSD was not a good "landing zone" for the 29-mm Sapien 3 transcatheter aortic valve. The patch shifted with the deployment of our first transcatheter valve leading to a significant paravalvular leak. Ultimately, placing a second transcatheter valve slightly deeper into the left ventricular outflow tract eliminated the paravalvular leak. At 30-day follow-up, TTE demonstrated no paravalvular leak and normal leaflet motion. At 1-year follow-up, the patient was doing well.

Key Points

- Tetralogy of Fallot is a rare congenital heart disease that involving multiple structural and valvular abnormalities and requires surgical correction earlier in life.
- With the ongoing experience and results of the TAVR procedure in adult AS patients, the indications can be extended to younger patients.
- The TAVR procedure may be a reasonable alternative therapeutic strategy for AS patients following surgically corrected congenital cardiac anomalies in selected high-risk patients.

References

1. Gilboa SM, Devine OJ, Kucik JE, Oster ME, Riehle-Colarusso T, Nembhard WN, et al. Congenital heart defects in the United States: estimating the magnitude of the affected population in 2010. Circulation. 2016;134(2):101–9. https://doi.org/10.1161/CIRCULATIONAHA.115.019307.
2. Ho KW, Tan RS, Wong KY, Tan TH, Shankar S, Tan JL. Late complications following tetralogy of Fallot repair: the need for long-term follow-up. Ann Acad Med Singap. 2007;36(11):947–53. https://annals.edu.sg/pdf/36VolNo11Nov2007/V36N11p947.pdf.
3. Karamlou T, McCrindle BW, Williams WG. Surgery insight: late complications following repair of tetralogy of Fallot and related surgical strategies for management. Nat Clin Pract Cardiovasc Med. 2006;3(11):611–22. https://www.nature.com/articles/ncpcardio0682.
4. Sanchez AM, Lozier MR, Alvardo HR, Sarkar A, Smith JM, Molina S, et al. When "blue babies" grow up: complications after surgical repair of tetralogy of Fallot. JACC Case Rep. 2020;2(11):1723–9. https://www.sciencedirect.com/science/article/pii/S2666084920308408.
5. Lillo R, Panaioli E, Graziani F, Delogu AB, Leone AM, Perri G, et al. Undiagnosed severe late complications of repaired tetralogy of fallot. Circ Cardiovasc Imaging. 2020;13(6):e010273. https://doi.org/10.1161/CIRCIMAGING.119.010273.
6. Waldmann V, Bouzeman A, Duthoit G, Koutbi L, Bessiere F, Labombarda F, et al. Long-term follow-up of patients with tetralogy of Fallot and implantable cardioverter defibrillator: the DAI-T4F nationwide registry. Circulation. 2020;142(17):1612–22. https://doi.org/10.1161/CIRCULATIONAHA.120.046745.
7. Sabate Rotes A, Connolly HM, Warnes CA, Ammash NM, Phillips SD, Dearani JA, et al. Ventricular arrhythmia risk stratification in patients with tetralogy of Fallot at the time of pulmonary valve replacement. Circ Arrhythm Electrophysiol. 2015;8(1):110–6. https://doi.org/10.1161/CIRCEP.114.001975.
8. Maury P, Sacher F, Rollin A, Mondoly P, Duparc A, Zeppenfeld K, et al. Ventricular arrhythmias and sudden death in tetralogy of Fallot. Arch Cardiovasc Dis. 2017;110(5):354–62. https://www.sciencedirect.com/science/article/pii/S1875213617300190.
9. Ammash NM, Dearani JA, Burkhart HM, Connolly HM. Pulmonary regurgitation after tetralogy of Fallot repair: clinical features, sequelae, and timing of pulmonary valve replacement. Congenit Heart Dis. 2007;2(6):386–403. https://pubmed.ncbi.nlm.nih.gov/18377431/.

10. Ishizaka T, Ichikawa H, Sawa Y, Fukushima N, Kagisaki K, Kondo H, et al. Prevalence and optimal management strategy for aortic regurgitation in tetralogy of Fallot. Eur J Cardiothorac Surg. 2004;26(6):1080–6. https://academic.oup.com/ejcts/article/26/6/1080/528983.
11. Warnes CA, Child JS. Aortic root dilatation after repair of tetralogy of Fallot: pathology from the past?: pathology from the past? Circulation. 2002;106(11):1310–1. https://doi.org/10.1161/01.cir.0000032580.69198.a5.
12. McRae ME, Coleman B, Atz TW, Kelechi TJ. Patient outcomes after transcatheter and surgical pulmonary valve replacement for pulmonary regurgitation in patients with repaired tetralogy of Fallot: a quasi-meta-analysis. Eur J Cardiovasc Nurs. 2017;16(6):539–53. https://pubmed.ncbi.nlm.nih.gov/28756698/.

Part II
Mitral Valve

Edge-to-Edge Mitral Valve Repair in a Patient with Situs Inversus

Ofir Koren, Robert Naami, and Sharon Shalom Natanzon

1 Clinical Presentation

A 77-year-old male with past medical history remarkable for systolic heart failure with reduced ejection fraction (NYHA Class III–IV symptoms), situs inversus, atrial fibrillation, diabetes mellitus, hyperlipidemia, chronic obstructive lung disease, chronic kidney disease, abdominal aortic aneurysm, hypertension, coronary disease, status-post bypass grafting (unknown grafts) followed by multiple percutaneous coronary interventions, aortic stenosis, status post recent transcatheter aortic valve replacement with 26-mm Sapien valve S3, presents to our center with cardiogenic shock secondary to severe mitral regurgitation.

2 Images and Supported Data

Chest X-ray upon admission demonstrates situs inversus with mild pulmonary vascular congestion, bilateral pleural effusions, and right internal jugular hemodialysis

Supplementary Information The online version contains supplementary material available at [https://doi.org/10.1007/978-3-031-05965-0_25].

O. Koren (✉)
Smidt Heart Institute, Cedars-Sinai Medical Center, Los Angeles, CA, USA

Faculty of Medicine, Technion, Israel Institute of Technology, Haifa, Israel
e-mail: Ofir.Koren@cshs.org

R. Naami
University Hospitals Cleveland Medical Center, Cleveland, OH, USA

S. S. Natanzon
Cedars Sinai Medical Center, Los Angeles, CA, USA

O. Koren et al. (eds.), *Complex Cases in Structural Heart Intervention*,
https://doi.org/10.1007/978-3-031-05965-0_25

catheter terminating in the right atrium (Fig. 1). Pre-procedural TEE demonstrated moderately depressed left ventricular systolic function, severe mitral regurgitation, and bioprosthetic stent-valve in the aortic position (Fig. 2, Videos 1 and 2).

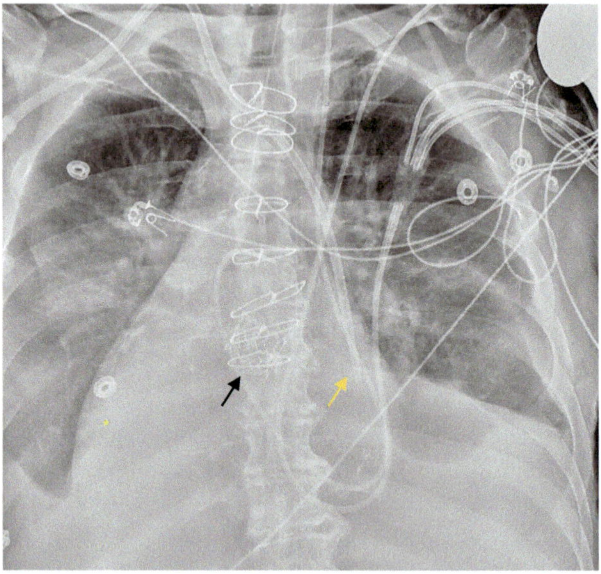

Fig. 1 Chest X-Ray upon admission demonstrates situs inversus with mild pulmonary vascular congestion and bilateral pulmonary effusions. Note the silhouette of the left ventricle protruding to the right side of the chest (yellow asterisk), the position and orientation of a prior transcatheter bioprosthetic heart valve (black arrow), and a right internal jugular hemodialysis catheter terminating at the right atrium (orange arrow)

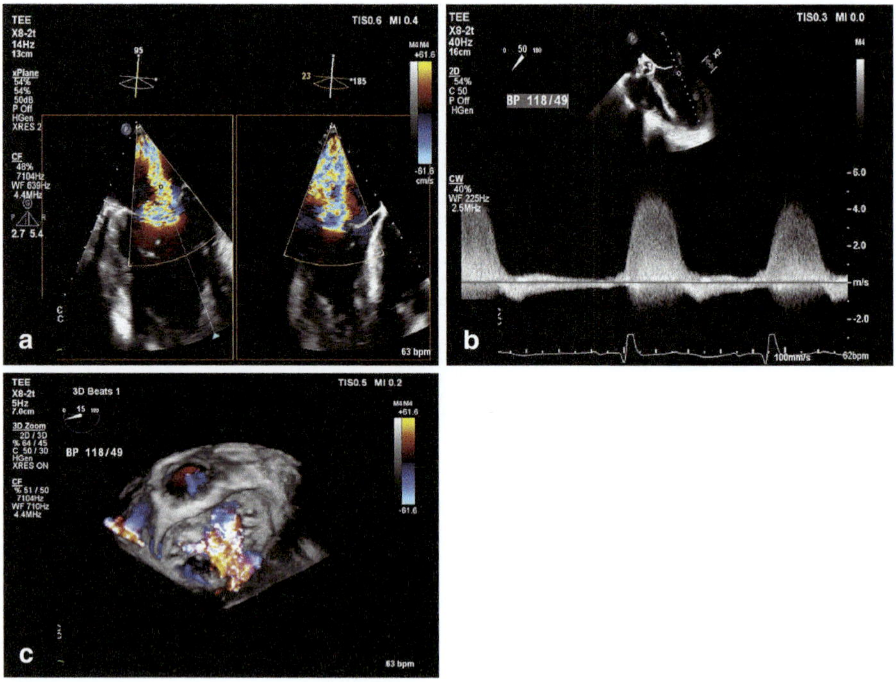

Fig. 2 TEE view of the MV TEER procedure indicating severe mitral regurgitation with central jet (**a**, **c**) and high velocity (**b**). The Blood pressure during the exam was 118/49 mmHg

3 Pre-Procedural Consideration: Pitfalls, Dilemmas, and Challenges

The patient was evaluated by a cardiac surgeon and was considered at prohibitive risk for surgical repair of the mitral valve and therefore referred for the percutaneous mitral valve repair using the MitraClip G4 NT device. Special consideration with both imaging and procedural guidance was taken, given the history of situs inversus.

4 Outcome and Follow-Up

Before the procedure, the patient was stabilized with various vasopressor agents, including phenylephrine, vasopressin, dobutamine, and continuous renal replacement therapy for volume removal.

Venous access was obtained from the left femoral vein. We then advanced our wire into the SVC and proceeded with transseptal puncture across the interatrial septum under echocardiography and fluoroscopic guidance. After advancing our wire into the left upper pulmonary vein, the Abbott MitraClip delivery steerable guide and MitraClip device were advanced into the left atrium (Fig. 3a, Video 3). The steerable deployment sheath was manipulated to optimize the positioning of the device. Following the closure of the MitraClip, TEE showed a well-seated clip and moderate mitral regurgitation (Video 4). The clip was then deployed under fluoroscopic and TEE guidance (Fig. 3b, c).

Due to significant residual mitral regurgitation, we decided to undergo additional clip (G4 NT) implantation. The next clip was prepped and advanced into the left atrium through the device deployment sheath. After carefully optimizing the device, the next clip was deployed under fluoroscopic and TEE guidance. Following the closure of the MitraClip, TEE showed a well-seated clip-on the A2P2 leaflets with a reduction of mitral regurgitation from severe to mild and favorable hemodynamics (Figs. 4 and 5, Video 5). A second clip was successfully released, and the delivery system was withdrawn (Fig. 6).

The remainder of the patient's hospitalization was unremarkable. The patient was treated with continuous renal replacement therapy for volume removal.

5 Discussion

Dextrocardia is a congenital cardiac anomaly in which the heart is located in the right hemithorax with the base-apex axis directed to the right and caudal position. While the precise mechanism of this malposition is not clearly understood, it is believed to stem from a communication aberrancy during embryologic development. It is estimated to occur in 1 in 8000 to 25,000 live births [1–4]. Dextrocardia

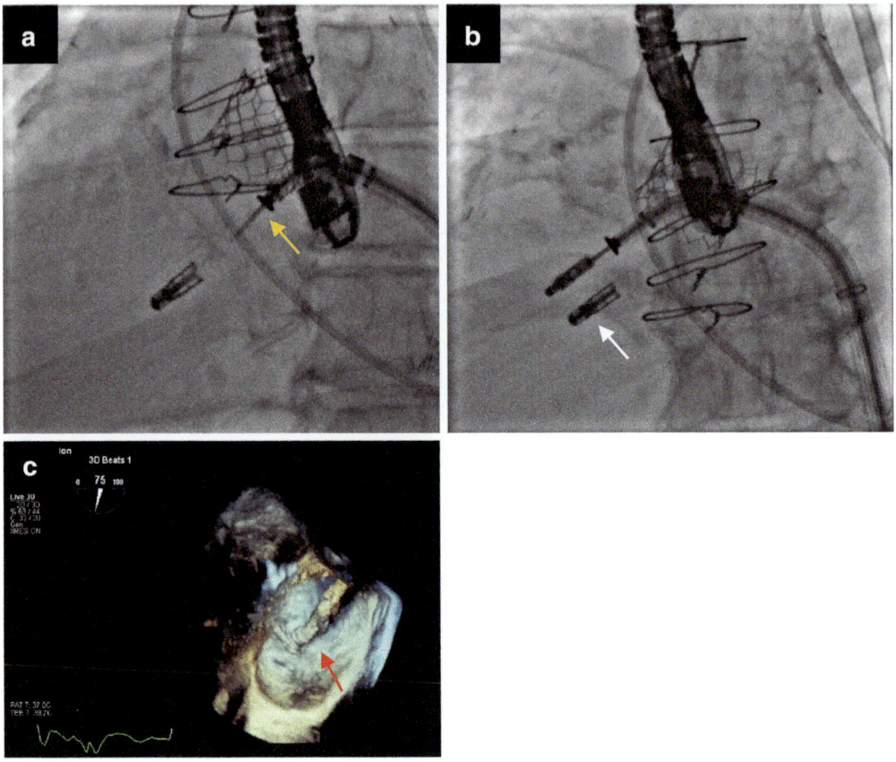

Fig. 3 Fluoroscopy views of the TEER procedure. Note the abnormal orientation of the mitral valve while crossing the left side during transeptal puncture (yellow arrow, **a**) and the deployment of MitraClips devices (white arrow on **b** and red arrow on **c**)

is commonly described in conjunction with anatomical situs, which refers to the configuration of the atria relative to the abdominal viscera and tracheobronchial tree. The most common distinct types of the situs anomaly are the solitus, the inversus, and the ambiguous. Most commonly associated with dextrocardia is situs inversus, where visceroatrial situs is a mirror image of normal. Dextrocardia also occurs with normal visceroatrial relationships (situs solitus) and inconsistent visceroatrial relationships (situs ambiguous) [5, 6]. While dextrocardia is often associated with other cardiac abnormalities, the frequency of these abnormalities varies based on the associated situs; 5% with situs inversus to 90% with situs solitus. The malformation type also varies according to the situs; situs solitus and inversus often demonstrate transposition of the great arteries, whereas ambiguous is most often remarkable for total anomalous pulmonary venous return [7].

Dextrocardia, with its associated situs, presents a unique challenge in patients requiring transcatheter interventions. Namely, operators must adjust their perspective and technical acumen to compensate for the opposite anatomy. In the current literature, coronary and structural heart interventions have successfully been

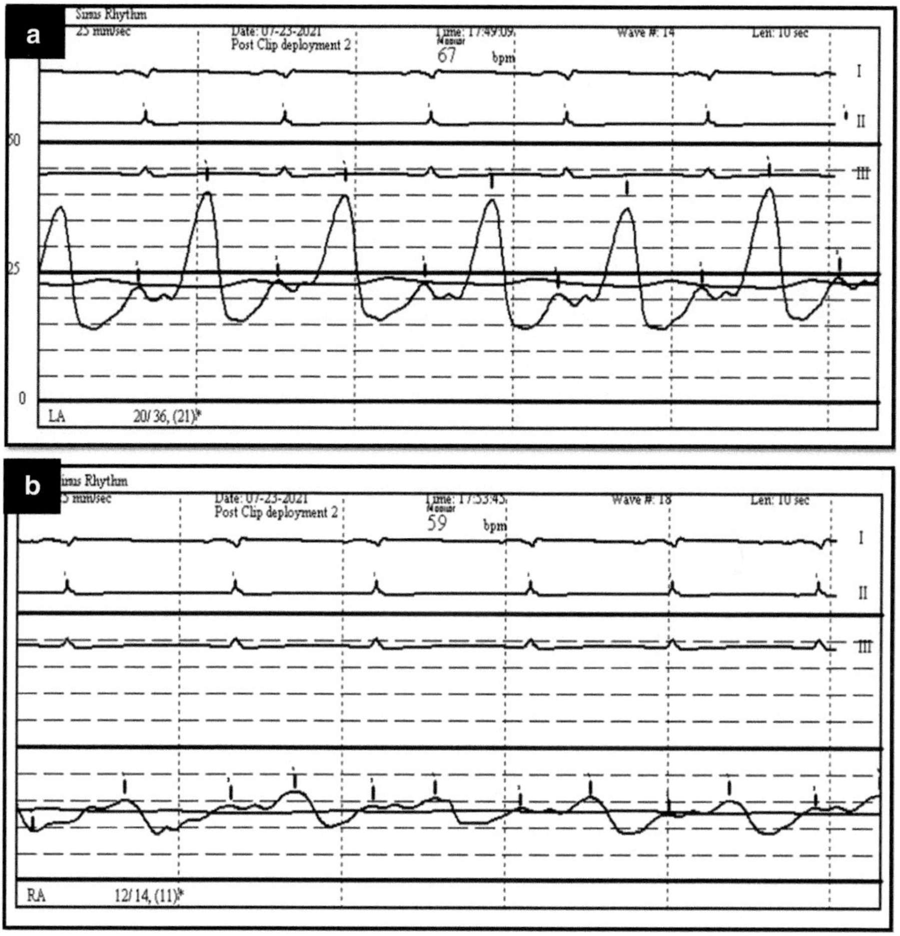

Fig. 4 Right Atrium pressure recording before (**a**) and after (**b**) the MV TEER procedure. Note the reduction in V wave (black arrow) following the deployment of two MitraClip

completed in patients with dextrocardia situs inversus. In the realm of coronary interventions, arterial access and equipment points remain unchanged. Major differences include catheter manipulation and angiographic interpretation [8–11]. Instead of the conventional torque, reverse torque is necessary to cannulate or engage the coronary vessels. For example, a guiding catheter rotated counterclockwise will cannulate the left anatomical RCA.

Additionally, mirror images are needed to aid operator orientation and visualization intraoperatively [12, 13]. A common technique is to reverse the right and left anterior oblique projections while maintaining the cranial and caudal tilt. As a result, right-sided views produce the usual left-sided images and vice versa. Thus, the LAO cranial position cameras yielded a mirror image of the RAO cranial view [14, 15].

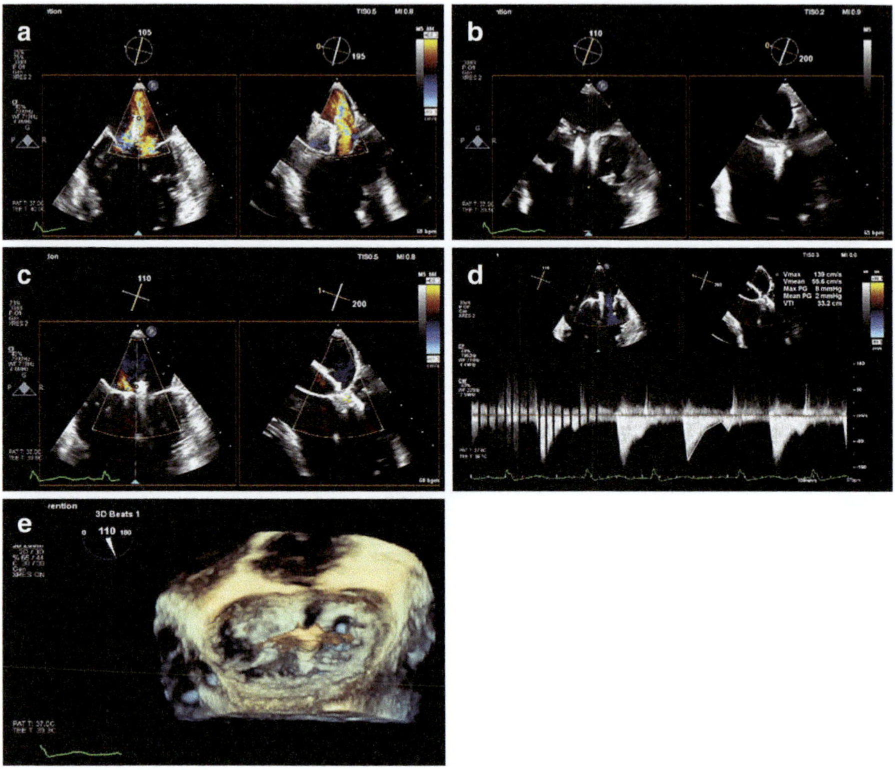

Fig. 5 TEE view before and during the MV TEER procedure. (**a**) Severe mitral regurgitation. (**b**) Two MitraClips attached to the mitral leaflets. (**c**) Color Doppler over the mitral valve following MitraClip procedure. (**d**) Pressure gradient over the MV following MitraClip procedure. (**e**) 3D TEE showing two MitraClips at the A2P2 position

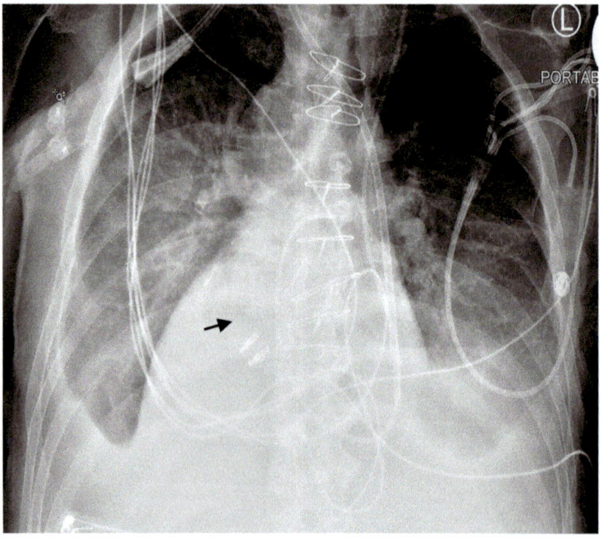

Fig. 6 Chest X-ray following the MV TEER procedure, with clips on the right side of the chest. This may be confused with Tricuspid valve clips (black arrow)

Regarding structural heart interventions, few studies demonstrate procedural success using a transfemoral or transapical approach; rather, they used a CT angiography to help delineate precise anatomy, such as the visceral organ laterality, cardiac apical position, and great vessel orientation [16–18]. Imaging also guides an operator's approach to catheter handling, proper angling for valve deployment, and selection of angiographic images [19, 20]. Operators often use a left-right reversed fluoroscopic image that flips the rotational orientation but does not affect catheter manipulation during valve insertion and pull-back. Other considerations include valve selection. The CoreValve Evolut R is a favorable choice as it can be recaptured and repositioned to achieve favorable positioning in complex anatomy. An additional consideration is the placement of the delivery system. Previous cases describe inserting and rotating the delivery system opposite of normal to allow the catheter to take the opposite direction, given the patient's right-sided aortic arch and anatomy [20, 21].

Key Points

- Dextrocardia presents a unique challenge to the interventional cardiologist.
- Planning interventional procedures in dextrocardia patients necessitates careful planning using multimodality imaging.
- MitraClip is feasible in dextrocardia patients.

References

1. Perloff JK, Marelli AJ. Perloff's clinical recognition of congenital heart disease. 6th ed. Philadelphia, PA: W.B. Saunders; 2012. p. 15–30.
2. Maldjian PD, Saric M. Approach to dextrocardia in adults: review. AJR. 2007;188:S39–49.
3. Perloff JK. The cardiac malpositions. Am J Cardiol. 2011;108:1352–61.
4. Buxton A, Morganroth J, Josephson M, Perloff J, Shelburne J. Isolated dextroversion of the heart with asymmetric septal hypertrophy. Am Heart J. 1976;92:785–90.
5. Walmsley R, Hishitani T, Sandor GG, Lim K, Duncan W, Tessier F, et al. Diagnosis and outcome of dextrocardia diagnosed in the fetus. Am J Cardiol. 2004;94:141–3.
6. Bernasconi A, Azancot A, Simpson JM, Jones A, Sharland GK. Fetal dextrocardia: diagnosis and outcome in two tertiary centres. Heart. 2005;91:1590–4.
7. Bohun C, Potts J, Casey B, Sandor G. A population-based study of cardiac malformations and outcomes associated with dextrocardia. AJC. 2007;100:305–9.
8. Hynes KM, Gau GT, Titus JL. Coronary heart disease in situs inversus totalis. Am J Cardiol. 1973;31:666–9.
9. Liem KL, ten Veen JH. Inferior myocardial infarction in a patient with mirror-image dextrocardia and situs inversus totalis. Chest. 1976;69:239–41.
10. Alzand BS, Dennert R, Kalkman R, Gorgels AP. Acute anteroseptal myocardial infarction in a patient with dextrocardia. J Electrocardiol. 2009;42:254–7.
11. Moreyra AE, Saviano GJ, Kostis JB. Percutaneous transluminal coronary angioplasty in situs inversus. Catheter Cardiovasc Diagn. 1987;13:114–6.
12. Dhanjal TS, Davison P, Cotton JM. Primary percutaneous coronary intervention for acute myocardial infarction in a patient with dextrocardia. Cardiol J. 2009;16:168–71.
13. Jauhar R, Gianos E, Kashifuddin B, Roethel M, Kaplan BM. Primary angioplasty in a patient with dextrocardia. J Interv Cardiol. 2005;18:127–30.

14. Macdonald JE, Gardiner R, Chauhan A. Coronary angioplasty via the radial approach in an individual with dextrocardia. Int J Cardiol. 2008;131:e10–1.
15. Goel PK. Double-inversion technique for coronary angiography viewing in dextrocardia. Catheter Cardiovasc Interv. 2005;66:281–5.
16. Bohun CM, Potts JE, Casey BM, Sandor GG. A population-based study of cardiac malformations and outcomes associated with dextrocardia. Am J Cardiol. 2007;100:305–9.
17. Alrifai A, Kabach M, Lovitz L, Rothenberg M, Nores M, Fanari Z. Severe aortic stenosis in dextrocardia with situs invertus and anomalous single coronary ostium treated with transcatheter aortic valve replacement. Cardiovasc Revasc Med. 2018;19:33–6.
18. Romaguera R, Roura G, Gómez-Hospital JA, Gómez-Lara J, Moris C, Cequier A. CoreValve aortic bioprosthesis implantation in a patient with situs inversus totalis with dextrocardia. Rev Esp Cardiol (Engl Ed). 2013;66:409–10.
19. Weich HS, van Wyk J, van Zyl W, Vivier R, Phillips A, Mabin T. First case of trans apical implantation of an aortic valve in a patient with dextrocardia. J Cardiothorac Surg. 2012;7:24.
20. Good RI, Morgan KP, Brydie A, Beydoun HK, Nadeem SN. Transfemoral aortic valve implantation for severe aortic stenosis in a patient with dextrocardia situs inversus. Can J Cardiol. 2014;30:1108.
21. Agrawal Y, Miller M, Pratt JW, Martin D, Kalavakunta JK, Saltiel F, et al. Transcatheter aortic valve replacement for severe aortic stenosis in dextrocardia with situs inversus: first reported case in the United States. Int J Cardiol. 2016;209:137–8.

Transcatheter Mitral Valve Replacement in a Patient with Severe Mitral Annular Calcification

Ofir Koren, Siamak Kohan, and Danon Kaewkes

1 Clinical Presentation

A 41-year-old female presented with a history of Systemic Lupus Erythematosus (SLE) treated with chronic immunosuppressive therapy, a history of pulmonary embolism, end-stage renal disease on hemodialysis and subclavian thrombosis status post stent complicated by occlusion, as well as thrombophlebitis treated with antibiotics, severe mitral stenosis, moderate mitral regurgitation due to significant mitral annulus calcification, and recent pacemaker implantation due to complete heart block. Presented with shortness of breath and daily functional limitations. The patient was classified as NYHA III upon admission.

2 Images and Supported Data

Preoperative workup with TTE (Videos 1, 2 and 3, Fig. 1) showed normal left ventricular function and severe mitral stenosis with a peak gradient of 14 mmHg and mean gradient of 10 mmHg. LHC (Videos 4 and 5, Fig. 2) showed normal coronary

Supplementary Information The online version contains supplementary material available at [https://doi.org/10.1007/978-3-031-05965-0_26].

O. Koren (✉)
Smidt Heart Institute, Cedars-Sinai Medical Center, Los Angeles, CA, USA

Faculty of Medicine, Technion, Israel Institute of Technology, Haifa, Israel
e-mail: Ofir.Koren@cshs.org

S. Kohan
Kaiser Permanente Los Angeles Medical Center, Los Angeles, CA, USA

D. Kaewkes
Department of Medicine, Faculty of Medicine, Khon Kaen University, Khon Kaen, Thailand

O. Koren et al. (eds.), *Complex Cases in Structural Heart Intervention*,
https://doi.org/10.1007/978-3-031-05965-0_26

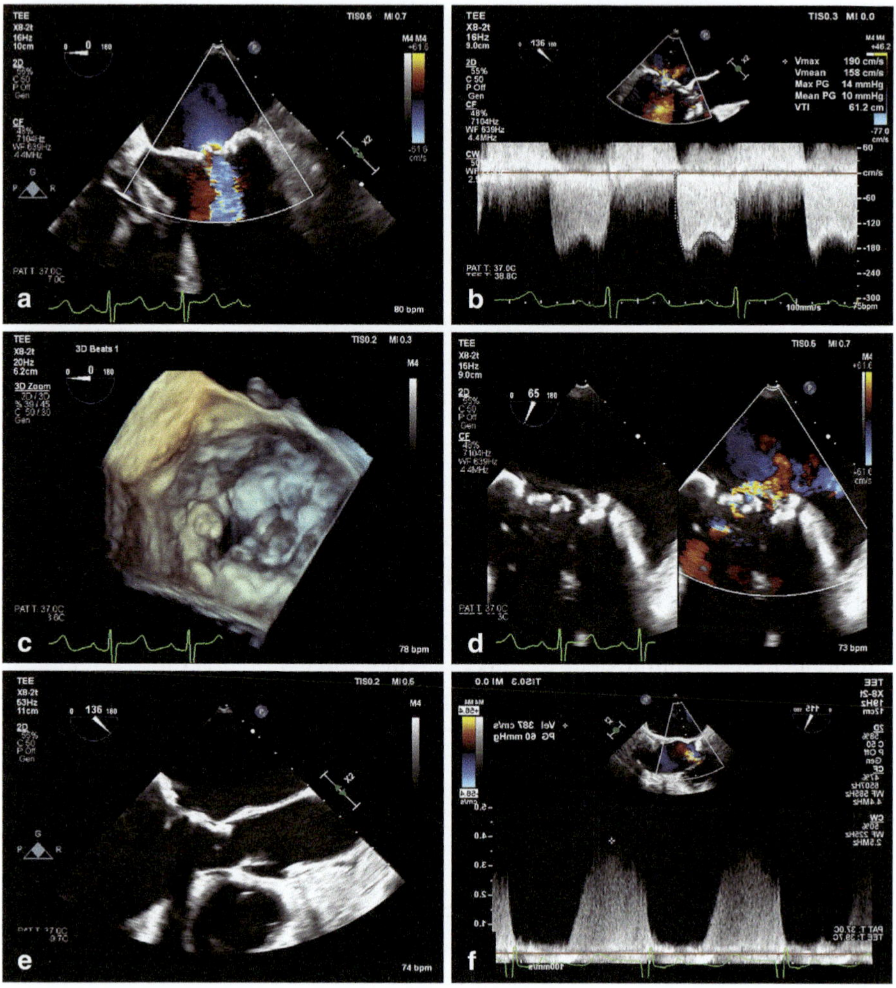

Fig. 1 Transesophageal echocardiography before the transcatheter mitral valve replacement procedure. (**a**) Color Doppler flow across the MV. (**b**) Flow velocity and pressure gradient across the MV. (**c**) 3D en face view of a calcified MV. (**d**) Severe mitral annulus with color Doppler. (**e**) Aortic valve during systole. (**f**) Flow velocity and pressure gradient across AV

arteries and severe mitral annulus calcification (MAC) and MV leaflet calcification. CT (Fig. 3) revealed a low risk of LVOT obstruction with a neo-LVOT area of 529 mm^2.

3 Pre-Procedural Consideration: Pitfalls, Dilemmas, and Challenges

A 6-French pigtail catheter was inserted into the left femoral artery. An 11-French sheath was placed into the right femoral vein, followed by a 7-French long

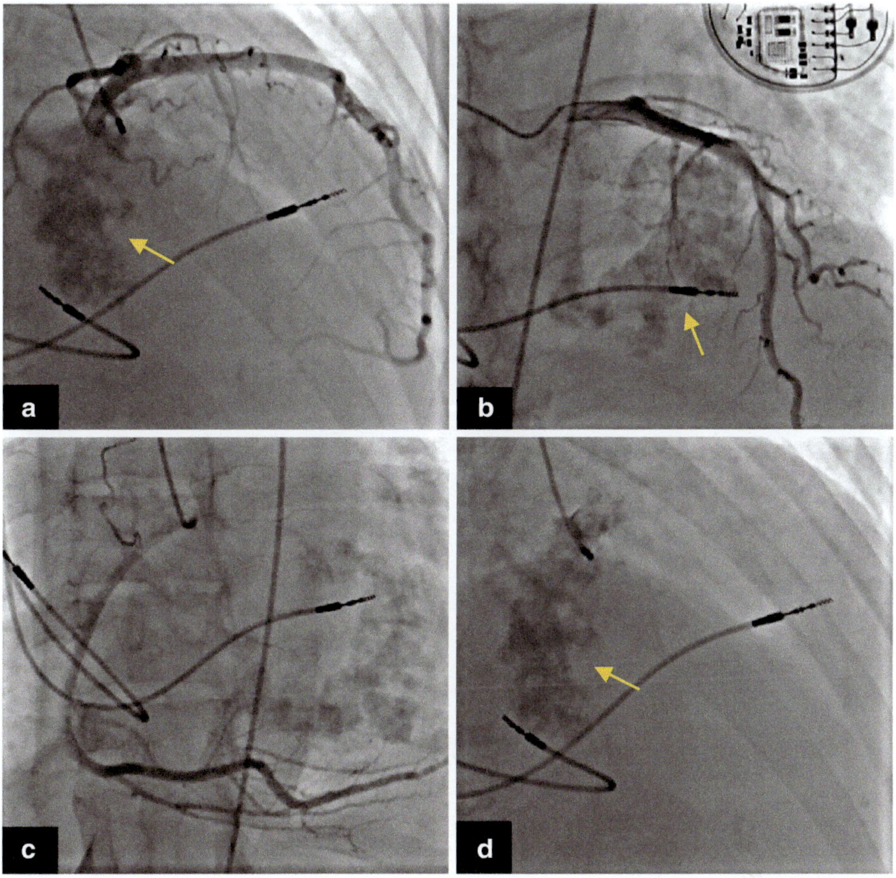

Fig. 2 Angiography of the coronary arteries indicating no obstructive lesions and severe mitral annular calcification (MAC). (**a**) LAO projection of severe MAC (yellow arrow). (**b**) RAO projection of severe MAC (yellow arrow). (**c**) RCA angiography. (**d**) Caudal view of severe MAC (yellow arrow)

introducer. Then, a 5-French balloon-tipped pacemaker wire was advanced to the right ventricle and atrium, where baseline pressures were recorded. Under fluoroscopy and TEE guidance, the transseptal puncture was performed with a BRK needle, and then an 8.5-French Baylis sheath was advanced transseptal to the left atrium. The patient was fully anticoagulated with heparin, and the ACT was monitored. The 6-French pigtail catheter in the femoral artery was advanced through the aorta and into the left ventricle. The baseline pressures were obtained from the left atrium, left ventricle, and aorta. Next, a 0.032 wire was advanced into the left upper pulmonary vein. The Baylis sheath was exchanged to the 8.5-French Agilis flex sheath, which was advanced to the left ventricle with the help of the pigtail catheter. The Safari extra small wire was advanced into the left ventricle. The pigtail catheter was removed, and then a transseptal septostomy was performed using a 12 × 40 mm Z-Med balloon with manual inflation.

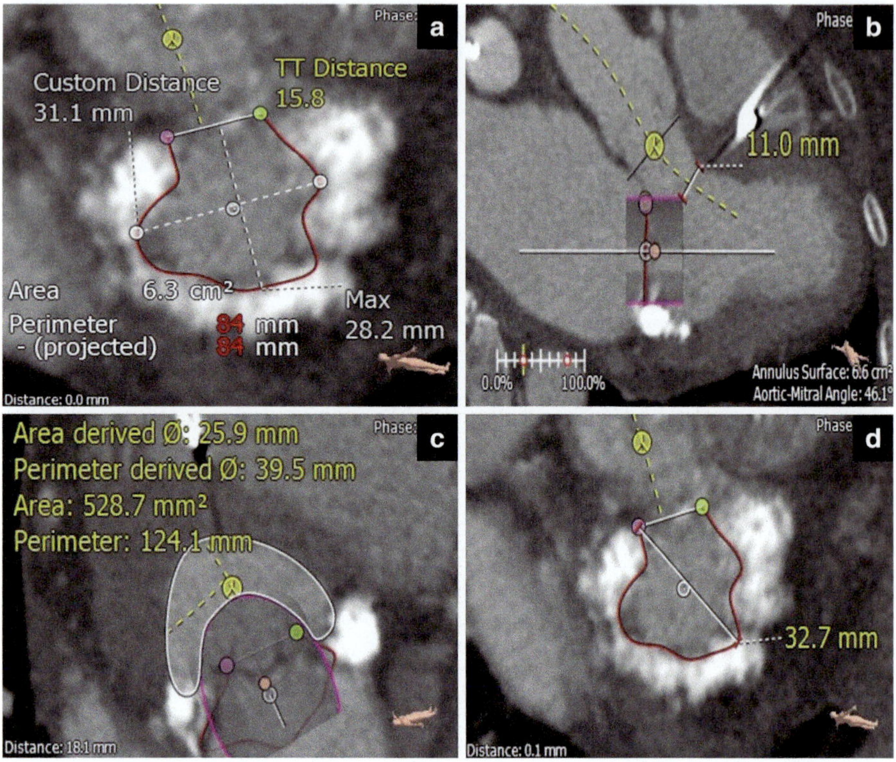

Fig. 3 Reconstructed CT before the TMVR procedure. (**a**) Mitral annular diameters of 31.1 × 28.2 mm, MV area of 6.3 cm^2, and a perimeter of 84 mm. (**b**) Aorto-mitral angle of 46.1°. (**c**) A neo-LVOT area of 528.7 mm^2 for Sapien S3 THV. (**d**) Extensive mitral annular calcification with a maximal diameter of 32.7 mm

A dedicated Sapien 3 (29 mm) bioprosthesis was prepped in the standard fashion. The Agilis catheter and 11-French sheath were removed over the Safari wire, and the 16-French sheath was inserted and advanced into the inferior vena cava. The Sapien system was advanced into the left atrium and left ventricle, being confirmed and guided by fluoroscopy and TEE. Under rapid ventricular pacing at 180 bpm, the balloon-expandable bioprosthesis was deployed with approximately 4 mL of contrast (Video 6). We optimized the positioning of the valve with post-dilation guided by fluoroscopy. The valve deployment system was removed from the body. Figure 4 depicts the TMVR procedure step-by-step. Post-procedural TEE (Videos 7 and 8, Fig. 5) showed acceptable results with a minimal paravalvular leak.

4 Outcome and Follow-Up

Post-procedure TEE and TTE confirmed the valve position with normal leaflet motion without leaks. The patient's hospitalization was unremarkable, and her symptoms significantly improved at 30 days.

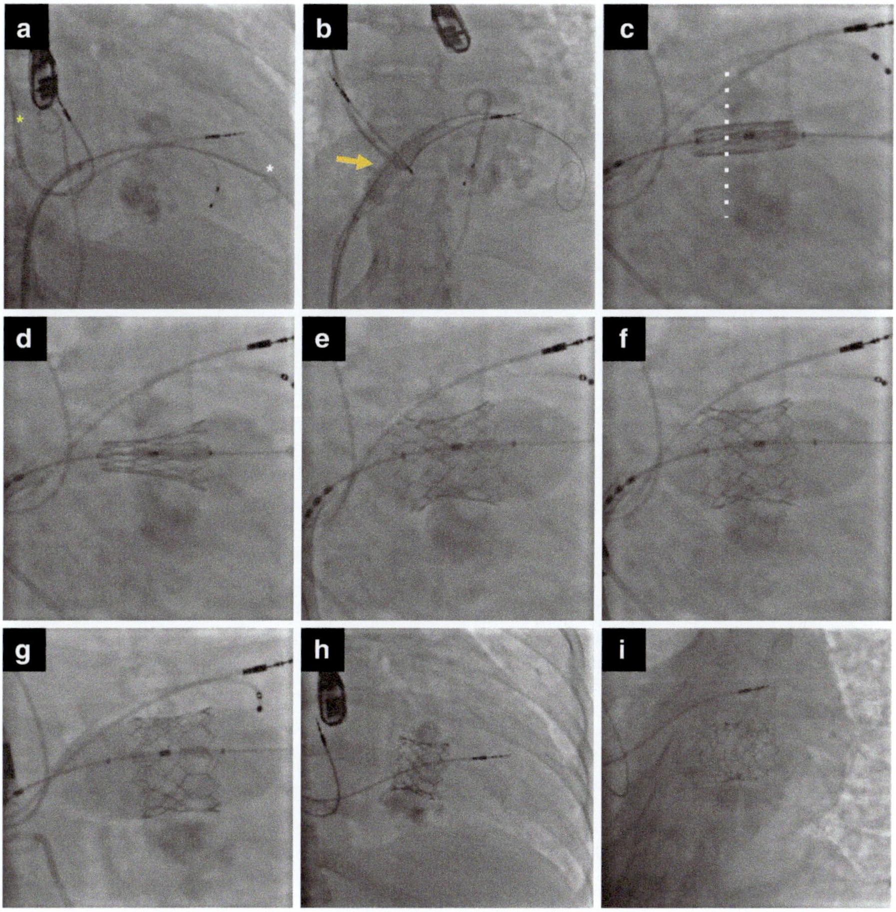

Fig. 4 Fluoroscopy views of the TMVR procedure (step-by-step). (**a**) LAO view of the mitral annulus for transeptal puncture with a pigtailed catheter on the left atrium crossing over the fossa ovalis (white asterisk) with BRK needle 8.5-French Baylis transcatheter transseptal sheath. The transeptal puncture was guided by TEE and fluoroscopy using a pigtailed catheter (yellow asterisk) on the ascending aorta as a marker. (**b**) Transseptal septostomy was performed using a 12 × 40 mm Z-Med balloon with manual balloon inflation (yellow arrow). (**c**) The deployment of a Sapien-3 THV over the mitral annulus (dashed white line) in a 3:7 manner (30% on the atrial side and 70% on the ventricle side). (**d**) Early phase of a bioprosthetic Sapien-3 mitral valve deployment. (**e**) Mid phase of valve deployment. (**f**) Final phase of valve deployment. (**g**) Post-positioning dilatation. (**h**) LAO view of the final result. (**i**) Cranial view of the THV

5 Discussion

The prevalence of mitral annulus calcification (MAC) is 8–15%. Risk factors for the development of MAC are similar to atherosclerosis and include age, hypertension, valvular heart disease, chronic kidney disease, and dialysis [1, 2]. Our patient had most of the risk factors. Usually, MAC is an asymptomatic and incidental finding discovered during cardiac evaluation. However, MAC may cause functional mitral

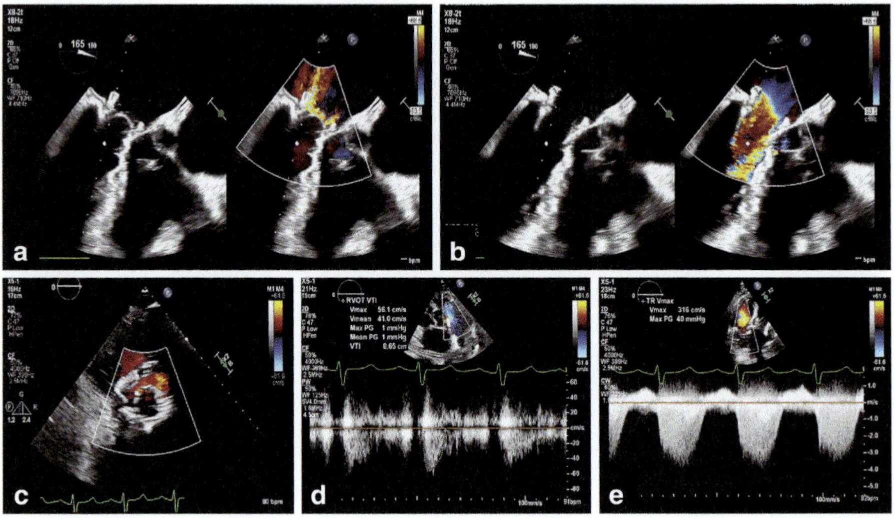

Fig. 5 TEE post TMVR procedure. (**a**) Color Doppler across the mitral valve during diastole. (**b**) Color Doppler across the mitral valve during diastole. (**c**) The positioning of the THV over the mitral valve. (**d**) Reduction in the pressure gradient across the mitral valve following TMVR. (**e**) Reduction in the pressure gradient across the tricuspid valve following TMVR indicates promising initial results of improving pulmonary artery pressure

stenosis (MS) or mitral regurgitation (MR) in certain cases. Limited studies reported MS prevalence of 6–8% and moderate to severe MR in 33% of MAC patients [3, 4]. In patients with MR, MAC was found in 12% of patients compared to 4% without MR [5].

Mitral valve (MV) intervention is indicated for symptomatic severe mitral stenosis or regurgitation [6]. MAC is a rare cause of severe, symptomatic MS. In these cases, the treatment is valve replacement rather than percutaneous MV balloon valvuloplasty due to poor procedural success. Valvuloplasty can be used in MS to retract commissural fusion, as done in rheumatic valve disease with mild regurgitation; however, this is not commonly done in MAC [7]. The mortality rate of a surgical MV replacement is significantly high, with a 30-day mortality rate of 27% for MAC patients vs. 7% for non-MAC patients [8, 9]. Circumflex artery injury, hemorrhage, thromboembolic events, atrioventricular disruption, and ventricular rupture are among the most common complications of MVR [9, 10]. Multiple strategies have been proposed to limit these complications.

In cases where the mitral annulus is adequately dilated, it is possible to remove a part of the valve and sew a prosthetic valve without the removal of calcium. In these cases, it is important to sew the prosthetic valve in pliable tissue instead of the calcium bar to avoid possible paravalvular leak and dehiscence [9]. In 36 patients who had an intraarterial insertion of a mitral prosthesis, the operative mortality was 36% and valve dehiscence rates were 17% [11]. An additional strategy includes decalcifying the mitral annulus before patch reconstruction and mitral valve replacement or repair. Various studies found in-hospital mortality rates of 3.3%, 30-day survival of 91%, 5-year survival of 73–79%, seven-year survival rates of 93%, and freedom from reoperation rates at 89–91% for five years among symptomatic MR and MS treated with this strategy [9, 10, 12]. Postoperative complications included low cardiac output syndrome (13%), myocardial infarction (5%), infection (5%), mediastinal bleeding (3%), AV block (3%), stroke (2%), and hemorrhage [10, 12].

The experience of transcatheter mitral valve replacements (TMVR) among patients with severe MAC has been limited given procedural and post-operative challenges, such as risks of paravalvular regurgitation and calcium embolization. Given these risks, severe MAC has been a contraindication for TMVR. There is limited data on the success and complications of TMVR. One multicenter registry (32 centers) retrospectively analyzed 64 patients who underwent TMVR with balloon-expandable valves. Results showed technical success rates in 72% of patients and 30-day all-cause mortality rates of 30%. Complications included a need for a second valve (17%), left ventricular tract obstruction with hemodynamic compromise (9%), embolization (6%), and perforation (3%) [13]. Another study reported 1-year outcomes of TMVR in 12 patients with severe MAC. Procedural success was reported in 67% of patients, and one-year survival rates were 57%. Complications included valve migration and instability requiring a second valve (17%), left ventricle outflow tract obstruction (17%), and paravalvular leak (9%) [14].

One large systemic review analyzed 27 studies that looked at both surgical and transcatheter MVR in MAC [15]. Patients undergoing surgical MVR had 30-day mortality rates of 6%, 1-year mortality rates of 16%, 5-year mortality rates of 39%, and 10-year mortality rates of 62%. Transcatheter approaches led to a median technical success rate of 11%, re-intervention rates of 17%, and major in-hospital bleeding rates of 5%. The outcomes of the transseptal TMVR revealed median in-hospital rates of 17%, 30-day mortality rates of 23%, and 1-year mortality rates of 43%. This review deduced that TMVR is preferred in patients with higher surgical risk from advanced age, comorbidities, or cardiac anatomy.

Key Points

- TMVR for MAC patients is usually reserved nowadays for very high risk or inoperable surgical patients.
- Assessing the annulus size in reconstructed CT analysis for MAC patients is challenging and may underestimate or overestimate the real dimensions.
- The high complications rate reported in MAC patients is believed to be associated with various factors such as atrial fibrillation, remodeling of the left sided heart chambers, obstruction of the LVOT by the anterior mitral leaflet, and paravalvular leak due to valve misalignment. All of these factors contribute to poor outcomes.

References

1. Abramowitz Y, Jilaihawi H, Chakravarty T, Mack MJ, Makkar RR. Mitral annulus calcification. J Am Coll Cardiol. 2015;66(17):1934–41.
2. Kanjanauthai S, Nasir K, Katz R, Rivera JJ, Takasu J, Blumenthal RS, Eng J, Budoff MJ. Relationships of mitral annular calcification to cardiovascular risk factors: the Multi-Ethnic Study of Atherosclerosis (MESA). Atherosclerosis. 2010;213(2):558–62.
3. Aronow WS, Schwartz KS, Koenigsberg M. Correlation of murmurs of mitral stenosis and mitral regurgitation with presence or absence of mitral anular calcium in persons older than 62 years in a long-term health care facility. Am J Cardiol. 1987;59(1):181–2.
4. Labovitz AJ, Nelson JG, Windhorst DM, Kennedy HL, Williams GA. Frequency of mitral valve dysfunction from mitral anular calcium as detected by Doppler echocardiography. Am J Cardiol. 1985;55(1):133–7.
5. Movahed MR, Saito Y, Ahmadi-Kashani M, Ebrahimi R. Mitral annulus calcification is associated with valvular and cardiac structural abnormalities. Cardiovasc Ultrasound. 2007;5(1):1–4.
6. Nishimura RA, Otto CM, Bonow RO, Carabello BA, Erwin JP, Fleisher LA, Jneid H, Mack MJ, McLeod CJ, O'Gara PT, Rigolin VH. 2017 AHA/ACC focused update of the 2014 AHA/ACC guideline for the management of patients with valvular heart disease: a report of the American College of Cardiology/American Heart Association Task Force on Clinical Practice Guidelines. J Am Coll Cardiol. 2017;70(2):252–89.
7. Falk V, Baumgartner H, Bax JJ, De Bonis M, Hamm C, Holm PJ, Iung B, Lancellotti P, Lansac E, Muñoz DR, Rosenhek R. 2017 ESC/EACTS guidelines for the management of valvular heart disease. Eur J Cardiothorac Surg. 2017;52(4):616–64.
8. Cammack PL, Edie RN, Edmunds LH Jr. Bar calcification of the mitral annulus: a risk factor in mitral valve operations. J Thorac Cardiovasc Surg. 1987;94(3):399–404.
9. Feindel CM, Tufail Z, David TE, Ivanov J, Armstrong S. Mitral valve surgery in patients with extensive calcification of the mitral annulus. J Thorac Cardiovasc Surg. 2003;126(3):777–81.
10. Papadopoulos N, Dietrich M, Christodoulou T, Moritz A, Doss M. Midterm survival after decalcification of the mitral annulus. Ann Thorac Surg. 2009;87(4):1143–7.
11. Nataf P, Pavie A, Jault F, Bors V, Cabrol C, Gandjbakhch I. Intraatrial insertion of a mitral prosthesis in a destroyed or calcified mitral annulus. Ann Thorac Surg. 1994;58(1):163–7.
12. Carpentier AF, Pellerin M, Fuzellier JF, Relland JY. Extensive calcification of the mitral valve annulus: pathology and surgical management. J Thorac Cardiovasc Surg. 1996;111(4):718–30.
13. Guerrero M, Dvir D, Himbert D, Urena M, Eleid M, Wang DD, Greenbaum A, Mahadevan VS, Holzhey D, O'Hair D, Dumonteil N. Transcatheter mitral valve replacement in native mitral valve disease with severe mitral annular calcification: results from the first multicenter global registry. J Am Coll Cardiol Interv. 2016;9(13):1361–71.
14. Eleid MF, Cabalka AK, Williams MR, Whisenant BK, Alli OO, Fam N, Pollak PM, Barrow F, Malouf JF, Nishimura RA, Joyce LD. Percutaneous transvenous transseptal transcatheter valve implantation in failed bioprosthetic mitral valves, ring annuloplasty, and severe mitral annular calcification. J Am Coll Cardiol Interv. 2016;9(11):1161–74.
15. Alexis SL, Malik AH, El-Eshmawi A, George I, Sengupta A, Kodali SK, Hahn RT, Khalique OK, Zaid S, Guerrero M, Bapat VN. Surgical and transcatheter mitral valve replacement in mitral annular calcification: a systematic review. J Am Heart Assoc. 2021;10(7):e018514.

Air Embolization During a MitraClip Procedure

Danon Kaewkes, Yonatan Moshkovits, and Michael M. Shenoda

1 Clinical Presentation

A 75-year-old male presented in our clinic with dyspnea upon exertion that developed two months prior. The patient's medical history was notable for hypertension, hyperlipidemia, atrial fibrillation, tricuspid regurgitation (TR), and mitral regurgitation (MR). He underwent coronary angiography one month prior at an outside hospital, which revealed no significant coronary obstruction. Subsequently, the patient underwent percutaneous mitral valve edge-to-edge repair with a single MitraClip (Abbott Laboratories, Abbott Park, IL). Despite undergoing the MitraClip procedure, his dyspnea upon exertion persisted.

2 Images and Supported Data

Transthoracic and transesophageal echocardiography (TTE and TEE) revealed moderately dilated left ventricular (LV) size and severely depressed LV systolic function with an LV ejection fraction of 25%. The right ventricle was moderately

Supplementary Information The online version contains supplementary material available at [https://doi.org/10.1007/978-3-031-05965-0_27].

D. Kaewkes (✉)
Department of Medicine, Faculty of Medicine, Khon Kaen University, Khon Kaen, Thailand
e-mail: Danon@kku.ac.th

Y. Moshkovits
Leviev Heart Center, Sheba Medical Center, Ramat-Gan, Israel

M. M. Shenoda
Interventional Cardiology and Structural Heart Disease, Santa Barbara Cottage Hospital, Santa Barbara, CA, USA

O. Koren et al. (eds.), *Complex Cases in Structural Heart Intervention*,
https://doi.org/10.1007/978-3-031-05965-0_27

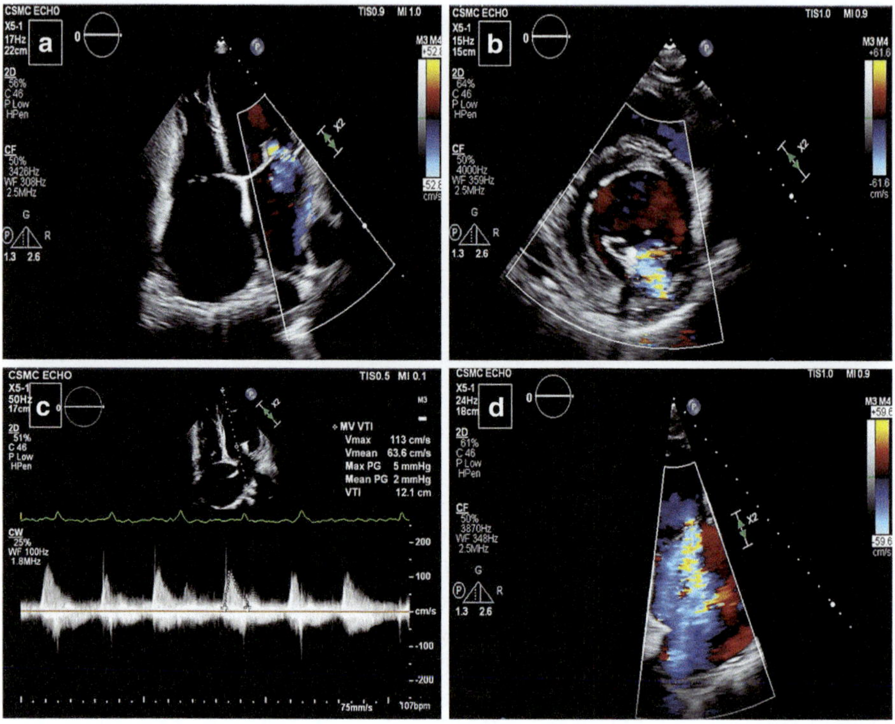

Fig. 1 Pre-procedural transthoracic echocardiography of the mitral valve. (**a**) Color Doppler across the MV in 4C TTE view. (**b**) Color Doppler across the MV in short axis TTE view with residual MR lateral to a previous implanted clip. (**c**) Flow velocity and pressure gradient over the MV. (**d**) Color Doppler of severe TR in RV inflow view

dilated with severely impaired systolic function (Videos 1, 2 and 3). One MitraClip was seen on the anterior and posterior leaflets of the mitral valve with residual moderate to severe MR lateral to the MitraClip and a mean transmitral pressure gradient of 2 mmHg (Fig. 1). There was also severe TR with an estimated pulmonary systolic pressure of 39 mmHg (Video 4).

3 Pre-Procedural Consideration: Pitfalls, Dilemmas, and Challenges

Given the significance of the patient's MR and TR, the pre-procedure consideration focused on which valve (mitral or tricuspid) should be treated first and which valve caused their residual symptoms. In general, left-sided valve pathology should be treated first, as this may improve the right-sided valve pathology by reducing pressure and volume load to the right side. Therefore, this patient was scheduled for another mitral valve repair using an additional MitraClip(s).

4 Technique

Following the placement of a 16F sheath, the transseptal puncture was performed under fluoroscopic and echocardiographic guidance. After crossing the interatrial septum, the patient was anticoagulated with heparin, and the 22F Abbott MitraClip Steerable delivery guide was advanced into the left atrium (Video 5). A MitraClip NTW was prepped in the standard fashion and was carefully advanced into the left atrium through the device deployment sheath under fluoroscopic and TEE guidance. The steerable deployment sheath was manipulated to optimize the positioning of the device lateral to the previously implanted clip over the MR jet. We noted some potential air bubbles in the left chambers at this stage (Videos 6 and 7, Fig. 2) and found that the three-way stop-cock on the clip introducer was turned in the wrong direction (Fig. 3). EKG monitoring showed transient ST-segment elevation in the inferior leads; however, the patient's hemodynamics were stable. We aspirated air from the system, restored the fluid column, and set the stop-cocks correctly. After careful optimization, the clip was deployed under fluoroscopic and TEE guidance (Videos 8 and 9). Following the closure of the MitraClip, TEE showed a well-seated clip and trivial MR (Fig. 4, Video 10). The clip was successfully released in the standard fashion, and the delivery system was withdrawn. TEE once more demonstrated a significant amount of air accumulated at the anterior aspect of the LV. We treated it by giving 100% oxygen, starting a dobutamine drip, and using a body shaking maneuver.

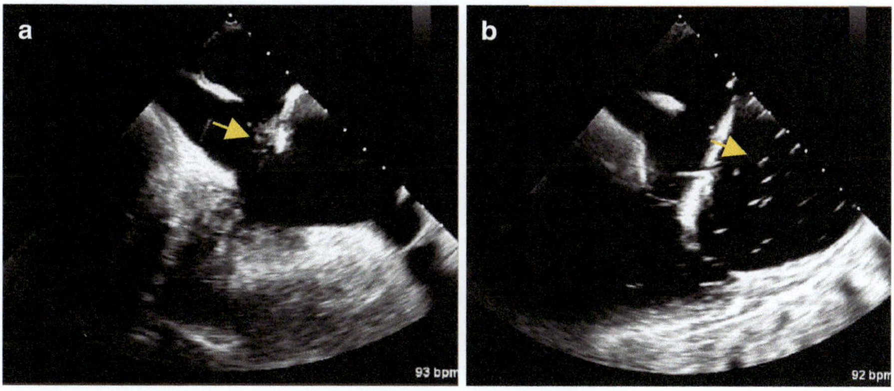

Fig. 2 Peri-procedural TEE. (**a**) Air bubbles (yellow arrow) coming out of the mitral clip introducer. (**b**) Air bubbles progressing into the LV cavity (yellow arrow)

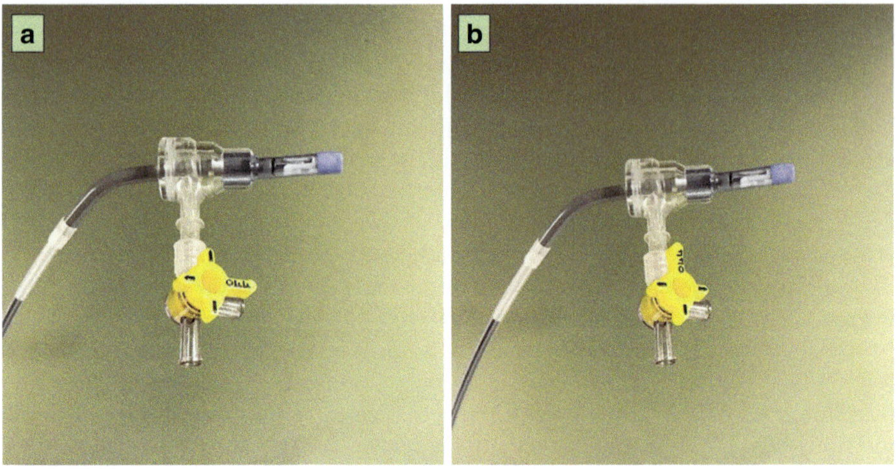

Fig. 3 Different directions of a three-way stop-cock on the clip introducer. (**a**) Wrong direction. (**b**) Correct direction

Fig. 4 Post-procedure TEE with color Doppler across the mitral valve with a residual mild MR (yellow arrow) after MitraClip implantation lateral to the previous clip (green arrow)

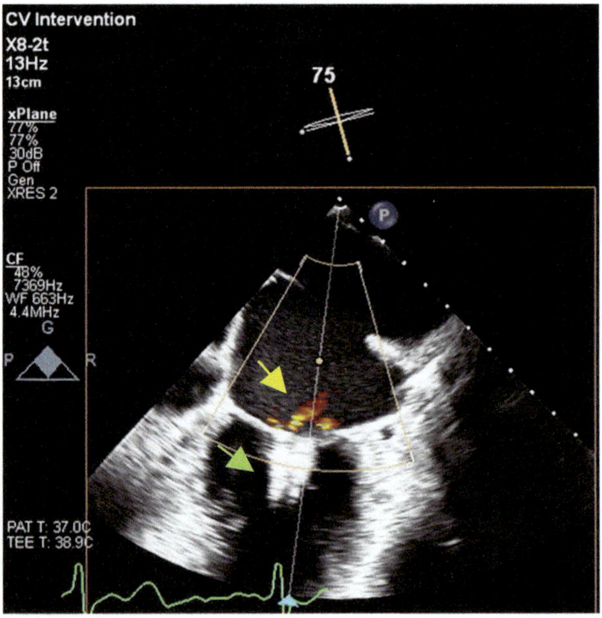

5 Outcome and Follow-Up

Predischarge TTE showed well-seated MitraClips with mild residual MR. The mean transmitral pressure gradient was 2 mmHg, and there was no residual air in the LV. The patient had no neurological deficit and was discharged on the next day in great condition.

6 Discussion

Air embolism is a rarely encountered but much-dreaded complication of endovascular procedures that results in significant morbidity and mortality [1]. The true incidence of air embolism is unknown because of the nonspecific clinical signs and the lack of comprehensive diagnosis documentation. Therefore, many instances go unreported. In this case, the air embolism occurred from the wrong direction of the three-way stop-cock on the clip introducer, allowing air into the system. Fortunately, the air embolism was detected early because the MitraClip procedure was performed under TEE. For the management of air embolism, the initial priority is to prevent further air embolism and resuscitation when necessary. Supportive measures such as administering 100% oxygen, catheter aspiration, increasing cardiac contractility, and body shaking maneuver have been proven to resolve air embolisms [2, 3]. Our case emphasizes the importance of paying close attention to details during every step of the procedure, as minor errors can lead to life-threatening complications. Understanding the available treatment options and the rapid institution of these measures can be lifesaving during inadvertent air embolization during the MitraClip procedure.

Key Points

- Paying close attention to details during every step of the MitraClip preparation and procedure reduces errors and complications such as an air embolism due to an erroneous three-way stop-cock direction.
- Early recognition and rapid treatment of air embolization during structural cases are imperative to avoid a catastrophic outcome.
- The initial steps in managing air embolization are to stop the source of air and support the patient.
- Effective treatments include administering 100% oxygen, catheter aspiration, increasing cardiac contractility via inotropic support, and body shaking maneuvers.

References

1. Bessereau J, Genotelle N, Chabbaut C, Huon A, Tabah A, Aboab J, Chevret S, Annane D. Long-term outcome of iatrogenic gas embolism. Intensive Care Med. 2010;36(7):1180–7.
2. McCarthy CJ, Behravesh S, Naidu SG, Oklu R. Air embolism: practical tips for prevention and treatment. J Clin Med. 2016;5(11):93.
3. Hadjadj S, Del Val D, Robert R, Beaudoin J, Rodés-Cabau J, Paradis JM. To take one's breath away: echocardiography-guided aspiration of an air embolism during a MitraClip procedure. CJC Open. 2021;3(1):115–7.

Left Ventricular Outflow Obstruction Following TMVR

Danon Kaewkes, Ofir Koren, Siamak Kohan, and Hezzy Shmueli

1 Clinical Presentation

An 87-year-old male presented in our clinic with dyspnea upon minimal exertion (5–10 steps) that developed one month prior. He was then recently hospitalized with congestive heart failure two weeks prior. The patient's medical history was notable for type 2 diabetes, hypertension, hyperlipidemia, atrial fibrillation, and chronic kidney disease stage 3. Fourteen years ago, he underwent mitral and tricuspid valve repair due to tricuspid regurgitation (TR) and mitral regurgitation (MR) using 30 mm Edward ETlogix annuloplasty ring and 34 mm CarboMedics annuloplasty ring, respectively. On current echocardiography, he was found to have recurrent severe MR and moderate to severe TR. The patient was at high surgical risk, and therefore, not suitable as a surgical candidate.

D. Kaewkes (✉)
Department of Medicine, Faculty of Medicine, Khon Kaen University, Khon Kaen, Thailand
e-mail: Danon@kku.ac.th

O. Koren
Smidt Heart Institute, Cedars-Sinai Medical Center, Los Angeles, CA, USA

Faculty of Medicine, Technion, Israel Institute of Technology, Haifa, Israel
e-mail: Ofir.Koren@cshs.org

S. Kohan
Kaiser Permanente Los Angeles Medical Center, Los Angeles, CA, USA

H. Shmueli
Cardiology Department, Soroka University Medical Center, Beer Sheva, Israel

O. Koren et al. (eds.), *Complex Cases in Structural Heart Intervention*,
https://doi.org/10.1007/978-3-031-05965-0_28

2 Images and Supported Data

Transthoracic and transesophageal echocardiography (TTE and TEE) revealed normal left ventricular (LV) size and hyperdynamic LV systolic function with an LV ejection fraction of 70%. Mitral and tricuspid valve rings were seen with severe MR and moderate to severe TR. The mean transmitral pressure gradient was 5 mmHg, and the estimated pulmonary systolic pressure was 67 mmHg. The aortic valve was mildly calcified with mild stenosis (Fig. 1). Cardiac computed tomography (CT) showed a complete mitral valve ring with a mitral annulus area of 400 mm^2. Neo-LV outflow tract (LVOT) area estimated for virtual 23 and 26 mm Sapien 3 were 315 and 264 mm^2, respectively. Direct 3D planimetry showed a mitral valve orifice area of 2.2 cm^2 (Fig. 2).

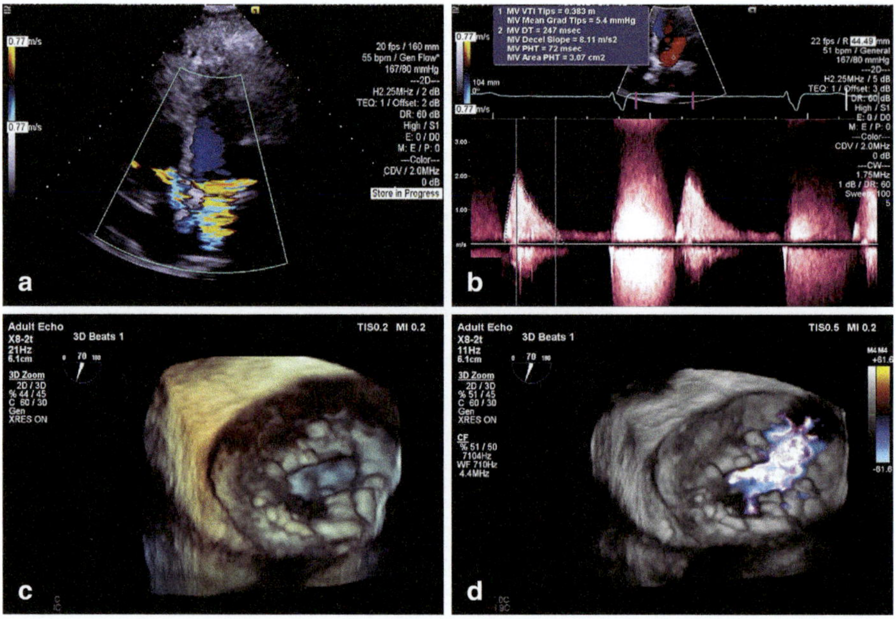

Fig. 1 Pre-procedural transthoracic and transesophageal echocardiography of the mitral and the tricuspid valves. (**a**) Color Doppler across the mitral and tricuspid valves indicates severe MR and moderate to severe TR. (**b**) Flow velocity and pressure gradient across the mitral valve indicate a transmitral mean gradient of 5.4 mmHg. (**c**) A 3D en face view of the mitral valve with a complete mitral valve ring. (**d**) Severe MR on 3D en face view

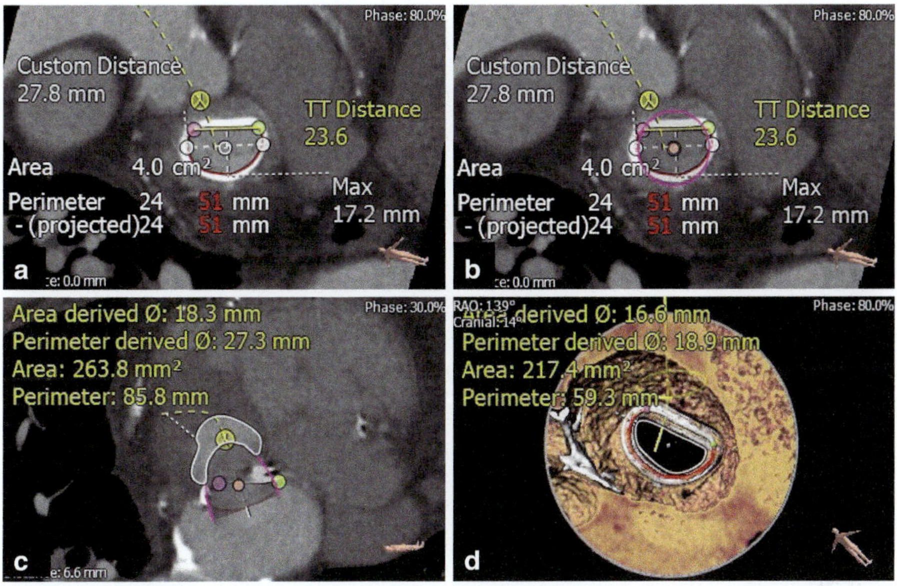

Fig. 2 Pre-procedure reconstructed CT analysis of the mitral valve. (**a**) Mitral annulus area and diameter. (**b**) Mitral valve annulus using a Virtual 26 mm Sapien 3 valve. (**c**) The neo-LVOT area after deploying a virtual 26 mm Sapien 3 valve. (**d**) Mitral valve orifice area by direct 3D planimetry

3 Pre-Procedural Consideration: Pitfalls, Dilemmas, and Challenges

Since the patient was not a candidate for redo mitral valve surgery, we focused on the treatment strategy for failed surgical valve rings with severe MR. The small mitral valve orifice area and the relatively high baseline trans-mitral pressure gradient made this patient, not a good case for transcatheter edge-to-edge repair. However, percutaneous treatments were considered. In this patient, the mitral annulus area and neo-LVOT were suitable and adequate for transcatheter mitral valve replacement (TMVR) with Sapien 3 valve. Therefore, TMVR in the surgical ring was scheduled for this patient.

4 Technique

Following the placement of an 11F sheath, the transseptal puncture was performed under fluoroscopic and echocardiographic guidance at the mid-portion and slightly posterior aspect of the right atrium. Then, the mitral valve was crossed with a Safari wire to the LV apex by using a pigtail inside an Agilis catheter. A balloon septoplasty was performed followed by a TMVR in the mitral valve ring using 26 mm Edward Sapien 3 Ultra. Post-procedural TEE revealed trivial paravalvular leakage

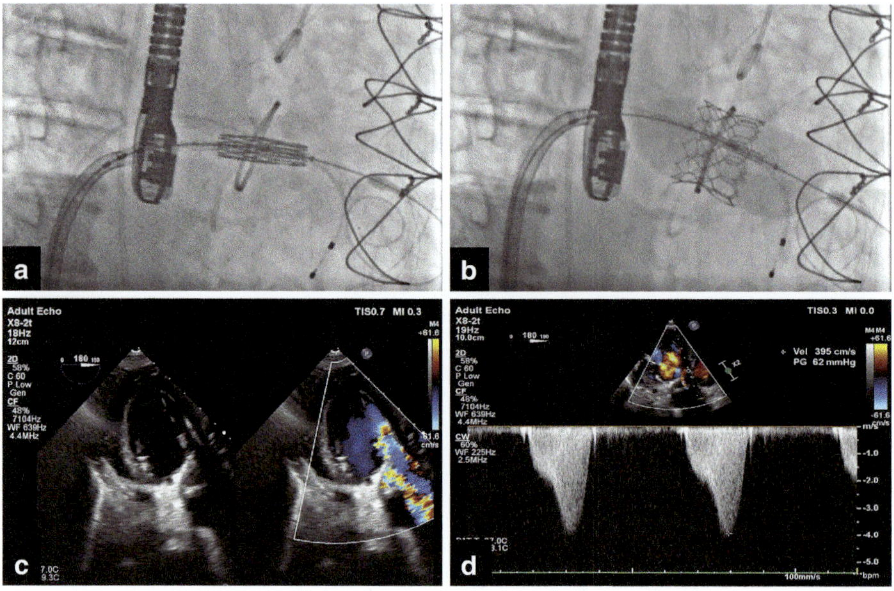

Fig. 3 Fluoroscopic images and peri-procedural TEE of transcatheter mitral valve replacement. (**a**) 26 mm Sapien 3 positioned over the mitral valve ring. (**b**) Deploying a 26 mm Sapien 3 valve across the mitral valve ring. (**c**) Accelerated flow at the LVOT area. (**d**) Flow velocity and pressure gradient across the LVOT with a typical dagger shaped appearance

and LVOT gradient up to 62 mmHg (Fig. 3). The patient was hemodynamically stable and was transferred to the post-intervention care unit. However, after the procedure, the patient developed hematuria, anemia, and acute kidney injury suggestive of intravascular hemolysis due to the high shearing stress at the LVOT. After discussion with the heart team, surgical treatment at this stage was deemed high risk, and the interventricular septum was too thin for an alcohol septal ablation. Thus, we performed transfemoral transcatheter aortic valve replacement (TAVR) using a 29 mm self-expandable Medtronic Evolut Pro. The valve was deployed low at the LVOT level to treat LVOT obstruction, but there was residual moderate paravalvular aortic regurgitation (AR) because of the low-positioned implantation. Thus, a 26 mm Edward Sapien 3 Ultra was deployed inside the Evolut valve at the aortic annulus level as a bailout treatment for paravalvular AR (Fig. 4).

5 Outcome and Follow-Up

The procedure was complicated by retroperitoneal bleeding and complete heart block, requiring permanent pacemaker implantation. The patient gradually improved and was discharged after 14 days of hospitalization. Pre-discharge TTE showed

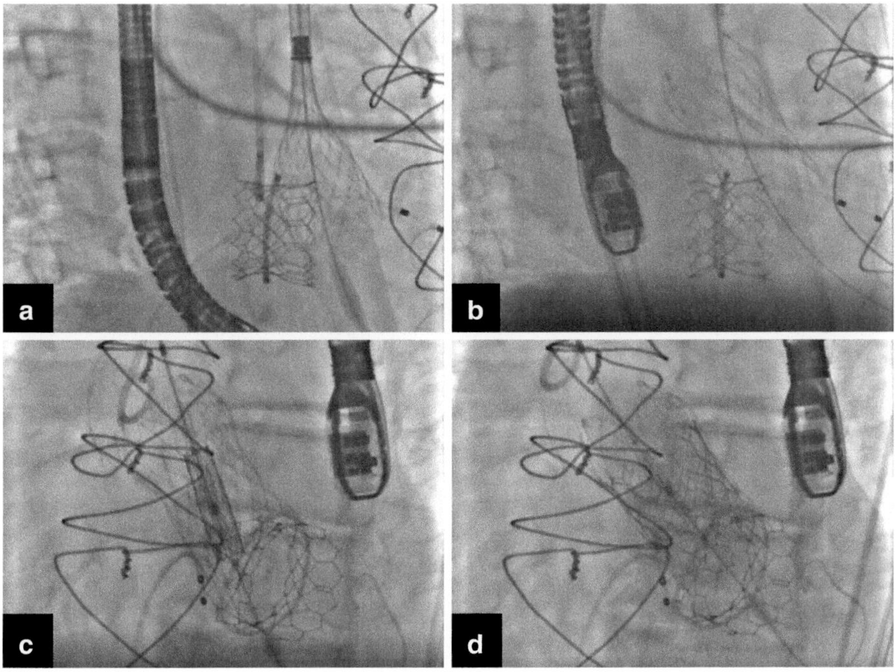

Fig. 4 Deployment of self-expandable and balloon-expandable valves. (**a** and **b**) The deployment of a 29 mm Evolut Pro valve at a low position across the aortic valve annulus. (**c** and **d**) Deploying a second 26 mm Sapien 3 Ultra valve over the 29 mm Evolut due to residual aortic regurgitation

good LV systolic function and no residual pressure gradient. Bioprosthetic stent valves were well-seated at mitral and aortic positions with good function. No significant paravalvular leakage or residual LVOT gradient was noted (Fig. 5).

6 Discussion

TMVR using balloon-expandable aortic transcatheter heart valves (THV) has emerged as an alternative treatment option for patients with severe MR due to failed surgical repair with annuloplasty rings and bad candidacy for conventional mitral valve surgery [1]. In a recent prospective study, the technical success rate of this procedure was 67%, and the mortality rates at 30 days and 1 year were 7% and 23%, respectively [2]. In this case, we successfully implanted the Edwards Sapien 3 Ultra valve in the previous annuloplasty ring; however, the patient developed acute hemolysis, which required blood transfusion due to LVOT obstruction. Patients with LVOT obstruction have significantly higher procedural mortality than those without LVOT obstruction. The estimated neo-LVOT area $\leq$170 mm^2 by pre-procedural CT was predictive of LVOT obstruction with a sensitivity of 96% and a

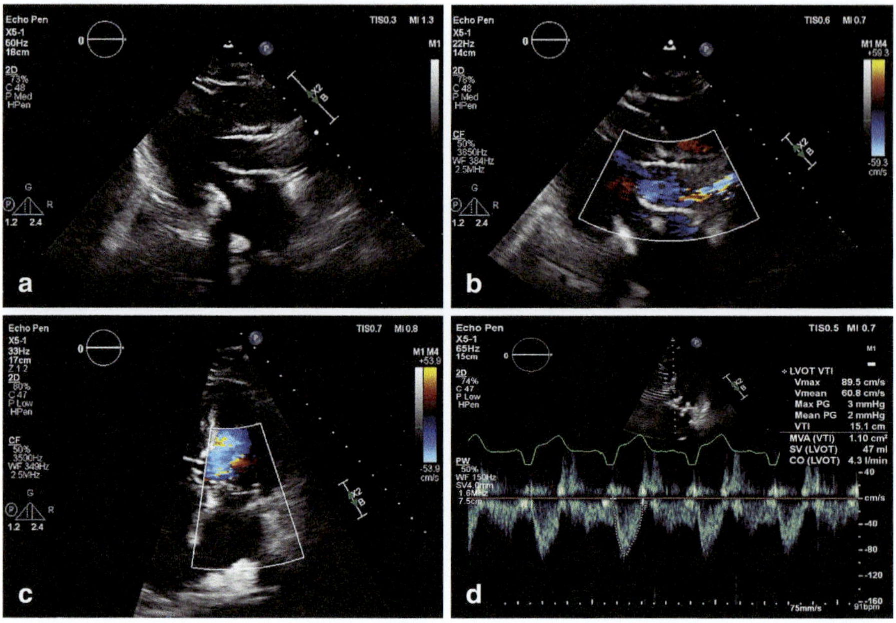

Fig. 5 Post-procedure TTE of the mitral and aortic valves. (**a**) Bioprosthetic valves can be seen at the mitral and the aortic positions. (**b**) Color Doppler over the aortic valve indicates no significant paravalvular leakage. (**c**) Color Doppler over the LVOT shows no accelerated flow. (**d**) Flow velocity and pressure gradient over the LVOT indicate no significant LVOT gradient

specificity of 92% [3]. In this patient, LVOT obstruction occurred even when the estimated neo-LVOT area was 264 mm^2 on pre-procedural CT. A possible explanation could be that the actual neo-LVOT area depends not only on the size of THV, but also on the implanting position, the valve size post-dilatation, the length of the anterior mitral leaflet, and hyperdynamic contraction of LV. We also demonstrated that deployment of a TAVR device deep into the LVOT can be a viable treatment option for LVOT obstruction after TMVR, specifically when surgery and alcohol septal ablation are unsuitable for the patient [4]. Our case demonstrated both the feasibility of TMVR in a previous mitral annuloplasty ring by using a balloon-expandable aortic THV, and the usefulness of self-expandable TAVR as a bailout treatment for LVOT obstruction following TMVR.

Key Points

- TMVR in a previous mitral annuloplasty ring by using a balloon-expandable aortic THV is feasible.
- LVOT obstruction is one of the complications following TMVR, which may be partially predictable by pre-procedural CT.
- TAVR with a self-expandable valve deployed deep into LVOT can be a treatment option for LVOT obstruction after TMVR.

References

1. Yoon SH, Whisenant BK, Bleiziffer S, Delgado V, Dhoble A, Schofer N, Eschenbach L, Bansal E, Murdoch DJ, Ancona M, Schmidt T. Outcomes of transcatheter mitral valve replacement for degenerated bioprostheses, failed annuloplasty rings, and mitral annular calcification. Eur Heart J. 2019;40(5):441–51.
2. Guerrero M, Wang DD, Pursnani A, Salinger M, Russell HM, Eleid M, Chakravarty T, Ng MH, Kodali SK, Meduri CU, Pershad A. Prospective evaluation of TMVR for failed surgical annuloplasty rings: MITRAL trial valve-in-ring arm 1-year outcomes. JACC Cardiovasc Interv. 2021;14(8):846–58.
3. Yoon SH, Bleiziffer S, Latib A, Eschenbach L, Ancona M, Vincent F, Kim WK, Unbehaum A, Asami M, Dhoble A, Silaschi M. Predictors of left ventricular outflow tract obstruction after transcatheter mitral valve replacement. J Am Coll Cardiol Interv. 2019;12(2):182–93.
4. Duncan A, Quarto C, Ernst S, Rigby M, Yadav R, Davies S. Transcatheter aortic valve replacement to treat left ventricular outflow tract obstruction and significant paravalvular leak following transcatheter mitral valve replacement. Case. 2019;3(3):90–9.

Clip Steerable Delivery System Malfunction

Ofir Koren, Troy Sanders, and Arvind Reddy Devanabanda

1 Clinical Presentation

The patient is a 70-year-old female with a past medical history of non-obstructive hypertrophic cardiomyopathy, pulmonary hypertension, chronic kidney disease stage III, paroxysmal atrial fibrillation on coumadin, ICD placement, hemothorax, and thoracotomy post defibrillator change, and severe symptomatic tricuspid regurgitation (NYHA class III). The patient has been referred to our center to determine whether she is appropriate for a tricuspid clip procedure. The patient endorses worsening fatigue, shortness of breath while speaking, and edema responsive to diuresis. She denies chest pain, palpitations, presyncope, syncope orthopnea, fevers, and chills.

Supplementary Information The online version contains supplementary material available at [https://doi.org/10.1007/978-3-031-05965-0_29].

O. Koren (✉)
Smidt Heart Institute, Cedars-Sinai Medical Center, Los Angeles, CA, USA

Faculty of Medicine, Technion, Israel Institute of Technology, Haifa, Israel
e-mail: Ofir.Koren@cshs.org

T. Sanders
David Geffen School of Medicine, University of California, Los Angeles, CA, USA

A. R. Devanabanda
Cedars Sinai Medical Center, Los Angeles, CA, USA

O. Koren et al. (eds.), *Complex Cases in Structural Heart Intervention*,
https://doi.org/10.1007/978-3-031-05965-0_29

2 Images and Supported Data

Pre-procedural TTE revealed normal left ventricular systolic function, severe bilateral atrial enlargement with significant right atrial pressures (>15 mmHg), mild aortic regurgitation, and severe tricuspid regurgitation (Fig. 1, Videos 1–4). Pre-procedural TEE further characterized the tricuspid valve as having a coaptation gap

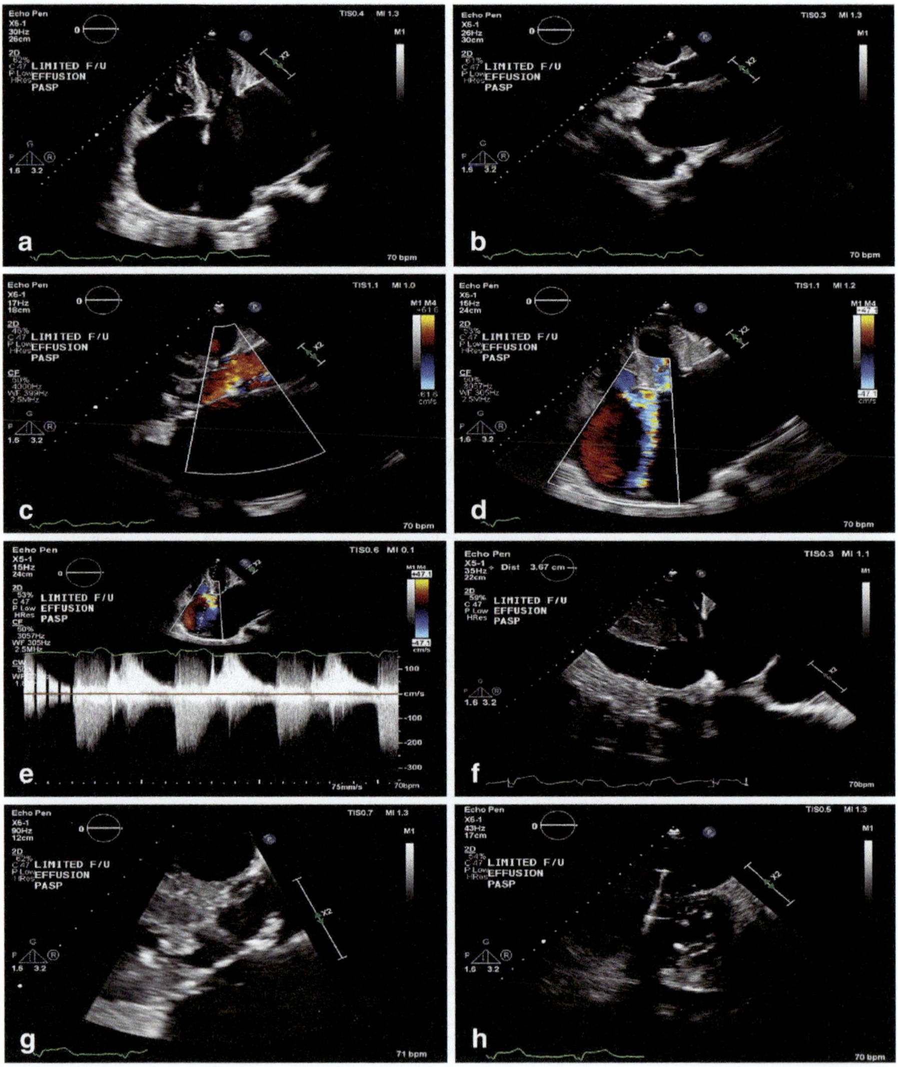

Fig. 1 TTE before the procedure. Severe bilateral atria enlargement is seen on the 4-chambers (**a**) and long-axis views (**b**). Color Doppler at aortic valve indicating mild aortic regurgitation (**c**) and severe tricuspid regurgitation (**d**). (**e**) Flow velocity over the tricuspid valve indicates a peak flow of over 3 ml/s (**f**). Dilated Inferior vena cava during systole shows high right atrial pressure due to pulmonary hypertension and severe TR. (**g**) A mobile mass attached to the basal septal wall near LVOT is most consistent with a non-obstructive membrane. (**h**) Pacemaker lead in the right ventricle on short-axis view

of 0.84 cm, an effective regurgitant orifice of 1.0 cm^2, and posterior leaflet length of 11.7 mm. The pacemaker lead restricted the septal leaflet. The right-ventricular volume was measured to be 75 ml (Fig. 2, Videos 5–8). Right-heart catheterization

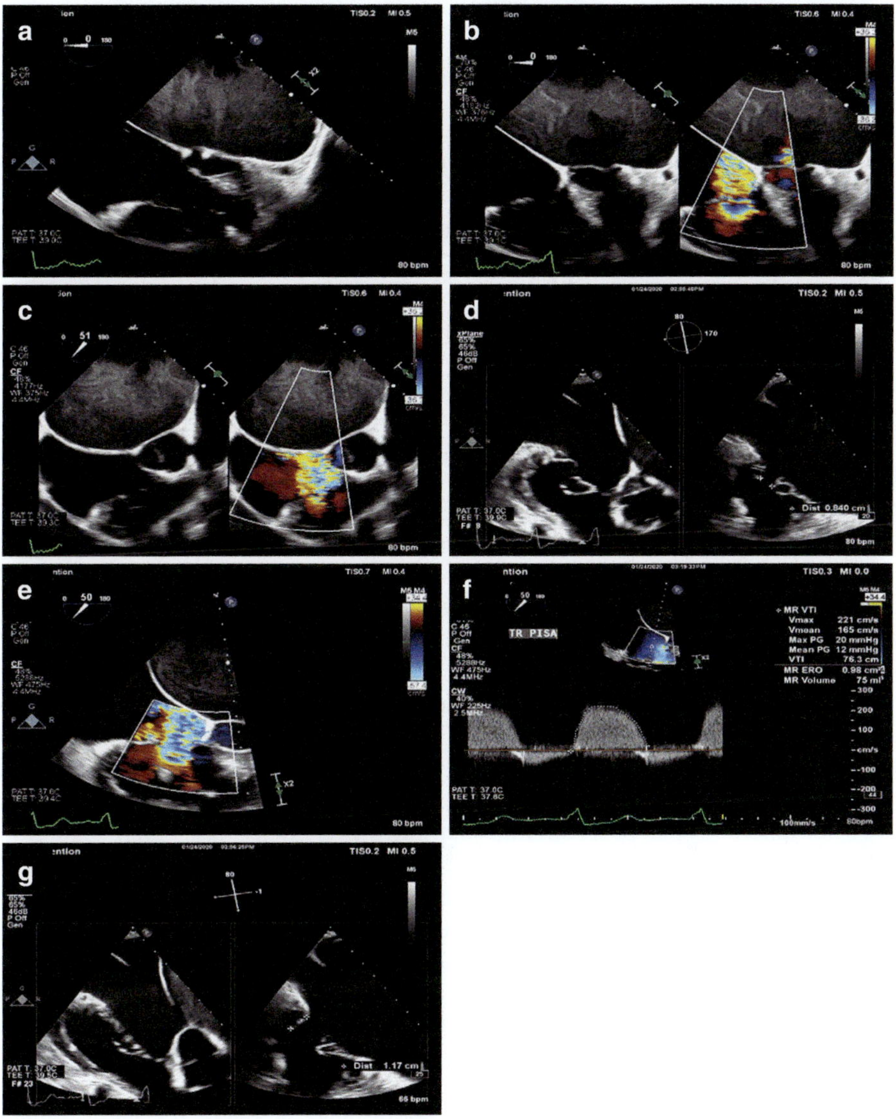

Fig. 2 TEE before the procedure. (**a**) Severely dilated left and right atria. (**b**) Color Doppler over the tricuspid valve indicates severe tricuspid regurgitation with a centraly directed jet during a systolic phase. (**c**) Tricuspid flow jet during the diastolic phase. (**d**) Malcoaptation of the tricuspid leaflets with a large coaptation gap of 0.84 cm. (**e**) Aligning Color Doppler flow jet for proximal isovelocity surface area (PISA) measurements. (**f**) Effective regurgitation orifice (ERO) calculation showing an ERO of 1.0 cm^2 and a RV volume of 75 ml. (**g**) Short axis on the tricuspid valve showing a posterior tricuspid leaflet length of 11.7 mm

revealed mean pulmonary artery pressure of 25 mmHg, normal cardiac out and index (CO: 5.38 L/min; CI: 3.01 L/min/m^2), and mildly elevated right and left-sided filling pressures.

3 Procedure and Outcome

The patient has severe symptomatic tricuspid regurgitation with signs and symptoms of right-sided heart failure. She is therefore a reasonable candidate for tricuspid clip implantation using the G4 MitraClip system. She underwent removal of her ICD lead with implantation of a leadless pacemaker. The procedure was complicated by pericardial effusion and cardiac tamponade, treated with pericardiocentesis (850 cc).

On the day of the procedure, femoral venous access was obtained, and a 6 French multipurpose catheter was advanced over a 0.035-in. J-tip guidewire into the superior vena cava (SVC). Then, a Boston 0.035-in. superstiff wire was advanced through the sheath and positioned in the SVC, followed by successful placement of 22F Abbott MitraClip delivery steerable system into the right atrium (Fig. 3a, b). The MitraClip was prepped in the standard fashion and was carefully advanced into the right atrium through the device deployment sheaths under fluoroscopy and TEE guidance. The steerable deployment sheath was manipulated to optimize the positioning of the device (Video 9). After careful optimization of positioning the device, the MitraClip was deployed under the fluoroscopy and TEE guidance (Fig. 3c–e).

Following the closure of the G4 XTR MitraClip in the septal, anterior position, TEE showed a well-seated clip and severe residual tricuspid regurgitation. The clip was successfully released in a standard fashion (Fig. 3f, g, Video 10).

Due to severe residual regurgitation, a second clip was deployed in the anterior septal position toward the commissure; there was no residual tricuspid regurgitation jet in the anterior septal position (Fig. 4a–d). However, there was a severe regurgitation jet in the septal posterior and center position of the valve due to a flail leaflet (Fig. 4e, f, Videos 11 and 12). Therefore, a third clip was prepped and advanced into the right atrium through the device deployment sheaths. While the third clip was being opened, the clip popped out of the delivery system due to a device malfunction (Fig. 5a, b).

At this point, the decision was made to snare the clip from the left femoral venous approach (Video 13). We advanced a 35 cm gooseneck snare and successfully snared the clip into the Gore seal sheath. The Gore dry seal sheath was then pulled back along with the clip toward the left femoral venous approach. We could pull out the sheath, but the clip was retained in the left femoral venous access site (Fig. 5c, d).

After reviewing the treatment options, we consulted a vascular surgeon to perform a surgical cutdown to the left femoral venous area and extract the retained

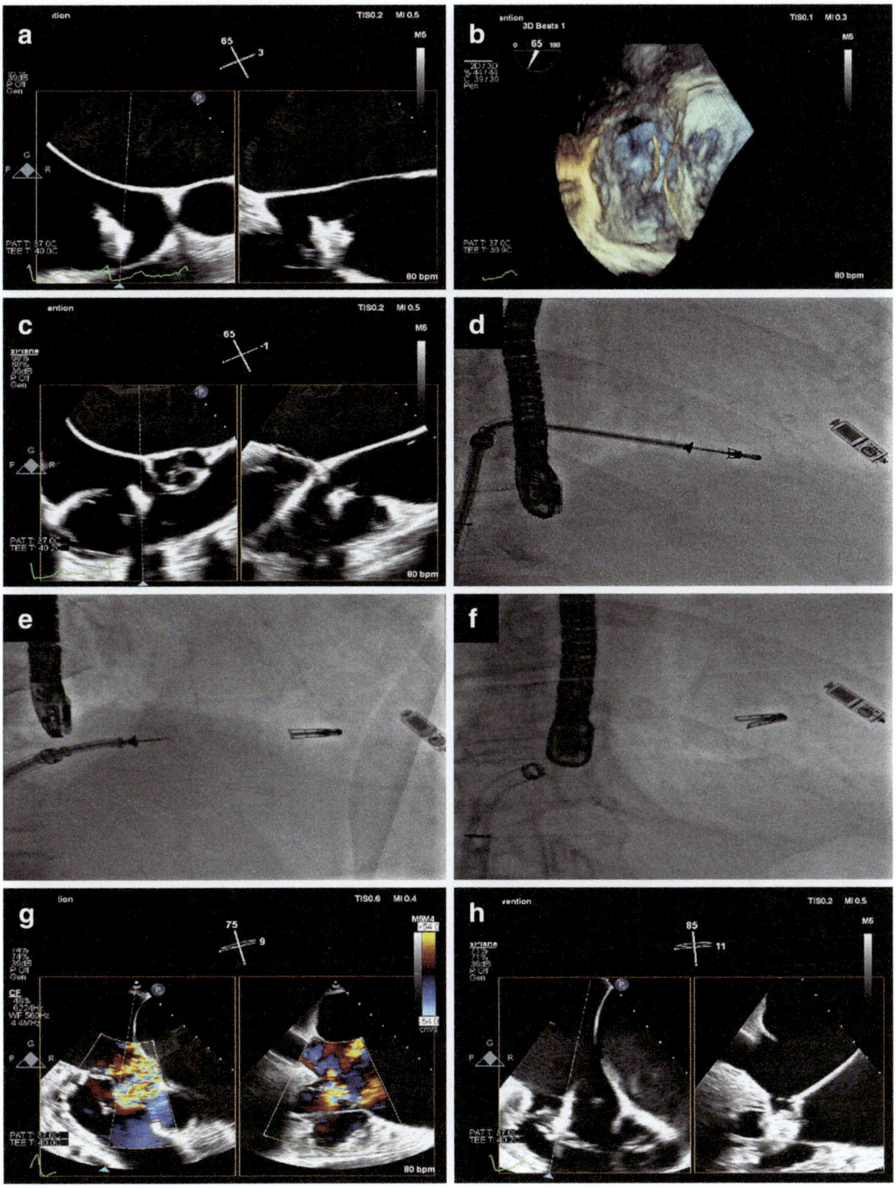

Fig. 3 Step-by-step edge-to-edge tricuspid repair using the MitraClip device system. (**a**) Long axis AV TEE view showing clip advanced to the right atrium. (**b**) Tricuspid valve 3D en face view of the delivery system in the right atrium. (**c**) Positioning the steerable device in the right atrium—TEE view. (**d**) Setting the steerable device in the right atrium—fluoroscopic view. (**e**) Detachment of the clip at the annular plane of the tricuspid valve. (**f**) Retrieval of the steerable delivery system. (**g**) Color doppler over the tricuspid valve indicates severe residual TR following the procedure. (**h**) Well seated clip with severe residual TR

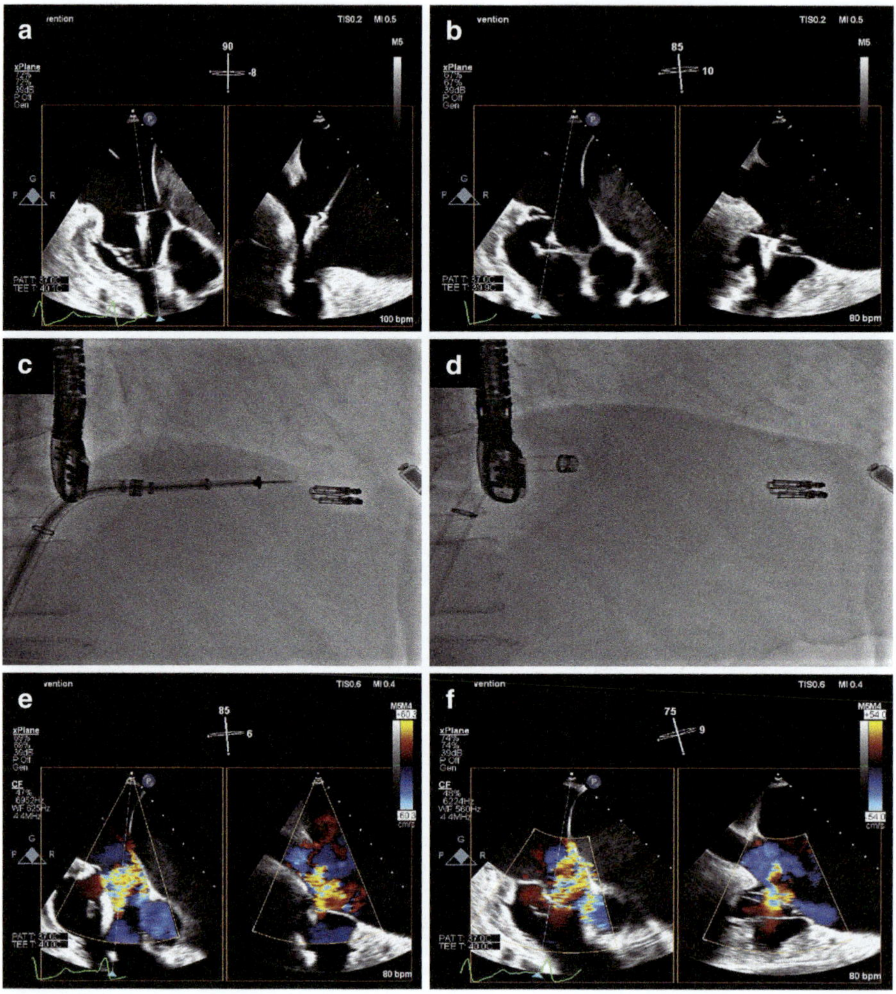

Fig. 4 Deployment of a second clip on the tricuspid valve. (**a**, **b**) Advancing the clip using the steerable delivery system and positioning it over the TV. (**c**) After careful optimization, the clip was deployed in the anterior septal position toward the commissure using the G4 XTR Mitra Clip steerable sheath. (**d**) Detachment of the clip and retrieval of the delivery system. (**e**, **f**) Residual TR in the septal posterior and the center of the valve due to flail leaflets

MitraClip device (Fig. 5e). Following removal of the MitraClip, the delivery sheath was removed from the right femoral venous access site, and hemostasis was achieved with the previously placed Perclose suture.

The patient, receiving aggressive diuresis, did well postoperatively. Post-op TTE revealed no changes in left ventricular ejection fraction and two MitraClips on the tricuspid valve with mild to moderate residual regurgitation (Video 14). She was

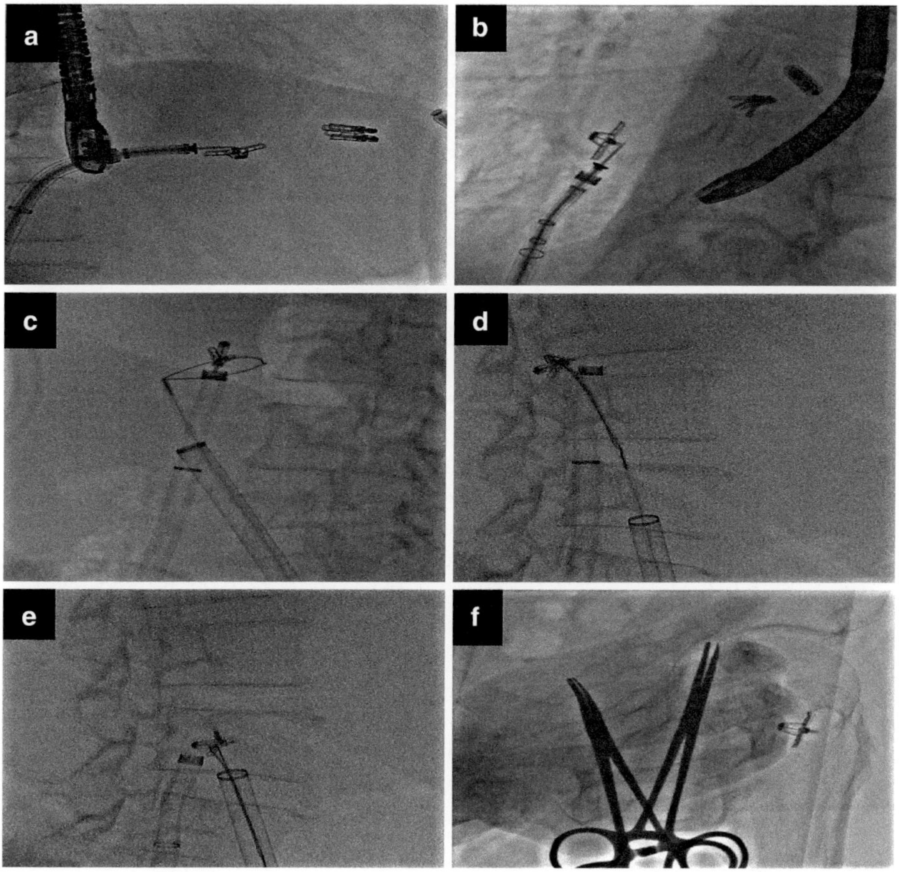

Fig. 5 Delivery system malfunction during the procedure. (**a**) Unintendedly opening of a third clip in the right atrium. (**b**) Attempts to retrieve the device failed. (**c**) The clip was successfully captured by a 35 cm gooseneck snare and advanced into the Gore seal sheath. (**d**, **e**) Failure to remove the clip and the sheath at the femoral vein level. (**f**) Surgical vascular cutdown was needed

stable and ambulating without shortness of breath on the day of discharge. On a 30-day post-discharge appointment, the patient endorsed feeling better since the procedure and improved to NYHA class I–II.

4 Discussion

Severe tricuspid regurgitation can be managed surgically at the same time as left-sided valve surgery or isolated in those with right-sided heart failure [1]. The use of a transcatheter device for those who are at high surgical risk is currently being evaluated for tricuspid treatment, and recent data indicates that procedural success rate were achieved in 62–81% of patients [2, 3]. The most common interventional technique used is the transcatheter tricuspid valve edge-to-edge repair (TTVR) with the MitraClip, as used in this case. The most recent development is the TriClip, shown in the TRILUMINATE trial, to treat symptomatic patients with moderate or greater tricuspid regurgitation who were deemed to be at high risk for surgery [4]. At 1 year, the tricuspid regurgitation of patients treated with the TriClip was reduced to moderate or less in 71% of subjects compared with 8% of patients at baseline [4]. All-cause mortality and overall major adverse event rates were 7.1% [4]. Thus far, there have been no case reports or literature showing delivery system malfunction during tricuspid repair; however, there have been reports of device malfunction using the MitraClip therapy for mitral valve repair [5]. Abbott recently recalled its XTR MitraClip in 2019, due to a physician error in proper device implantation that caused the clip to open unexpectedly due to excessive force during clip positioning, [6]. This recall status was terminated after the release of a new NTR MitraClip, which included more specific instructions for placement. In 2016, the FDA classified an Abbott recall as Class 1 due to unclear instructions, which lead to user error and to nine reports of malfunctions, as well as one death from the clip [7]. Another Class 1 device recall occurred in 2019 for Portico's Solo ReCollapsible Access System, whose tip had the potential of breaking off [8]. In 2015, Medtronic required Class 1 recall of its EnVeo R Loading System used during TAVR for eight reports of particulates in the system [9]. One case describes another very rare event in which placement of a third MitraClip resulted in its embolization from the anterior leaflet and lodged in her axilla, which was noticed 1 year after her procedure [10]. It is unclear to the authors of this case study whether this was due to operator error or a possible increased risk of clip detachment with multiple clips. Companies are constantly working to make devices more user-friendly and safer for their patients. Still, the cases described here serve an important role in educating physicians to prepare for all rare complications.

Key Points

- Device malfunction is a rare phenomenon in structural heart interventions, yet poses a serious complication and requires challenging solutions.
- There is no way to anticipate device malfunction.
- The operator should be aware of the possibility of device malfunction and be familiar with techniques to overcome it.

References

1. Otto CM, Nishimura RA, Bonow RO, Carabello BA, Erwin JP III, Gentile F, Jneid H, Krieger EV, Mack M, McLeod C, O'Gara PT. 2020 ACC/AHA guideline for the management of patients with valvular heart disease: executive summary: a report of the American College of

Cardiology/American Heart Association Joint Committee on Clinical Practice Guidelines. J Am Coll Cardiol. 2021;77(4):450–500.
2. Besler C, Orban M, Rommel KP, Braun D, Patel M, Hagl C, Borger M, Nabauer M, Massberg S, Thiele H, Hausleiter J. Predictors of procedural and clinical outcomes in patients with symptomatic tricuspid regurgitation undergoing transcatheter edge-to-edge repair. J Am Coll Cardiol Interv. 2018;11(12):1119–28.
3. Taramasso M, Hahn RT, Alessandrini H, Latib A, Attinger-Toller A, Braun D, Brochet E, Connelly KA, Denti P, Deuschl F, Englmaier A. The International Multicenter TriValve Registry: which patients are undergoing transcatheter tricuspid repair? J Am Coll Cardiol Interv. 2017;10(19):1982–90.
4. Lurz P, von Bardeleben RS, Weber M, Sitges M, Sorajja P, Hausleiter J, Denti P, Trochu JN, Nabauer M, Tang GH, Biaggi P. Transcatheter edge-to-edge repair for treatment of tricuspid regurgitation. J Am Coll Cardiol. 2021;77(3):229–39.
5. Mkalaluh S, Szczechowicz M, Karck M, Weymann A. Failed MitraClip therapy: surgical revision in high-risk patients. J Cardiothorac Surg. 2019;14(1):1–4.
6. Class 2 device recall Abbott MitraClip XTR clip delivery system [Internet]. accessdata.fda.gov. https://www.accessdata.fda.gov/scripts/cdrh/cfdocs/cfRes/res.cfm?ID=172622.
7. Jibrell A. Abbott's clip delivery system recall deemed class 1 [Internet]. FDAnews 2016. https://www.fdanews.com/articles/175783-abbotts-clip-delivery-system-recall-deemed-class-1.
8. Class 1 Device Recall Portico Solo ReCollapsible Access System [Internet]. accessdata.fda.gov. https://www.accessdata.fda.gov/scripts/cdrh/cfdocs/cfRes/res.cfm?ID=172423.
9. Class 1 Device Recall Medtronic EnVeo R Loading System [Internet]. accessdata.fda.gov. https://www.accessdata.fda.gov/scripts/cdrh/cfdocs/cfres/res.cfm?id=138827.
10. Bilge M, Alsancak Y, Ali S, Duran M, Biçer H. An extremely rare but possible complication of MitraClip: embolization of clip during follow-up. Anatol J Cardiol. 2016;16(8):636.

TMVR Valve Dislodgement

Vivek Patel, Daniel Zumerkorn Hassan, and Muhammad Zubair

1 Clinical Background

The patient is an 85-year-old male with a history of stage-III chronic kidney disease, aortic stenosis status post TAVR using 29-mm PORTICO valve, chronic atrial fibrillation/flutter on warfarin, status post pacemaker implantation, coronary artery disease status, coronary artery bypass grafting, hypertension, hyperlipidemia, chronic diastolic heart failure (NYHA Class IV), abdominal aortic aneurysm status post endovascular aneurysm repair, and chronic myelomonocytic leukemia. He comes to the clinic for evaluation and possible repair of the mitral valve. The patient's main complaint is shortness of breath at rest and minimal exertion over the past six months. Also, during this period, he was admitted several times for hypoxia and acute decompensated heart failure in the setting of worsening known mitral valve stenosis and regurgitation.

Supplementary Information The online version contains supplementary material available at [https://doi.org/10.1007/978-3-031-05965-0_30].

V. Patel (✉)
Smidt Heart Institute, Cedars-Sinai Medical Center, Los Angeles, CA, USA
e-mail: vivek.patel@cshs.org

D. Zumerkorn Hassan
Interventional Cardiology, Cedars-Sinai Medical Center, Los Angeles, CA, USA

M. Zubair
Cedars Sinai Medical Center, Los Angeles, CA, USA

O. Koren et al. (eds.), *Complex Cases in Structural Heart Intervention*,
https://doi.org/10.1007/978-3-031-05965-0_30

2 Imaging

Workup included TEE demonstrating normal left ventricular systolic function. It was also remarkable for severe, eccentric, and posteriorly directed mitral valve regurgitation associated with a vena contracta of 0.8 and pulmonary vein systolic flow reversal (Videos 1, 2 and 3). Additionally, the mitral apparatus contained severe annular calcification with restricted coaptation of the posterior leaflets and moderate mitral stenosis (mitral valve area 1.8–1.9 cm^2, mean transmitral gradient 3 mmHg, peak transmitral gradient 10 mmHg). A bioprosthetic valve was present in the aortic position and demonstrated normal leaflet motion and no paravalvular aortic regurgitation. Pre-procedural TTE confirmed these findings (Fig. 1). Cardiac reconstructed CT showed a mitral annular area of 7.2 cm^2 and a perimeter of 71 mm (Fig. 2). The following distances were also measured: the anterior to posterior leaflet was 24.3 mm, between the commissures was 37.6 mm, and trigone to trigone was 30.3 mm. In addition, the neo-left-ventricular outflow tract (neo-LVOT) was analyzed as part of the feasibility assessment for transcatheter mitral valve replacement (TMVR) as LVOT obstruction remains a primary concern in this procedure. The NEO LVOT was measured to have a perimeter of 132.4 mm and an area of 366.0 mm^2. The optimal deployment angle was estimated at RAO 36° and Caudal 31° (Fig. 3).

3 Pre-Procedural Considerations, Dilemmas, and Challenges

The patient was evaluated by cardiothoracic (CT) surgery and deemed a high-risk, inoperable surgical candidate. The patient, therefore, underwent transseptal mitral valve replacement using a 29-mm Edward Sapien S3 bioprosthesis.

4 Procedure, Outcome, and Follow-Up

The atrial septal puncture was performed under fluoroscopy and TEE guidance. After achieving right femoral venous access, a regular 0.032-in. guidewire was advanced into the superior vena cava, and the transseptal sheath was passed through an 11F sheath. An 18-G puncture needle was advanced into the introducer with the tip inside the guiding sheath. Under TEE and fluoroscopic guidance, the sheath was slowly and carefully pulled back into the right atrium. We repeated the procedure several times until we identified an optimal site of septal puncture at the midportion and slightly posterior aspect of the right atrium into the left atrium (Fig. 3a–c).

The sheath was then advanced into the left atrium. At this point, the patient was anticoagulated with heparin, and activated clotting time was then intermittently monitored and maintained in the therapeutic range. Then this sheath was exchanged

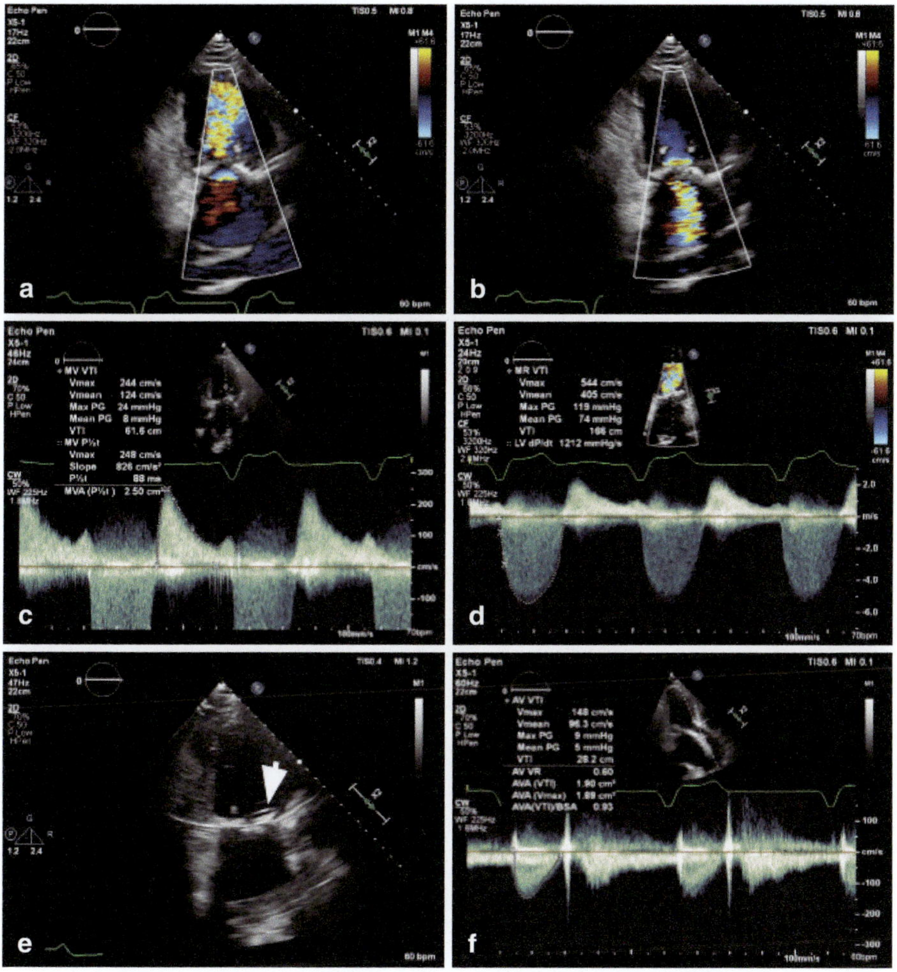

Fig. 1 Pre-procedural TTE images across the mitral and aortic valves. (**a**) Color Doppler over the mitral valve during diastole indicates moderate mitral stenosis. (**b**) Color Doppler over the mitral valve during systole indicates severe mitral regurgitation. (**c**) Flow velocity and pressure gradient over the mitral valve. (**d**) Continuous-wave Doppler spectral recording showing a VTI of 166 cm consistent with severe MR. (**e**) Severe mitral Annular calcification (white arrow). (**f**) The mean transaortic gradient of 8 mmHg was measured across the transcatheter valve

for the 8.5 Agilis catheter over a Protrak wire. The Agilis dilator and wire were removed, and the catheter was directed down to the mitral valve. A long 6F pigtail catheter was used to cross the mitral valve, which was exchanged for a Safari wire and positioned in the left ventricular apex. An atrial balloon septoplasty was then performed using a 14-mm × 4.0-cm balloon. The balloon and Agilis catheter were removed, and an Edwards 16F Sheath was introduced over this wire. The Edwards 29-mm S3 valve was then advanced over the wire and positioned across the mitral

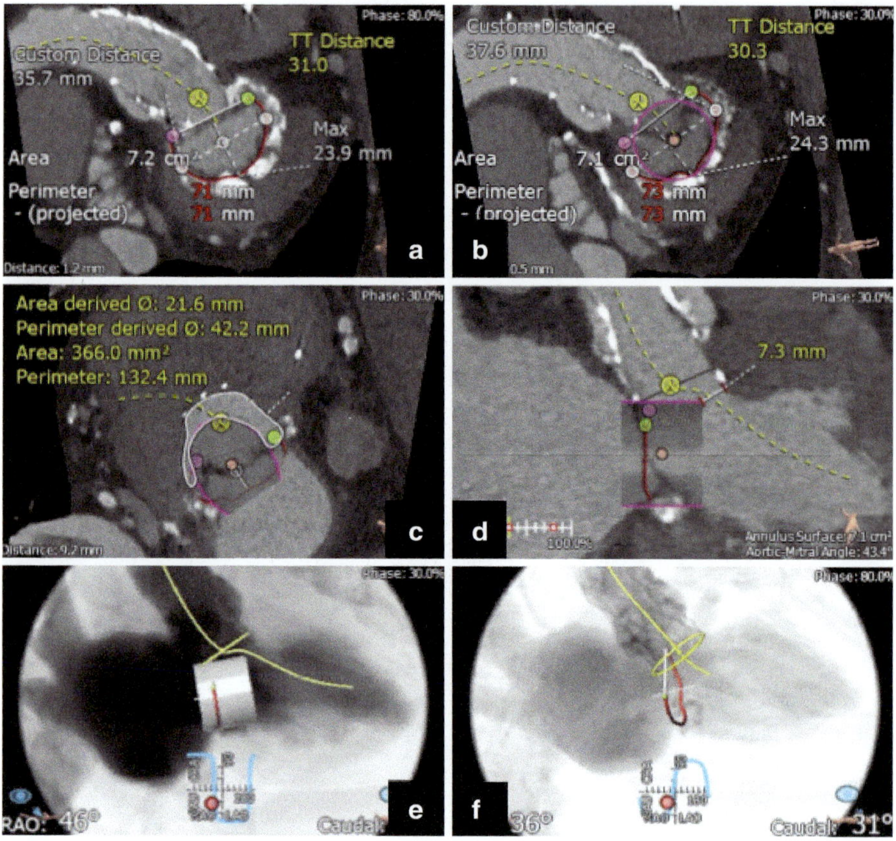

Fig. 2 Reconstructed cardiac CT analysis of the mitral valve and the neo-LVOT area. (**a**) Mitral valve annulus dimensions. (**b**) The position and dimension of a virtual Sapien-3 valve placed at mitral valve annulus. (**c**) The expected neo-LVOT area following deployment of 29 mm Sapien-3. (**d**) The diameter at the narrowest place from the valve and the LVOT. (**e**) Angiographic view of the neo-LVOT following 29 mm Sapien-3 valve deployment. (**f**) Deployment angle

valve in standard fashion with +5 cc (Fig. 3d, Video 4). Positioning was ascertained mainly by TEE guidance as fluoroscopic guidance showed calcification predominately below the annulus. During rapid pacing, it was then deployed (Fig. 4a, b).

A post-procedure TEE revealed a mild paravalvular leak. As the patient's blood pressure improved, the 29 mm S3 valve embolized into the left atrium (Fig. 3e–i, Videos 5, 6, 7 and 8). Our safari wire was still through the valve. We placed an Agilis catheter over an MPA2 which secured the valve. We then placed a second transseptal system, which happened to pass through the first transseptal puncture. We used the Agilis, a 6F JR4 diagnostic catheter, and a 260 cm stiff Terumo angled glidewire to cross the valve. We then removed the Agilis and diagnostic catheter. A 25 mm Amplatzer PFO occluder was advanced over a 10F Torqvue delivery system and attempted to pin the valve against the wall of the interatrial septum. However,

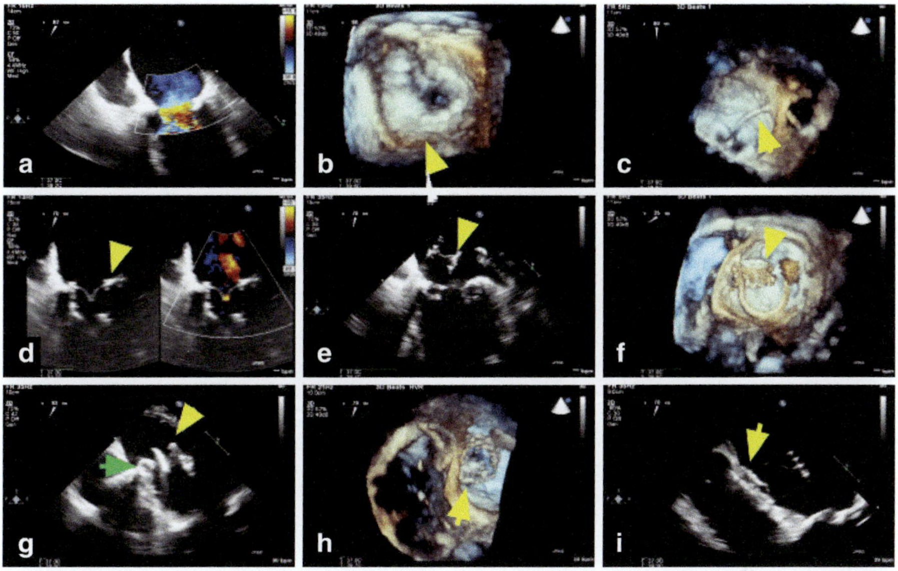

Fig. 3 TEE images of the TMVR during valve deployment, valve embolization, and treatment. (**a**) Color Doppler over the mitral valve indicates moderate to severe mitral stenosis. (**b**) En face 3D view of the MV showing severe mitral valve calcification, especially on the posterior segment (yellow arrow). (**c**) Sheath was advanced through the puncture site at the midportion and posterior aspect of the RA into the LA (yellow arrow). (**d**) The Sapien-3 valve can be seen in the mitral position (yellow arrow). (**e**) Sapien-3 valve can be seen floating in LA (yellow arrow). (**f**) Sapien-3 balloon-expandable valve was secured through Agilis catheter in Left Atrium (yellow arrow). (**g**) 25 mm Amplatzer patent foramen ovale (PFO) occluder was advanced over a guide crossing the THV struts (green arrow). (**h**) Successful deployment of PFO occluder over the Sapien-3 valve struts (yellow arrow). (**i**) Sapien-3 valve was pinned against the intertrial septum (yellow arrow)

it was unsuccessful as we had not crossed a stent strut (Video 9). The occluder was removed along with the first Agilis catheter. We again used an Agilis, a 6F JR4 diagnostic catheter, and a 260 cm stiff Terumo angled glidewire to cross a stent strut successfully. The 25 mm Amplatzer PFO occluder over a 10F Torqvue delivery system was advanced through the Agilis and was successfully deployed, pinning the Sapien valve against the interatrial septum (Fig. 3e, f, Videos 10, 11 and 12). After confirming stability, the Amplatzer was deployed (Fig. 4c–f, Video 13). We elected not to place another valve as the mitral annular calcification was not robust enough to hold the valve. A post-procedural TTE revealed the Sapien valve to be securely pinned to the interatrial septum in the left atrium (Fig. 5, Videos 14 and 15). After a comprehensive evaluation of the patient's surgical risk, the heart team decided that surgical extraction of the device and replacing the mitral valve would be too risky. We decided to initiate anticoagulation due to the high risk of developing stroke and the low bleeding risk. The patient died several days following the procedure.

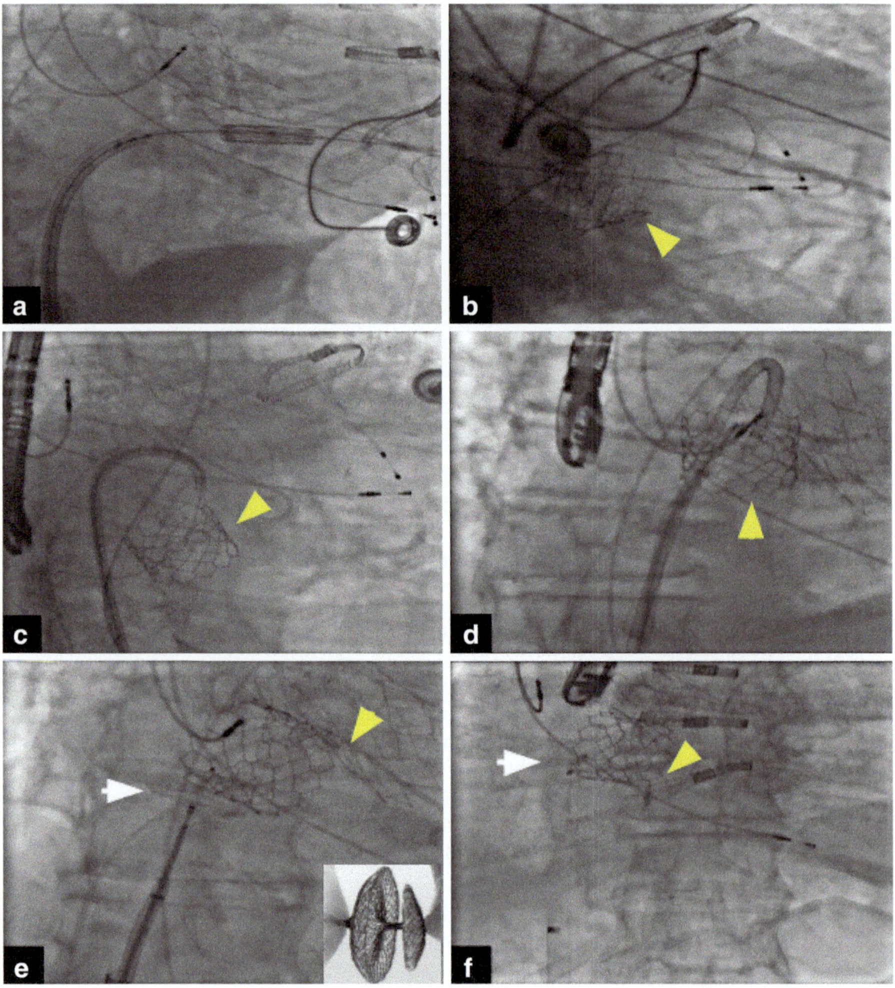

Fig. 4 Procedural fluoroscopic view of TMVR using balloon-expandable valve. (**a**) Transcatheter Sapien-3 valve was advanced across the mitral valve annulus. (**b**) The valve was positioned and deployed over the native mitral valve. (**c**) Sapien-3 displaced and floated free in the left atrium. (**d**) 260 cm stiff Terumo angled glidewire was successfully crossed over Sapien-3 valve stent strut. (**e**) 25 mm Amplatzer PFO occluder (lower right image) was delivered through a 10F Torqvue delivery system (white arrow) across Sapien-3 valve stent strut (yellow arrow). (**f**) Sapien-3 valve (yellow arrow) can be seen stable by the deployment of Amplatzer PFO occlude (white arrow) against the interatrial septum

5 Discussion

Severe mitral annular calcification (MAC) causing mitral valve dysfunction is often found in elderly patients having several cardiovascular comorbidities. The high surgical risk in this patient population presents a unique challenge in terms of

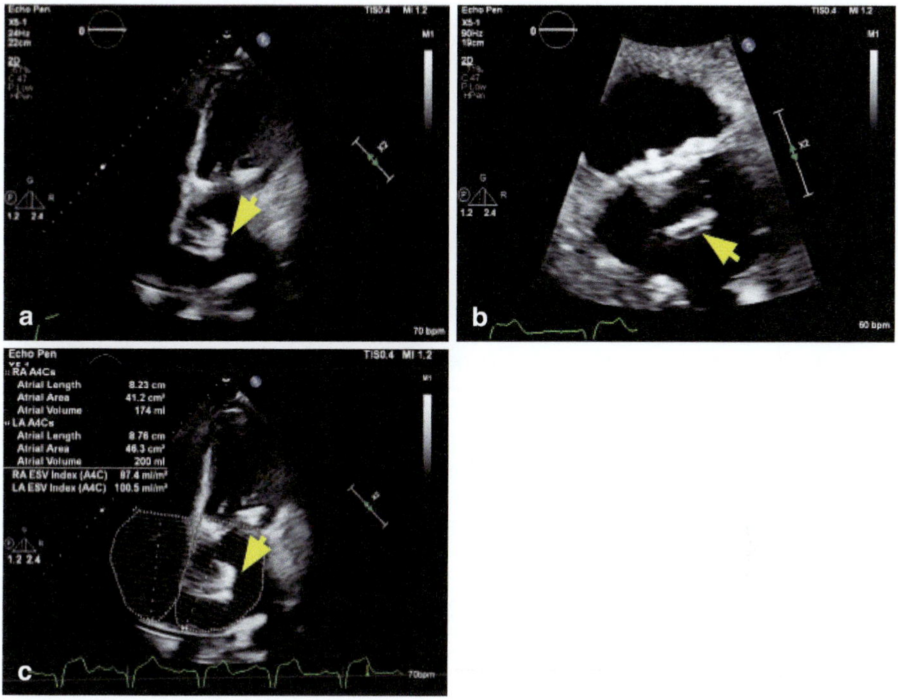

Fig. 5 Post-procedural TTE of the embolized valve anchored to the left atrium. (**a**) Sapien-3 valve well anchored in the left atrium (yellow arrow). (**b**) Sapien-3 valve is pinned across the intra-atrial septum between the right and left. (**c**) Right and left atria dimensions

acceptable mechanical interventions [1, 2]. TMVR, or transcatheter mitral valve replacement, is a relatively new therapy choice that minimizes the invasive measures of conventional surgery [3, 4]. TMVR had an overall 72% procedural success in extremely high-risk surgical patients in one large multicenter study, as defined by the Mitral Valve Academic Research Consortium (MVARC) [5]. However, despite its feasibility, serious complications may still arise. These include dissection at entry sites, left ventricular outflow tract obstruction, and valve embolization [6]. Significant factors contributing to valve embolization are directly related to THV sizing and require two main considerations. First, the valve must be properly anchored in the annulus, especially in the case of MAC. Secondly, a small neo-LVOT area (<200 mm^2) may be associated with a high risk for LVOT obstruction and high regurgitation flow. Therefore, if the annulus dimension is suitable for two THV sizes, choosing the valve according to the estimated neo-LVOT could serve a better outcome. Valve embolization was reported in 6% of cases [5]. Operator responses to embolization included surgical extraction in three cases and occluder device stabilization in one case [7]. In the latter case, surgical extraction was not performed, given the patient's high surgical risk. The patient died three weeks later. Therefore, as demonstrated in this report, it seems that the percutaneous bailout technique is a bridging therapy.

Key Points

- Transcatheter mitral valve dislodgment is a devastating complication that requires, in most cases, surgical extraction.
- The percutaneous bailout technique may serve as a bridge solution and an urgent open surgery alternative.
- Operators should be familiar with the technique and the complications involved.

References

1. Fox CS, Vasan RS, Parise H, Levy D, O'Donnell CJ, D'Agostino RB, Benjamin EJ. Mitral annular calcification predicts cardiovascular morbidity and mortality: the Framingham Heart Study. Circulation. 2003;107(11):1492–6.
2. Fox CS, Larson MG, Vasan RS, Guo CY, Parise H, Levy D, Leip EP, O'Donnell CJ, D'Agostino RB, Benjamin EJ. Cross-sectional association of kidney functions with valvular and annular calcification: the Framingham Heart Study. J Am Soc Nephrol. 2006;17(2):521–7.
3. Hasan R, Mahadevan VS, Schneider H, Clarke B. First in human transapical implantation of an inverted transcatheter aortic valve prosthesis to treat native mitral valve stenosis. Circulation. 2013;128(6):e74–6.
4. Himbert D, Bouleti C, Iung B, Nejjari M, Brochet E, Depoix JP, Ghodbane W, Fassa AA, Nataf P, Vahanian A. Transcatheter valve replacement in patients with severe mitral valve disease and annular calcification. J Am Coll Cardiol. 2014;64(23):2557–8.
5. Stone GW, Vahanian AS, Adams DH, Abraham WT, Borer JS, Bax JJ, Schofer J, Cutlip DE, Krucoff MW, Blackstone EH, Généreux P. Clinical trial design principles and endpoint definitions for transcatheter mitral valve repair and replacement. Part 1: Clinical trial design principles: a consensus document from the mitral valve academic research consortium. Eur Heart J. 2015;36(29):1851–77.
6. Sinning JM, Mellert F, Schiller W, Welz A, Nickenig G, Hammerstingl C. Transcatheter mitral valve replacement using a balloon-expandable prosthesis in a patient with calcified native mitral valve stenosis. Eur Heart J. 2013;34(33):2609.
7. Guerrero M, Wang DD, O'Neill W. Percutaneous rescue of an embolized valve after transcatheter mitral valve replacement. JACC Cardiovasc Interv. 2017;10(6):627–9.

Multiple Edge-to-Edge Percutaneous Repairs for Severe Mitral and Tricuspid Regurgitation

Ofir Koren, Troy Sanders, and Mohamed Hassanein

1 Clinical Presentation

The patient is an 83-year-old female with end-stage renal disease treated on dialysis, ischemic heart disease status post coronary artery bypass grafting (saphenous venous graft to the right coronary, left anterior descending, diagonal, and obtuse marginal), status post automatic implantable cardiac defibrillator placement, heart failure with reduced ejection fraction (NYHA Class III–IV, LVEF 35%), and severe mitral and tricuspid regurgitation. She previously had a MitraClip procedure for both the mitral and tricuspid valve due to prohibitive high mortality risk for cardiac surgery.

The patient has been experiencing worsening heart failure symptoms and was referred to our center for a redo percutaneous repair of both valves using the MitraClip device. Furthermore, the iatrogenic atrial septal defect that facilitated the first MitraClip procedure resulted in a bidirectional shunt with intermittent hypoxia.

Supplementary Information The online version contains supplementary material available at [https://doi.org/10.1007/978-3-031-05965-0_31].

O. Koren (✉)
Smidt Heart Institute, Cedars-Sinai Medical Center, Los Angeles, CA, USA

Faculty of Medicine, Technion, Israel Institute of Technology, Haifa, Israel
e-mail: Ofir.Koren@cshs.org

T. Sanders
David Geffen School of Medicine, University of California, Los Angeles, CA, USA

M. Hassanein
Cedars Sinai Medical Center, Los Angeles, CA, USA

O. Koren et al. (eds.), *Complex Cases in Structural Heart Intervention*,
https://doi.org/10.1007/978-3-031-05965-0_31

2 Images and Supported Data

Baseline TEE before the intervention revealed severe mitral and tricuspid regurgitation as well as moderately depressed left and right ventricular function (Fig. 1, Video 1). TEE following the first percutaneous mitral valve repair demonstrated two MitraClips deployed successfully in P3 and A3 segments with residual moderate mitral regurgitation (Fig. 2, Video 2). TEE illustrated two MitraClips on the septal and anterior leaflets with mild to moderate residual regurgitation (Fig. 3, Video 3). In addition, there was mild to moderate mitral regurgitation.

TEE before the third percutaneous procedure revealed moderately depressed left ventricular systolic function. The mitral valve showed moderate regurgitation, two MitraClips positioned on the anterior and posterior leaflets, and multiple regurgitant jets surrounding and between the clips. The tricuspid valve demonstrated severe regurgitation and the presence of two MitraClips on the tricuspid leaflets (Fig. 4). Additionally, there was an atrial septal defect with bidirectional shunting (Video 4).

3 Procedure and Outcome

The NT MitraClip was prepped in the standard fashion and advanced into the left atrium through the device deployment sheaths under fluoroscopy and TEE guidance. The steerable deployment sheath was manipulated to optimize the positioning of the device lateral to the previously deployed clips. After careful optimization, the clip was deployed to the A2-P2 leaflets under fluoroscopic and TEE guidance. Following the closure of the MitraClip, TEE showed a well-seated clip and traced mitral regurgitation (Fig. 5e, f, Video 5).

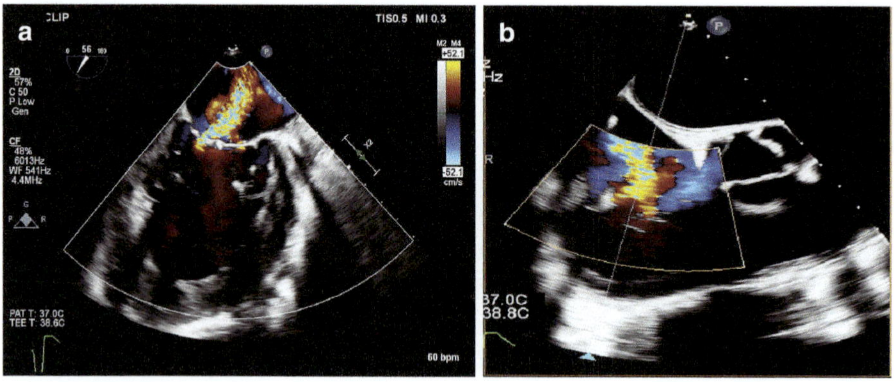

Fig. 1 Significant mitral and tricuspid regurgitation on ME two-chamber TEE view (**a**) and ME AV short axis view (**b**)

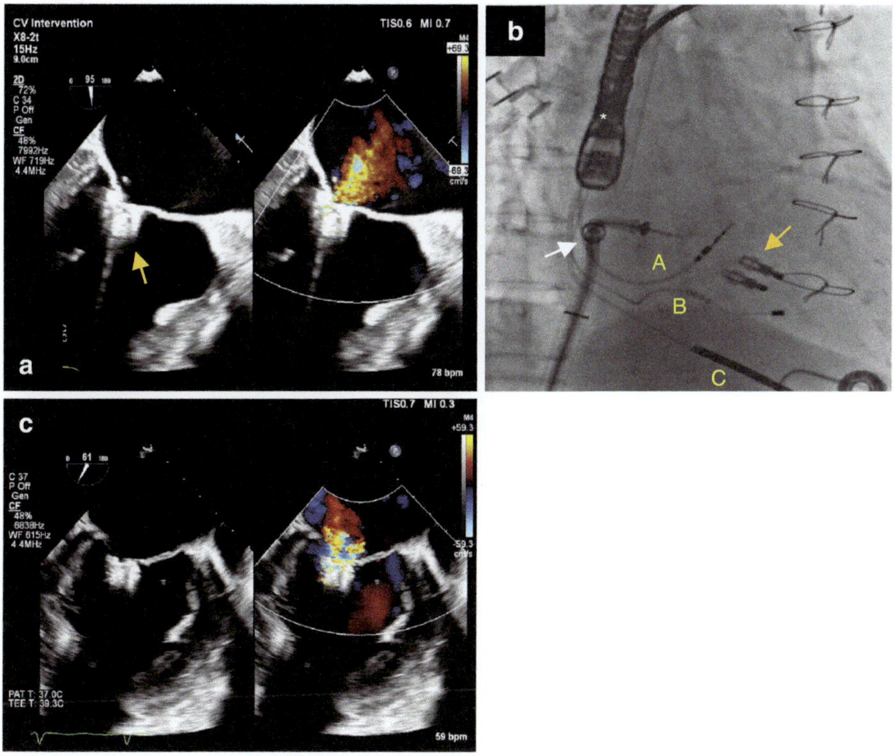

Fig. 2 Percutaneous edge-to-edge mitral valve repair. (**a**) Two MitraClips are attached to the P3 and the A3 segments of the mitral valve (yellow arrow)—TEE view. (**b**) MitraClip delivery system (white arrow) advanced via the interatrial septum using TEE (white asterisk). Note the previous clips over the MV (yellow arrow) and the ICD leads located on the right atrium (A), the right ventricle (B), and the left ventricles (C). (**c**) Color Doppler over the mitral valve indicates a reduction in the MV regurgitation flow following the MitraClip repair

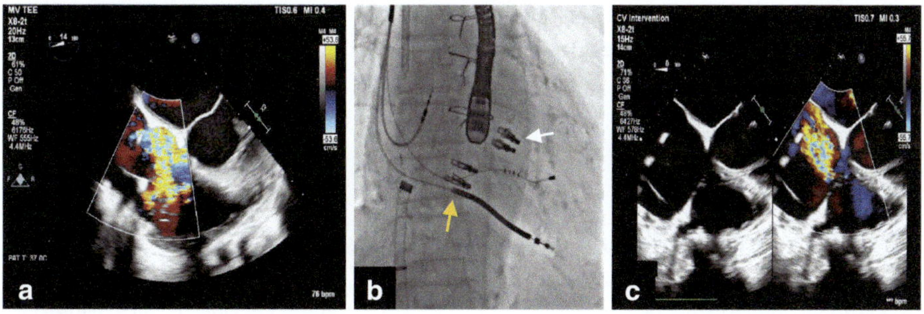

Fig. 3 Percutaneous edge-to-edge tricuspid repair. (**a**) Color Doppler over the tricuspid valve indicates severe TR. (**b**) Two MitraClips are attached to the septal and the anterior leaflets (yellow arrow), with two previously attached MitraClips on the mitral valve (white arrow). (**c**) Modest reduction in the regurgitation flow

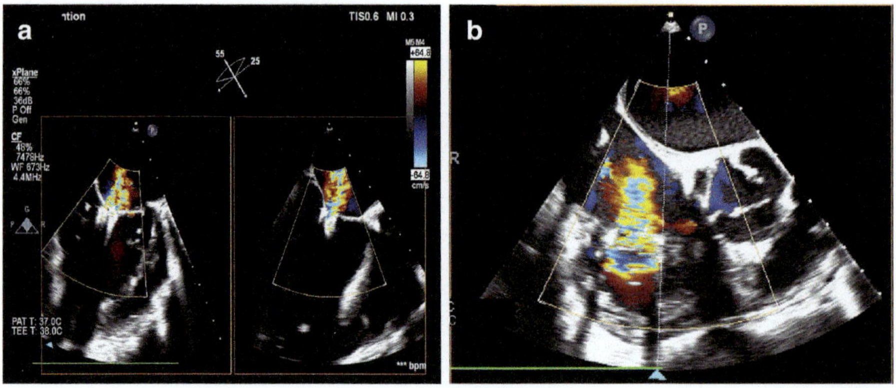

Fig. 4 Post-edge-to-edge mitral and tricuspid repair echocardiography. (**a**) Color Doppler over the mitral valve indicates residual moderate mitral regurgitation. (**b**) Color Doppler over the tricuspid valve shows severe tricuspid regurgitation

Next, an XTW clip was prepped in the standard fashion and carefully advanced into the right atrium through the device deployment sheaths under fluoroscopic and TEE guidance. The clip was deployed to the septal-anterior leaflets, and subsequent TEE showed a well-seated clip despite moderate-to-severe tricuspid regurgitation. The clip was successfully released in the standard fashion, and the delivery system was withdrawn. Due to significant residual tricuspid regurgitation, we proceeded with another clip to the septal-anterior leaflets (Fig. 5a). Following closure, TEE showed a well-seated second clip and moderate tricuspid regurgitation (Fig. 5c, d).

The iatrogenic ASD demonstrated bidirectional shunting with a positive bubble test. We attempted to close the defect with a 30 mm Gore Cardioform occluder device. The ASD was crossed with a diagnostic MPA catheter and a standard J-wire. A super-stiff wire was placed in the left upper pulmonary vein. The occluder device was prepped and advanced through the sheath and over the super-stiff wire. Under TEE and fluoroscopic guidance, the septal occluder device was successfully deployed in the standard fashion (Fig. 5b, Video 6).

The patient had no immediate complications following the procedure.

4 Discussion

Chronic secondary MR is a well-established cause of worsening heart failure symptoms. When considering a patient's chronic MR, a TTE should be the physician's first step to determine MR mechanism and severity. Severe secondary MR is defined as an ERO $\geq$40 mm^2, but outcomes are worse than those without, even in those with a moderate MR of ERO $\geq$20 mm^2 [1].

Patients with severe secondary MR refractory to medical treatment should be considered (if anatomic and morphologically appropriate) for percutaneous intervention. TEE's utilization during mitral clip placement is an essential key to guide

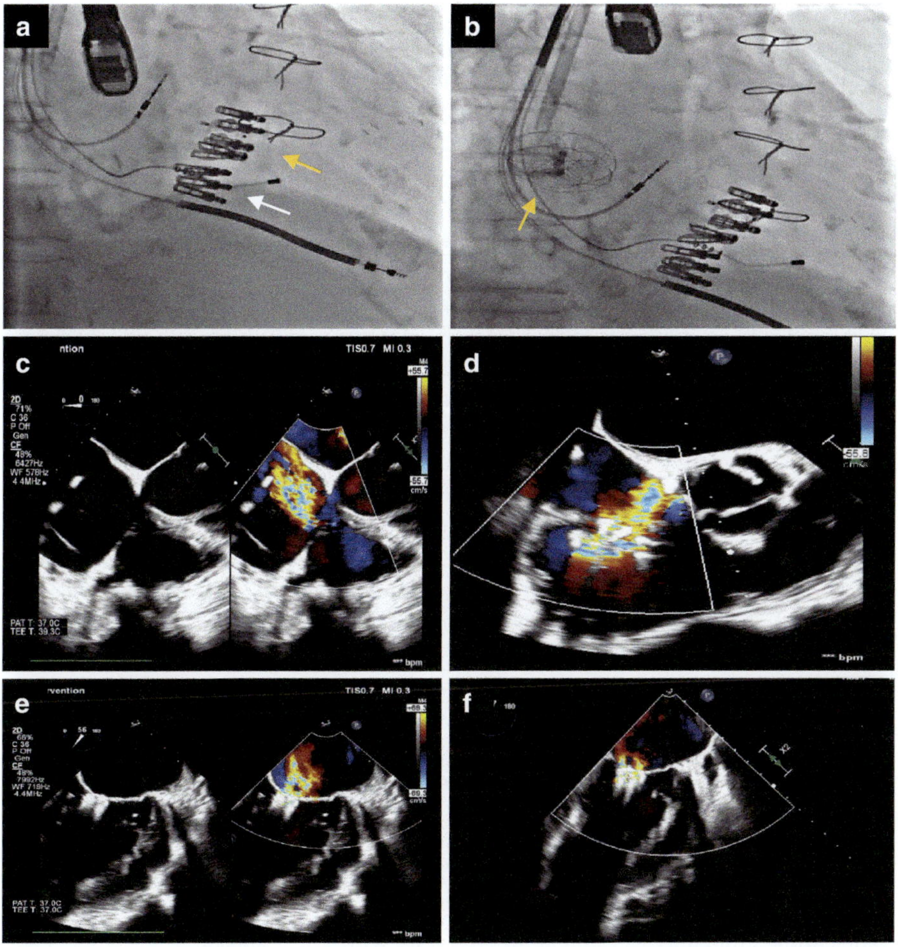

Fig. 5 Mitral valve repair using the MitraClip and APV II vascular plug devices. (**a**) Multiple clips and AVP II devices deployed to the A2-P2 leaflets (yellow arrow) and two MitraClips XTW deployed to the septal-anterior leaflets of the tricuspid valve (white arrow). (**b**) Fluoroscopic view of iatrogenic atrial septal defect closure device using the Gore Cardioform 30 mm device (yellow arrow). (**c**) Color Doppler over the tricuspid valve before the procedure. (**d**) Color Doppler over the tricuspid valve following the procedure. (**e**) Color Doppler over the mitral valve before the procedure. (**f**) Color Doppler over the mitral valve following the procedure

clip positioning, determining MR reduction, determining the necessity of multiple clips, and elucidating clip-induced MS. The AHA inclusion criteria for TEER include LVEF between 20–50%, LVESD ≤70 mm, and pulmonary artery systolic pressure ≤70 mm Hg. Both the COAPT and the EVEREST trials demonstrated similar exclusion criteria which the AHA has adopted for transcatheter mitral valve interventions, including evidence of calcification in grasping area of A2 or P2 scallops, presence of a significant cleft of A2 or P2 scallops, lack of primary and secondary chordal support, and vertical coaptation length <2 mm in valves with leaflet tethering [2 , 3]. The COAPT trial showed that TEER status post-medical treatment optimization improved survival, symptoms, hospitalization, and QOL for secondary MR patients compared to the conservative therapy arm [2]. For those patients who fall into Stages C and D for severe secondary MR, mitral valve surgery is reasonable according to AHA guidelines. At the same time, CABG intervention is ongoing for myocardial ischemia. Mitral valve surgery should also be considered for patients with chronic secondary MR due to atrial annular dilation with LVEF ≥50% with persistent NYHA class III or IV symptoms despite appropriate HF and associated AF therapies [4]. AHA notes that chordal-sparing mitral valve replacement may be a more appropriate option for chronic severe secondary MR with LVEF <50% who have persistent severe NYHA class III or IV symptoms while on optimal GDMT for HF (Stage D) [5].

While no defined features indicate the need for multiple mitral clip implantation, clinicians should be prepared for multiple clip installations if one mitral clip does not adequately reduce MR. Concerns have been raised about the possibility of multiple clips increasing the probability of elevated mitral valve gradient. In the EVEREST II randomized trial, 42% of patients were treated with two MitraClips. It demonstrated that a more severe MR is a good predictor of the necessity of >1 MitraClip [6]. A similar result of 37% was found in the ACCESS EU registry [7]. It has been shown in clinical trials that the necessity of multiple clips is equally safe and effective if >1 MitraClip is required for MR treatment [8]. Another study showed no independent correlation between clips number and postoperative MV orifice area or MV pressure gradient [9]. Studies have attempted to define the criteria for the necessity of using multiple clips. One study showed that multiple clips on a mitral valve should be indicated for patients with a wide regurgitant jet on TEE (≥7.5 mm of vena contracta) [10].

Treating both TR and MR simultaneously is a highly controversial debate. Concomitant TR is a common comorbidity in patients requiring MV surgery (MVS). Worldwide, the frequency of concomitant TR and MVS ranges from 7% to 65%. While some clinicians would tend to intervene with TR alongside MVS when TR is severe (grade III/IV) or rapidly progressive, others take a more aggressive approach and treat the TR during MVS given the increased morbidity and mortality of TVS status post-MVS. One meta-analysis found no difference in late or 30-day mortality between patients with tricuspid valve repair during MVS and those with only MVS [11]. A retrospective analysis of 1357 patients looking at long-term outcomes of concomitant TV repair in patients undergoing MVS showed no difference in death rates within 30 days, stroke, MI, or repeat MVS in those with or without concomitant TV repair [12]. It is important to note that simultaneous TV repair is a lengthy procedure with a higher probability of complications. The combined procedure should be planned carefully and discussed in a multi-disciplinary fashion with the patient.

Key Points

- Transcatheter edge-to-edge mitral valve repair with MitraClip is a safe and efficient therapy for selected patients with good anatomical criteria.

- The good results and the technology from the MitraClip extend to treating patients with severe TR.
- As presented in our case, combined mitral and tricuspid intervention is feasible. The operator should be familiar with the pros and cons of the procedure.

References

1. Zoghbi WA, Adams D, Bonow RO, Enriquez-Sarano M, Foster E, Grayburn PA, Hahn RT, Han Y, Hung J, Lang RM, Little SH. Recommendations for noninvasive evaluation of native valvular regurgitation: a report from the American Society of Echocardiography developed in collaboration with the Society for Cardiovascular Magnetic Resonance. J Am Soc Echocardiogr. 2017;30(4):303–71.
2. Stone GW, Lindenfeld J, Abraham WT, Kar S, Lim DS, Mishell JM, Whisenant B, Grayburn PA, Rinaldi M, Kapadia SR, Rajagopal V. Transcatheter mitral-valve repair in patients with heart failure. N Engl J Med. 2018;379(24):2307–18.
3. Feldman T, Wasserman HS, Herrmann HC, Gray W, Block PC, Whitlow P, St. Goar F, Rodriguez L, Silvestry F, Schwartz A, Sanborn TA. Percutaneous mitral valve repair using the edge-to-edge technique: six-month results of the EVEREST Phase I Clinical Trial. J Am Coll Cardiol. 2005;46(11):2134–40.
4. Velazquez EJ, Lee KL, Deja MA, Jain A, Sopko G, Marchenko A, Ali IS, Pohost G, Gradinac S, Abraham WT, Yii M. Coronary-artery bypass surgery in patients with left ventricular dysfunction. N Engl J Med. 2011;364(17):1607–16.
5. Otto CM, Nishimura RA, Bonow RO, Carabello BA, Erwin JP III, Gentile F, Jneid H, Krieger EV, Mack M, McLeod C, O'Gara PT. 2020 ACC/AHA guideline for the management of patients with valvular heart disease: executive summary: a report of the American College of Cardiology/American Heart Association Joint Committee on Clinical Practice Guidelines. J Am Coll Cardiol. 2021;77(4):450–500.
6. Armstrong EJ, Rogers JH, Swan CH, Upadhyaya D, Viloria E, McCulloch C, Slater J, Qureshi M, Williams J, Whisenant B, Feldman T. Echocardiographic predictors of single versus dual MitraClip device implantation and long-term reduction of mitral regurgitation after percutaneous repair. Catheter Cardiovasc Interv. 2013;82(4):673–9.
7. Maisano F, Franzen O, Baldus S, Schäfer U, Hausleiter J, Butter C, Ussia GP, Sievert H, Richardt G, Widder JD, Moccetti T. Percutaneous mitral valve interventions in the real world: early and 1-year results from the ACCESS-EU, a prospective, multicenter, nonrandomized post-approval study of the MitraClip therapy in Europe. J Am Coll Cardiol. 2013;62(12):1052–61.
8. Gooden SC, Hatoum H, Zhang W, Boudoulas KD, Dasi LP. Multiple MitraClips: the balancing act between pressure gradient and regurgitation. J Thorac Cardiovasc Surg. 2022;163:P1319–27.
9. Paranskaya L, D'Ancona G, Bozdag-Turan I, Akin I, Kische S, Turan GR, Divchev D, Rehders T, Westphal B, Schubert J, Nienaber CA. Percutaneous mitral valve repair with the mitraclip® system. Catheter Cardiovasc Interv. 2013;81(7):1224–31.
10. Alegria-Barrero E, Chan PH, Foin N, Syrseloudis D, Tavazzi G, Price S, Lindsay AC, Duncan A, Moat N, Di Mario C, Franzen OW. Concept of the central clip: when to use one or two MitraClips®. EuroIntervention. 2014;9(10):1217–24.
11. Tam DY, Tran A, Mazine A, Tang GH, Gaudino MF, Calafiore AM, Friedrich JO, Fremes SE. Tricuspid valve intervention at the time of mitral valve surgery: a meta-analysis. Interact Cardiovasc Thorac Surg. 2019;29(2):193–200.
12. Cetinkaya A, Ganchewa N, Hein S, Bramlage K, Bramlage P, Schönburg M, Richter M. Long-term outcomes of concomitant tricuspid valve repair in patients undergoing mitral valve surgery. J Cardiothorac Surg. 2020;15(1):210.

Transcatheter Tricuspid and Mitral Valve Replacement in a Patient with Cardiogenic Shock

Ofir Koren, Danon Kaewkes, Bar Naiberg, and Siddharth Singh

1 Clinical Presentation

A 55-year-old female patient with a history of moderate mitral stenosis, severe mitral regurgitation status post mitral valve replacement with 29 mm Magna valve, and severe tricuspid regurgitation status post tricuspid valve replacement with 25 mm Magna valve presented with NYHA class IV symptoms. The patient was in cardiogenic shock requiring vasopressor support, had bilateral large pleural effusions, and had acute kidney injury. She was evaluated by the cardiac surgeon and deemed to be a high-risk candidate for redo open-heart surgery.

2 Images and Supported Data

Transesophageal echocardiography (TEE) at admission showed normal left ventricular (LV) function and mildly calcific stenotic native trileaflet aortic valve with

Supplementary Information The online version contains supplementary material available at [https://doi.org/10.1007/978-3-031-05965-0_32].

O. Koren (✉)
Smidt Heart Institute, Cedars-Sinai Medical Center, Los Angeles, CA, USA

Faculty of Medicine, Technion, Israel Institute of Technology, Haifa, Israel
e-mail: Ofir.Koren@cshs.org

D. Kaewkes
Department of Medicine, Faculty of Medicine, Khon Kaen University, Khon Kaen, Thailand

B. Naiberg
Santa Monica High School, CA, USA

S. Singh
Cedars Sinai Medical Center, Los Angeles, CA, USA

O. Koren et al. (eds.), *Complex Cases in Structural Heart Intervention*,
https://doi.org/10.1007/978-3-031-05965-0_32

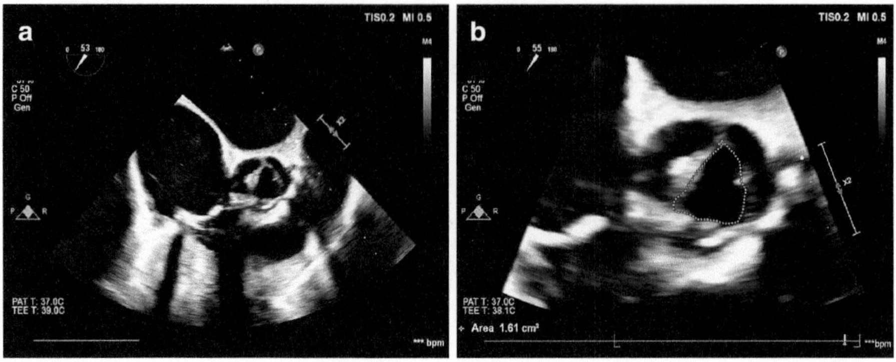

Fig. 1 Peri-procedural TEE. (**a**) Mildly calcified and stenotic tricuspid aortic valve. (**b**) Tricuspid valve area of 1.61 cm^2 measured by planimetry in short-axis view

an aortic valve area (by planimetry) of 1.61 cm^2 (Fig. 1). The tricuspid and the mitral bioprosthesis valves were severely stenotic with severe leaflet restriction. The peak and mean transmitral gradient were 12 and 8 mmHg, respectively. Mitral pressure half-time was 244 ms, and the mitral valve area was 0.9 cm^2 (Videos 1, 2 and 3). There was severe bioprosthetic tricuspid stenosis with mild tricuspid regurgitation. The mean pressure gradient across the tricuspid valve was 10 mmHg with a peak velocity of 2.2 m/s (Fig. 2, Videos 4, 5, 6 and 7). The patient did not undergo cardiac CT due to her clinical state and the urgency of the procedure.

3 Pre-Procedural Consideration: Pitfalls, Dilemmas, and Challenges

The patient presented with an acute decompensated cardiogenic shock, along with multiple and severe valvular diseases. Due to her condition, the heart team denied an open-heart surgical treatment, and concluded that transcatheter is the only treatment option due to the urgent nature of the procedure and the high surgical risk of the patient. We treated the tricuspid valve from a procedural concern and urgency before doing an atrial septal puncture and approaching the mitral valve. We couldn't accurately assess the mitral annular dimensions or the neo-LVOT as CT was not performed. Therefore, the annular size and the neo-LVOT area were estimated using a TEE and relied on the size of the surgical valve.

4 Procedure and Outcome

A 16F Edwards sheath was placed over an extra-stiff wire in the right femoral vein. An 8.5 Fr Agilis catheter was advanced into the right atrium and directed to the tricuspid valve. A 6 Fr pigtail catheter was used to cross the tricuspid valve and

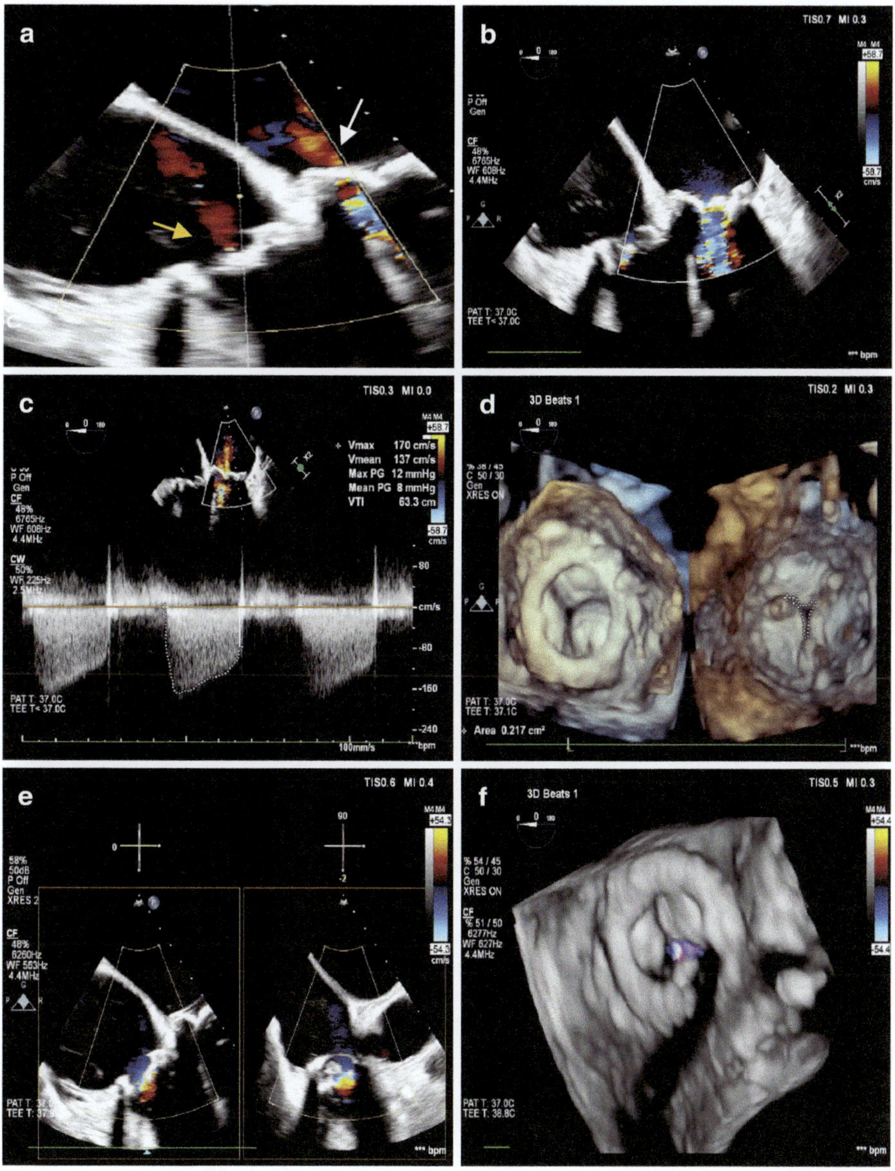

Fig. 2 Transesophageal echocardiography at admission in a state of cardiogenic shock. (**a**) Bioprosthetic valves at the mitral (white arrow) and the tricuspid (yellow arrow) valve positions. (**b**) Color Doppler over the mitral valve indicates significant mitral bioprosthetic dysfunction. The mitral valve prosthetics appear well seated with a very severe leaflets restriction. (**c**) Flow velocity and pressure gradient over the mitral valve shows a peak transmitral gradient of 12 mmHg, and a mean of 8 mmHg. (**d**) 3D En face view of the tricuspid valve shows a severe bioprosthetic tricuspid with an area of 0.217 cm^2 by planimetry. (**e**) Color Doppler over the tricuspid valve shows significant stenosis with mild regurgitation. (**f**) 3D En face view of the mitral valve shows severe bioprosthetic stenosis

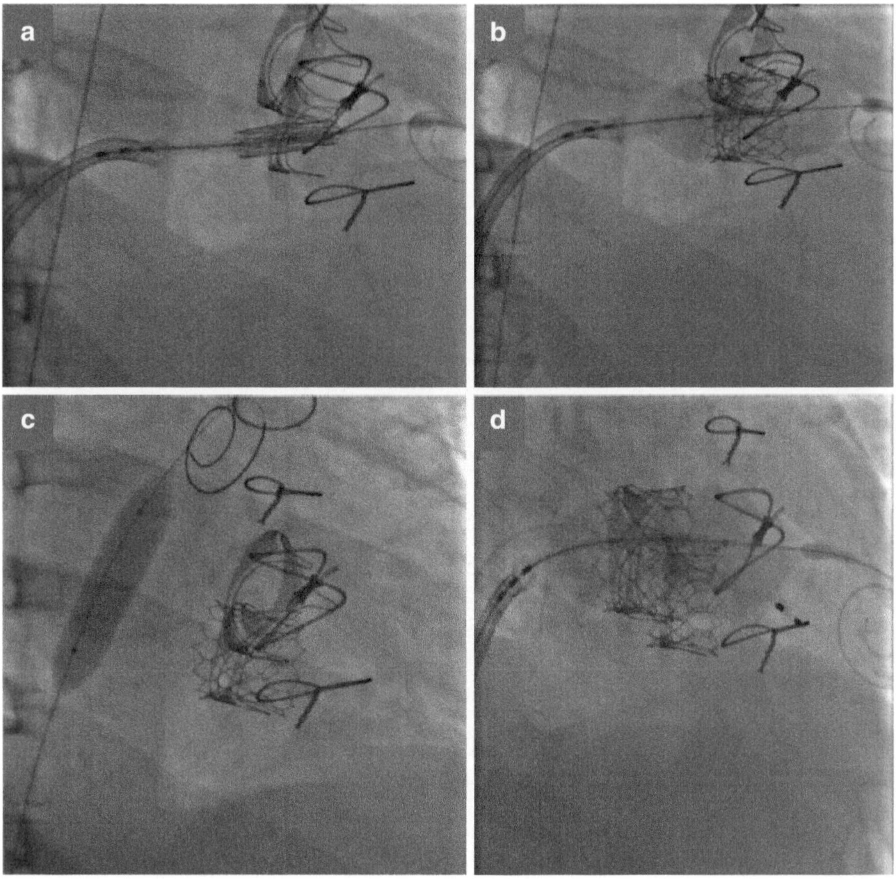

Fig. 3 Transcatheter mitral and tricuspid valves were deployed in prior bioprosthetic valves during cardiogenic shock. (**a**) Crossing the tricuspid valve with a 26 mm Sapien-3 delivery system. (**b**) Position the THV on the stenotic bioprosthetic tricuspid valve. (**c**) Following the successful deployment of the tricuspid THV an atrial balloon septoplasty was then performed using a 14 mm × 4 cm balloon. (**d**) Deployment of a 26 mm Sapien-3 THV over a stenotic bioprosthetic mitral valve

exchanged for a Safari wire positioned in the right ventricular (RV) apex. The Edwards 26 mm S3 Ultra valve was then positioned across the tricuspid valve and deployed during rapid pacing over the Safari wire (Fig. 3a, b, Video 8).

Next, the atrial septal puncture was performed with fluoroscopy and TEE guidance using a 0.035-in. VersaCross RF wire through the Baylis sheath (Fig. 3c, Video 9). Balloon atrial septoplasty was performed using a 14 mm × 4 cm balloon. Then, an 8.5 Fr Agilis catheter was introduced into the left atrium over the wire, and the catheter was directed down to the mitral valve. A long 6 Fr pigtail catheter crossed the mitral valve and was exchanged for a Safari wire positioned in the LV apex. The Edwards 29 mm S3 Ultra valve was then positioned across the mitral valve and

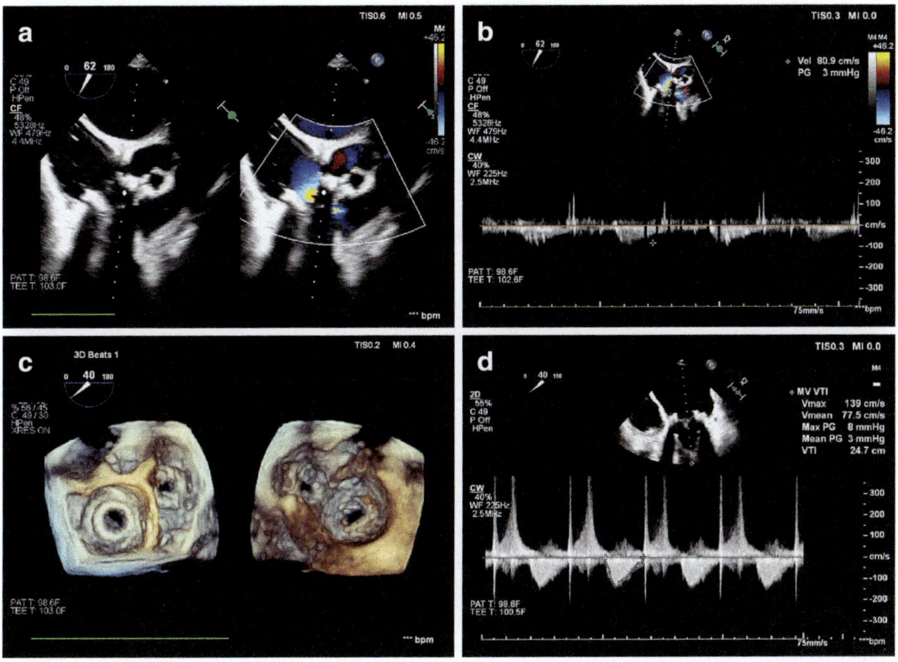

Fig. 4 TEE following double THVs deployment. (**a**) Color Doppler over the tricuspid valve indicates a well-seated bioprosthetic valve with normal leaflets motion. (**b**) Flow velocity over the tricuspid valve shows normal pressure gradient and only trivial regurgitation. (**c**) 3D en face view of the tricuspid and the mitral valves shows wide opening leaflets. (**d**) The mitral valve's flow velocity and pressure gradient indicate a peak gradient of 8 mmHg and mean of 3 mmHg (**d**)

deployed during rapid pacing, performed through a transvenous pacemaker placed in RV (Fig. 3c, d, Video 10).

Postprocedural TEE revealed no leak and good valve function (Fig. 4, Videos 11, 12 and 13).

Central venous pressure decreased from 22 to 11 mmHg. The patient was able to be weaned off vasopressors. Access sites healed well, and the patient could ambulate the next day. No significant bleeding occurred.

5 Discussion

Transcatheter treatment of valvular disease has emerged as the preferred treatment option for symptomatic severe aortic stenosis patients for a high- and intermediate-risk profile. The initial results from the TAVR studies led to the expansion of this technology for other valves and for various patients, such as those with degenerative MV disease and MAC and for those following surgical ring or valve implantation [1–3].

While most TMVRs performed are successful, all-cause mortality rates still tend to be quite high. In one systematic review, 308 patients were analyzed, and overall technical success was 91.7%, but all-cause and cardiovascular mortality at 10 months was 27.6% and 23.3%, respectively [4]. Other studies have shown worldwide experience with TMVR 30-day mortality rates of 25–40% [3]. These deaths were attributed primarily to sepsis, multiorgan failure, device thrombosis, and access site complications [5]. However, in older patients in a higher risk category for surgical interventions, TMVR showed significantly lower in-patient mortality of 0.7% to SMVR's 3.1% [6].

LVOT obstruction is the most catastrophic complication after TMVR, mainly due to the small ventricular cavity, the size and depth of transcatheter valve implantation, aortomitral angle, and the preservation of the anterior mitral leaflet. The neo-LVOT area is an estimated area, using a virtual transcatheter valve in preprocedural CT analysis that can assist in identifying patients at high risk for LVOT obstruction. Other methods, such as TEE, are considered unreliable and not accurate [7–9].

All-cause mortality of TMVR was highest in patients who underwent valve-in-MAC, followed by valve-in-ring and, lowest for valve-in-valve (native valve) [10].

The role of TMVR in cardiogenic shock is still unclear. The vast majority of studies conducted in a remote and single-center support the feasibility and safety use of TMVR. A recent review from a multicenter experience showed short and intermediate mortality benefits from TMVR in severe cardiogenic patients [11–13].

Transcatheter tricuspid valve replacement (TTVR) is a new therapeutic option conducted mostly in ongoing studies for patients with severe tricuspid regurgitations [14]. Data on TTVR in cardiogenic shock or simultaneous TMVR and TTVR have not been reported.

Key Points

- The transcatheter replacement of a failed surgical bioprosthetic mitral and tricuspid valves using a balloon-expandable THV is feasible.
- In suitable anatomy, less invasive mitral and tricuspid valve replacements may be appropriate in patients with high surgical risk.
- Long-term outcome studies are needed for transcatheter mitral and tricuspid valve replacement.

References

1. Leon MB, Smith CR, Mack M, Miller DC, Moses JW, Svensson LG, et al. Transcatheter aortic-valve implantation for aortic stenosis in patients who cannot undergo surgery. N Engl J Med. 2010;363(17):1597–607.
2. Smith CR, Leon MB, Mack MJ, Miller DC, Moses JW, Svensson LG, et al. Transcatheter versus surgical aortic-valve replacement in high-risk patients. N Engl J Med. 2011;364(23):2187–98. Epub 2011 Jun 5. PMID: 21639811. https://doi.org/10.1056/NEJMoa1103510.
3. Testa L, Popolo Rubbio A, Casenghi M, Pero G, Latib A, Bedogni F. Transcatheter mitral valve replacement in the transcatheter aortic valve replacement era. J Am Heart Assoc. 2019;8(22):e013352.

4. von Ballmoos MC, Kalra A, Reardon MJ. Complexities of transcatheter mitral valve replacement (TMVR) and why it is not transcatheter aortic valve replacement (TAVR). Ann Cardiothorac Surg. 2018;7(6):724.
5. Sarkar K, Reardon MJ, Little SH, Barker CM, Kleiman NS. Transcatheter mitral valve replacement for native and failed bioprosthetic mitral valves. Methodist Debakey Cardiovasc J. 2017;13(3):142.
6. Del Val D, Ferreira-Neto AN, Wintzer-Wehekind J, Dagenais F, Paradis JM, Bernier M, O'Connor K, Beaudoin J, Freitas-Ferraz AB, Rodés-Cabau J. Early experience with transcatheter mitral valve replacement: a systematic review. J Am Heart Assoc. 2019;8(17):e013332.
7. Bapat V, Buellesfeld L, Peterson MD, Hancock J, Reineke D, Buller C, Carrel T, Praz F, Rajani R, Fam N, Kim H. Transcatheter mitral valve implantation (TMVI) using the Edwards FORTIS device. EuroIntervention. 2014;10(Suppl U):U120–8.
8. Malik AH, Zaid S, Yandrapalli S, Shetty S, Aronow WS, Ahmad H, Tang GH. Trends and outcomes with transcatheter versus surgical mitral valve repair in patients ≥80 years of age. Am J Cardiol. 2020;125(7):1083–7.
9. Niikura H, Gössl M, Kshettry V, Olson S, Sun B, Askew J, Stanberry L, Garberich R, Tang L, Lesser J, Bae R. Causes and clinical outcomes of patients who are ineligible for transcatheter mitral valve replacement. J Am Coll Cardiol Interv. 2019;12(2):196–204.
10. Yoon SH, Makkar R. Transcatheter mitral valve replacement in patients with severe mitral annular calcification. Interv Cardiol Clin. 2019;8(3):301–12. https://doi.org/10.1016/j.iccl.2019.02.008.
11. Sun F, Liu H, Zhang Q, Lu F, Zhan H, Zhou J. Impact of atrial fibrillation on outcomes of patients treated by transcatheter mitral valve repair: a systematic review and meta-analysis. Medicine (Baltimore). 2020;99(40):e22195. https://doi.org/10.1097/MD.0000000000022195.
12. Flint K, Brieke A, Wiktor D, Carroll J. Percutaneous edge-to-edge mitral valve repair may rescue select patients in cardiogenic shock: findings from a single center case series. Catheter Cardiovasc Interv. 2019;94(2):E82–7. https://doi.org/10.1002/ccd.28089.
13. Pleger ST, Chorianopoulos E, Krumsdorf U, Katus HA, Bekeredjian R. Percutaneous edge-to-edge repair of mitral regurgitation as a bail-out strategy in critically ill patients. J Invasive Cardiol. 2013;25(2):69–72.
14. Goldberg YH, Ho E, Chau M, Latib A. Update on transcatheter tricuspid valve replacement therapies. Front Cardiovasc Med. 2021;8:619558. Published 2021 Feb 15. https://doi.org/10.3389/fcvm.2021.619558.

Part III
Miscellaneous

Apical Aneurysm Closure

Ofir Koren, Edmund Naami, and Wen Cheng

1 Clinical Presentation

The patient is a 65-year-old African American male with an extensive cardiovascular medical history of hypertension, hyperlipidemia, rheumatoid arthritis, paroxysmal atrial fibrillation (on Xarelto), Marfan syndrome, obstructive sleep apnea, sickle cell trait, recurrent gastrointestinal bleeds, deep vein thrombosis, descending aortic aneurysm complicated by type A aortic dissection requiring Bentall procedure using #27 pericardial Magna valve and a #32 Hemashield graft. The patient had incidentally postoperative lower extremity paraplegia and a left ventricular apical pseudoaneurysm. He presents to our center to discuss percutaneous options to treat his expanding left ventricular aneurysm. The patient feels well, denying chest pain, palpitations, dyspnea on exertion, paroxysmal nocturnal dyspnea, lightheadedness, and syncope; he endorses bilateral extremity edema. His primary complaint is fatigue.

Supplementary Information The online version contains supplementary material available at [https://doi.org/10.1007/978-3-031-05965-0_33].

O. Koren (✉)
Smidt Heart Institute, Cedars-Sinai Medical Center, Los Angeles, CA, USA

Faculty of Medicine, Technion, Israel Institute of Technology, Haifa, Israel
e-mail: Ofir.Koren@cshs.org

E. Naami
University of Illinois College of Medicine, Chicago, IL, USA

W. Cheng
Cedars Sinai Medical Center, Los Angeles, CA, USA

O. Koren et al. (eds.), *Complex Cases in Structural Heart Intervention*,
https://doi.org/10.1007/978-3-031-05965-0_33

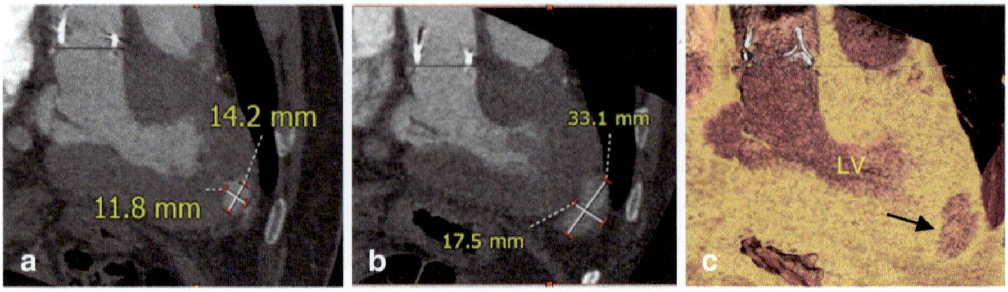

Fig. 1 Progression of the left ventricular pseudoaneurysm using reconstructed CT images. (**a**) Initial dimensions of the pseudoaneurysm. (**b**) Dimension of the pseudoaneurysm during 18 months of follow-up. (**c**) 3D volume-rendered view of an apical pseudoaneurysm (black arrow) along the lateral/posterior aspect of the left ventricle

2 Images and Supported Data

Preoperative TTE demonstrated preserved systolic function (ejection fraction 63%), akinesis of the basal inferior wall, and hypokinesis of the mid inferior wall. Additionally, contrast was detected lateral to the inferolateral, apical segment suggesting an aneurysm or pseudoaneurysm. Cardiac tomography and 3D reconstruction demonstrated a pseudoaneurysm of the left ventricular apical lateral wall at the left ventricular outflow tract (Fig. 1, Video 1). Additionally, a minimal luminal diameter of the right and left iliofemoral arteries was measured to be 11.4 × 12.1 and 6.4 × 16.8 mm, respectively. Dissections were present in the abdominal aorta, continuing to the left iliofemoral artery, as well as the ascending, continuing into the left subclavian and carotid arteries.

3 Pre-Procedural Consideration: Pitfalls, Dilemmas, and Challenges

A review of previous imaging demonstrated progression in the size of the aneurysm. The cardiovascular heart team repaired the pseudoaneurysm via a percutaneous closure with increasing concern for rupture. A transfemoral arterial access strategy was devised to access the LV via retrograde crossing of the surgical aortic valve. However, passage through the aortic root repeatedly proved unviable due to aortic tortuosity and the presence of a false lumen. We then converted to a transseptal approach. After gaining access to the left ventricle via transseptal puncture, a long balance 0.014″ wire was passed through the neck into the pseudoaneurysm. A JR4 could not be advanced due to the defect. We used telescoped 0.018″ and 0.035″ microcatheters to pass into the defect. We then withdrew the 0.018″ and balance wire. We attempted to wire the defect with an Amplatzer extra-stiff wire with a pigtail curve, but this withdrew the microcatheter into the LV. Our next attempt was to exchange the balance wire for an 0.018″ platinum plus wire. This time, we attempted to close the defect with an AVP4 8 mm device through the 0.035″ microcatheter. Although this was pulled flush with the exterior neck of the defect, it proceeded to collapse and slip into the ventricle, resulting in a loss of access again to the pseudoaneurysm.

Multiple microcatheter and wire combinations were next used, but we could not secure access with this approach. The limiting factors were the stability of the catheter and wire combinations, and limited reach due to the long length of the Agilis sheath. We had to terminate this closure attempt due to contrast dye usage.

One month later, the procedure was repeated using newer, longer transeptally and transapically fashioned catheters.

First, a transseptal puncture was successfully performed at the midportion and slightly posterior aspect of the right atrium into the left atrium. The 8.5 French sheaths were advanced into the left atrium (Fig. 2a). We then advanced a pigtail catheter into the LV and exchanged this for an 8F JR4. With the JR4 guide, we used contrast injection to identify the defect (Fig. 2b).

Through the chest wall, We then used a micropuncture needle to access the pseudoaneurysm through the chest wall and then wired a long balance 0.014″ wire through the defect into the LV. An En-Snare catheter was then passed through the JR4 guide into the LV and captured the balance wire (Fig. 2c, d, Video 2). The wire was then retrieved and externalized through the JR4 catheter—exiting the right femoral vein.

With a rail wire externalized, we passed a long 6F MP guide catheter through the 8F JR4 catheter, over this rail wire, and into the pseudoaneurysm. The rail wire was then removed. The position of the MP was confirmed angiographically. We passed a 12-mm AVP2 plug through the MP guide (Fig. 2e). The distal disc was deployed into the pseudoaneurysm. The plug was then withdrawn, and the proximal disc was deployed in the LV. The plug was released (Video 3). The MP catheter was exchanged for a pigtail catheter. Left ventriculography was then done, which verified plug placement and sealing of the defect (Video 4). The patient tolerated the procedure well without immediate complications and left the cardiac catheterization laboratory to the telemetry floor in stable condition. CT 6 months following the second procedure demonstrated resolution of the left ventricular pseudoaneurysm (Fig. 3a, b).

4 Discussion

Left ventricular pseudoaneurysm (LVPSA) is a rupture of the left ventricular wall contained by the pericardium. The true incidence of LVPSA is unknown; however, it most commonly occurs after myocardial infarction or cardiac surgery. Mitral valve replacements, in particular, have been associated with LVPSAs [1–6]. While untreated aneurysms have a high incidence of rupture, approximately 40%, surgical

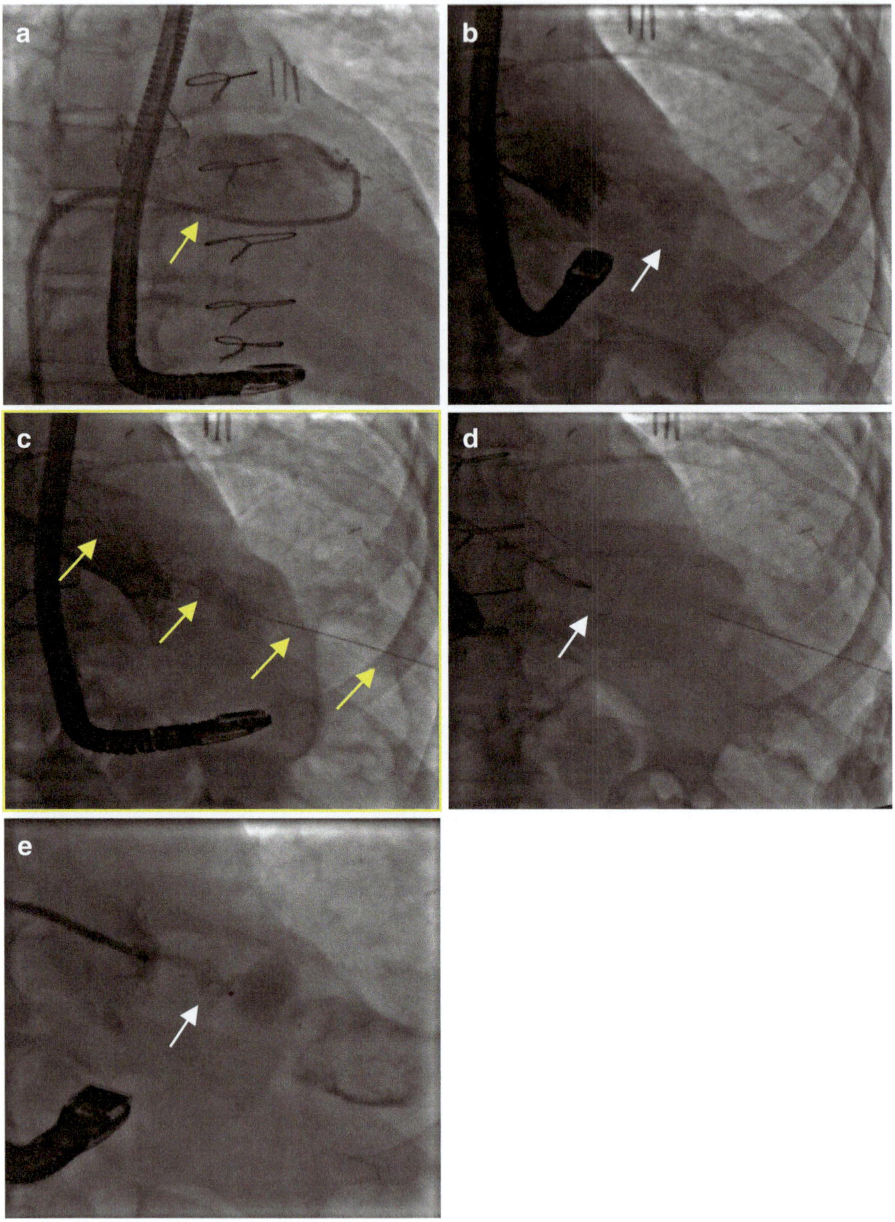

Fig. 2 Transcatheter closure of an apical pseudoaneurysm, step-by-step using fluoroscopic images. (**a**) Transseptal puncture was performed at the midportion and posterior aspect of the atrial septum with an 8.5 French sheath passing through the right atrium toward the left atrium. (**b**) Contrast from a pigtailed catheter marked the location and dimension of the pseudoaneurysm (white arrow). (**c**) Long balance wire was advanced through the chest wall via the pseudoaneurysm into the left ventricle (yellow arrows). (**d**) An en snare was used to capture the balance wire (white arrow). (**e**) 12 mm AVP2 was used to close the neck of the pseudoaneurysm (white arrow)

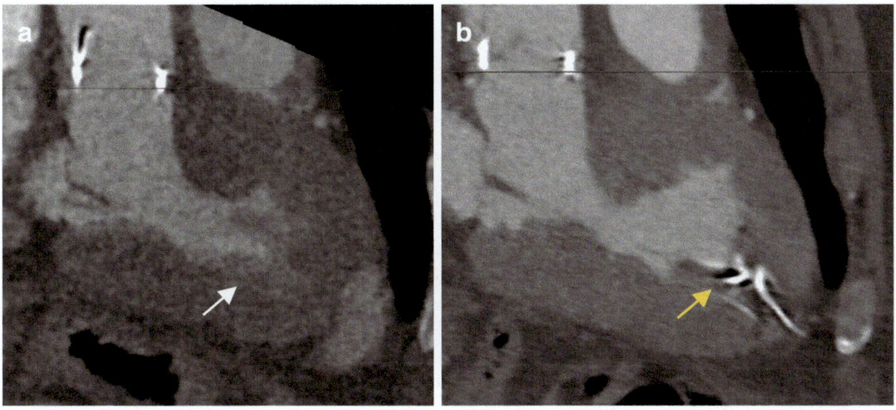

Fig. 3 Reconstructed CT images of the apical pseudoaneurysm before and after the procedure. (**a**) The pseudoaneurysm before the transcatheter closure (white arrow). (**b**) The pseudoaneurysm 6 months following the procedure with a resolution of the LV pseudoaneurysm (yellow arrow)

and medical treatments remain largely imperfect. Both therapy options carry a substantially high mortality risk. Surgical repair is associated with a 20–40% mortality rate, while medical treatment is higher at 50%. Recent studies and advancements in percutaneous technology allow transcatheter repair for high-risk surgical candidates [7]. In this procedure, a closure device is implanted at the orifice of the pseudoaneurysm, therefore, separating ventricular and aneurysmal cavities. As to methodology and device selection, no standardized guidelines have been published. In part, this stems from the variability of LVSPAs; cavity shape, overall size, neck length, and location that can differ between each patient [8]. Therefore, a large part of the workup involves 2D and 3D imaging characterization. Specifically, 3D echocardiography and volume-rendered computed-tomographic angiography can help navigate 2D imaging. Together with intraoperative TEE, these imaging modalities guide intraoperative fluoroscopy, select the appropriate closure device, and assess procedural success. Commonly used devices include occluder or vascular plugs. One significant factor in device selection is the type of access used to complete the procedure [9, 10]. A transfemoral arterial approach is more commonly used than a transseptal or transapical approach. However, multiple access sites or a hybrid approach may be required in rare circumstances [11].

Key Points

- Pseudoaneurysm is a rare cardiac complication that most commonly occurs after myocardial infarction or cardiac surgery.
- Surgical correction is currently the standard of care.
- Recently, a percutaneous approach has been proven safe and feasible for selected high surgical risk patients.
- Operators should be aware of all therapeutic techniques for pseudoaneurysm.

References

1. Van Tassel RA, Edwards JE. Rupture of heart complicating myocardial infarction: analysis of 40 cases including nine examples of left ventricular false aneurysm. Chest. 1972;61:104–16.
2. Vlodaver Z, Coe JI, Edwards JE. True and false left ventricular aneurysms: propensity for the alter to rupture. Circulation. 1975;51:567–72.
3. Yeo TC, Malouf JF, Oh JK, Seward JB. Clinical profile and outcome in 52 patients with cardiac pseudoaneurysm. Ann Intern Med. 1998;128:299–305.
4. Pretre R, Linka A, Jenni R, Turina MI. Surgical treatment of acquired left ventricular pseudoaneurysms. Ann Thorac Surg. 2000;70:553–7.
5. Figueras J, Alcalde O, Barrabes JA, Serra V, Alguersuari J, Cortadellas J, Lidon RM. Changes in hospital mortality rates in 425 patients with acute ST-elevation myocardial infarction and cardiac rupture over a 30-year period. Circulation. 2008;118:2783–9.
6. Frances C, Romero A, Grady D. Left ventricular pseudoaneurysm. J Am Coll Cardiol. 1998;32:557–61.
7. Clift P, Thorne S, de Giovanni J. Percutaneous device closure of a pseudoaneurysm of the left ventricular wall. Heart. 2004;90:e62.
8. Sakai K, Nakamura K, Ishizuka N, Nakagawa M, Hosoda S. Echocardiographic findings and clinical features of left ventricular pseudoaneurysm after mitral valve replacement. Am Heart J. 1992;124:975–82.
9. Dudiy Y, Kliger C, Jelnin V, Elisabeth A, Kronzon I, Ruiz CE. Percutaneous transapical access: current status. EuroIntervention. 2014;10 Suppl U:U84–U89. https://doi.org/10.4244/EIJV10SUA12.
10. Dudiy Y, Jelnin V, Einhorn BN, Kronzon I, Cohen HA, Ruiz CE. Percutaneous closure of left ventricular pseudoaneurysm. Circ Cardiovasc Interv. 2011;4:322–6.
11. Martinez CA, Rosen R, Cohen H, Ruiz CE. A novel method for closing the percutaneous transapical access tract using coils and gelatin matrix. J Invasive Cardiol. 2010;22:E107–9.

Closure of Subvalvular Fistula and Occlusion of Right Coronary Artery During TAVR

Ofir Koren, Mattan Arazi, and Yigal Abramowitz

1 Clinical Background

The patient is an 86-year-old female with a past medical history of aortic stenosis complicated with aortic valve endocarditis six months prior and was treated with an antibiotics regimens. She also has atrial fibrillation on warfarin and congestive heart failure with preserved ejection fraction. She underwent an evaluation of aortic stenosis to discuss treatment options.

The patient endorses dyspnea on exertion while performing activities of daily living (laundry, walking around the house). She is fragile, with at least five falls in the past 6 months. She has been admitted to the hospital for heart failure exacerbation on multiple occasions, most recently in the last month.

Supplementary Information The online version contains supplementary material available at [https://doi.org/10.1007/978-3-031-05965-0_34].

O. Koren (✉)
Smidt Heart Institute, Cedars-Sinai Medical Center, Los Angeles, CA, USA

Faculty of Medicine, Technion, Israel Institute of Technology, Haifa, Israel
e-mail: Ofir.Koren@cshs.org

M. Arazi
Goldschleger Eye Institute, Sheba Medical Center, Ramat Gan, Israel

Y. Abramowitz
Cardiology Department, Soroka University Medical Center, Beer Sheva, Israel

O. Koren et al. (eds.), *Complex Cases in Structural Heart Intervention*,
https://doi.org/10.1007/978-3-031-05965-0_34

2 Imaging

Pre-procedural TTE demonstrated severe aortic valve leaflet calcification with a mean transaortic gradient of 68 mmHg, peak transaortic gradient of 105 mmHg, and aortic valve area of 0.5 cm^2 via the continuity equation (Fig. 1a, b, Video 1). In addition, TTE demonstrated moderate aortic regurgitation, moderate-to-severe mitral regurgitation with a mean trans-mitral gradient of 5 mmHg, moderate tricuspid

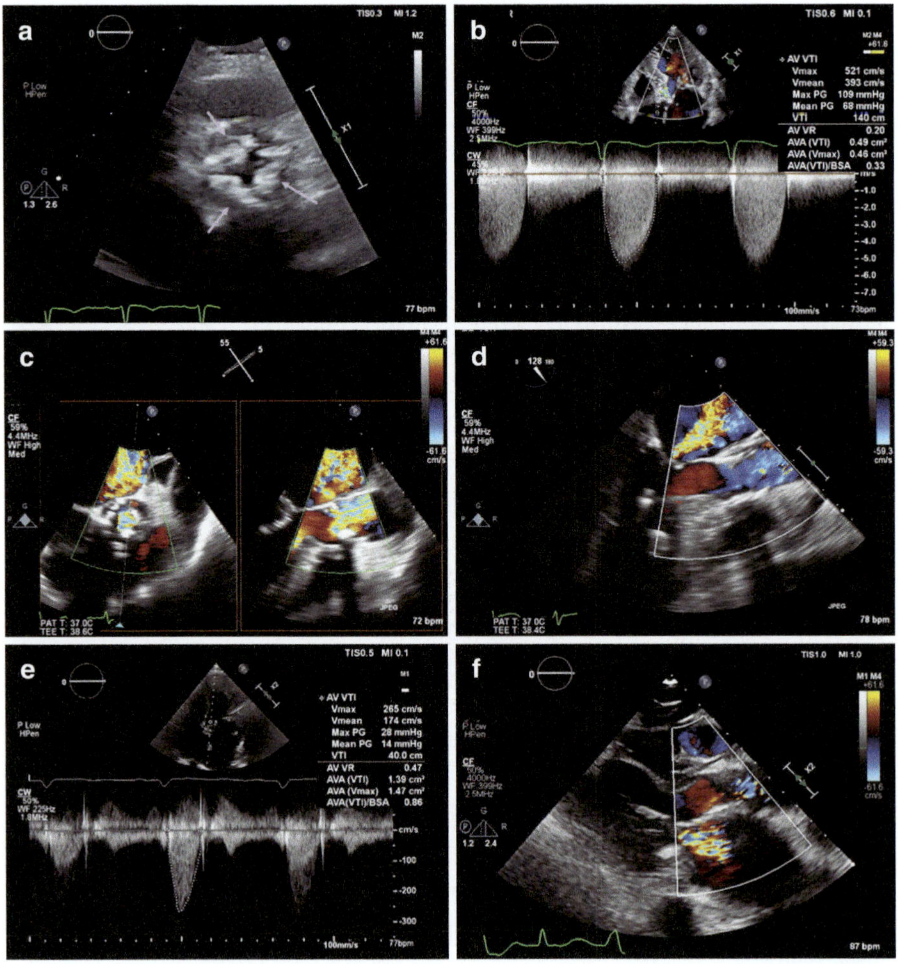

Fig. 1 Pre- and post-procedural echocardiography. (**a**) The short axis view indicates severe AV leaflet calcification. (**b**) Flow velocity and pressure gradient over the aortic valve indicated a mean gradient of 68 mmHg. (**c**) Color Doppler view shows mild to moderate mitral regurgitation. (**d**) Post-procedural TEE demonstrates a well-seated bioprosthetic valve and preserved flow across the AV. (**e**) Flow velocity and pressure gradient over the mitral valve show a flow reduction following the procedure. (**f**) Color Doppler at 30-day follow-up at the mitral and aortic valves were consistent with the postoperative findings

regurgitation, and estimated pulmonary artery pressure of 70 mmHg (Video 2). Cardiac reconstructed CT indicates an annular mean internal diameter of 22.3 mm, area of 384.8 mm^2, and perimeter of 71.0 mm. The right coronary artery was 11.9 mm above the annular plane, and the left coronary artery ostium was estimated 10.4 mm above the annular plane (Fig. 2a, d). CT also demonstrated a

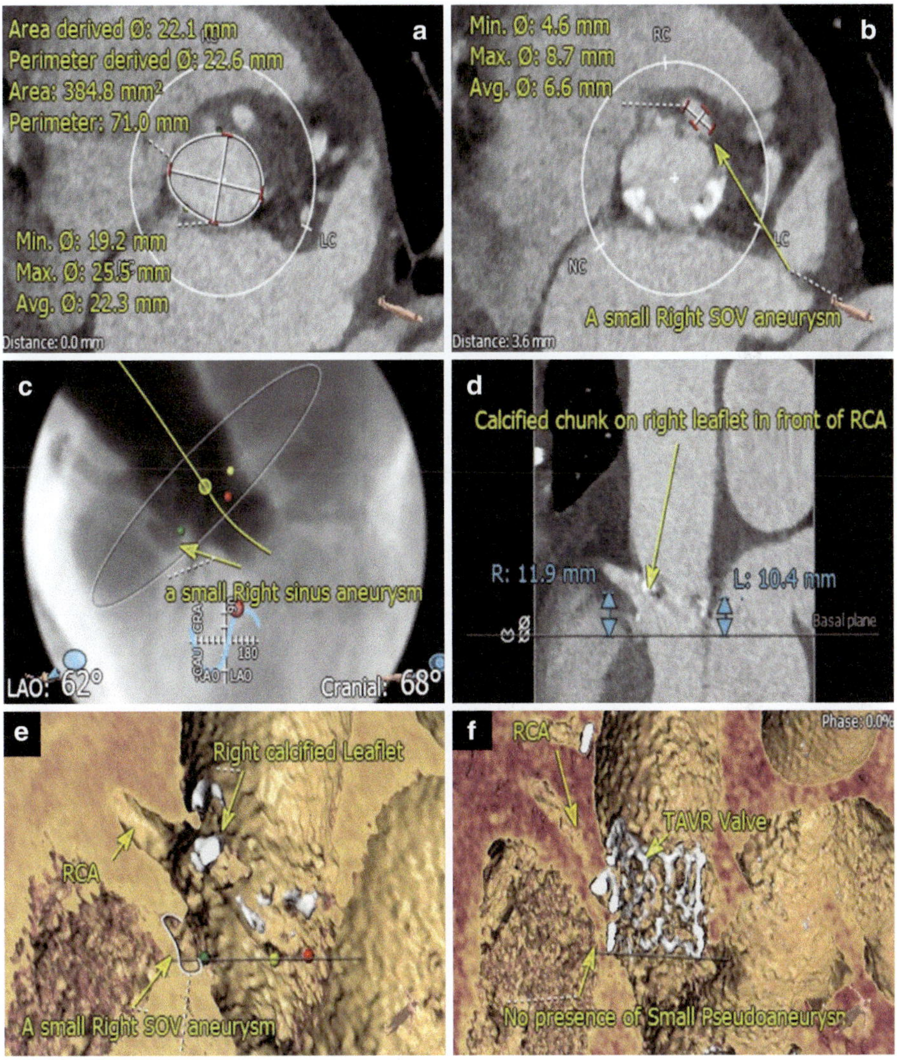

Fig. 2 Reconstructed cardiac CT imaging before the procedure. (**a**) Aortic valve annulus measurements. (**b**) Small pseudoaneurysm with a minimum diameter of 6.6 mm located on the right sinus of Valsalva (yellow arrow). (**c**) Angiographic view of the pseudoaneurysm (yellow arrow). (**d**) Calcified chunk on right coronary cusps (yellow arrow) is notable very close to right coronary ostia. (**e**) Volume rendering reconstruction image showing a small right sinus of Valsalva pseudoaneurysm. (**f**) The distance of the pseudoaneurysm to the transcatheter heart valve following the TAVR procedure

pseudoaneurysm on the right sinus of Valsalva, measuring a minimum diameter of 6.6 mm. The presence and location of the pseudoaneurysm were further supported on CT angiography, and the volume-rendered CT image before intervention (Fig. 2b, c, e). Pre-procedural coronary angiogram demonstrated non-obstructive coronary artery disease (Video 3).

3 Pre-Procedural Considerations, Dilemmas, and Challenges

The heart team evaluated the patient and found him an unsuitable candidate due to frailty and very high surgical risk with a Society of Thoracic Surgeons (STS) score of 7. The sub-valvular fistula connected the right sinus of Valsalva to the right atrium. This added increased risk to the percutaneous approach.

The patient was followed by an infectious disease (ID) specialist, given her diagnosis of endocarditis in the previous six months. She was cleared for a valvular intervention. She was deemed stable for a valvular intervention if she remained infection-free for three months.

4 Procedure, Outcome, and Follow-Up

Procedural TEE demonstrated severe aortic stenosis and mild-to-moderate mitral regurgitation consistent with previous imaging (Fig. 1c, Video 4). A 23-mm Edwards Sapien S3 valve delivery system was positioned across the stenotic aortic valve (Video 5) and deployed with rapid pacing at 180 beats per minute (−1 cc in the inflation device). A post-procedure TEE revealed no central aortic regurgitation, no perivalvular regurgitation, and reduced stenosis (Fig. 1d, Video 6).

The pigtail catheter was then advanced, and an aortic root angiography was performed, which showed high-grade occlusion of the right coronary ostium (Fig. 3a–c, Video 7). The patient was noted to have ECG changes with ST elevations in the inferior leads. A 6F JR guide catheter was placed through the RFA. We attempted to recross into the RCA multiple times with different coronary wires and catheters, including a Balance, Confianza Pro 12 Astato in different sizes and Fielder XT. Ultimately it was unsuccessful. We decided to place the patient on cardiopulmonary bypass using the 14F arterial Edwards sheath and the venous cannula in the right femoral artery. We placed a 6F AR1 in the LFA sheath and engaged the right cusp. A 6F XBLAD 3.5 guide catheter was placed in the right radial sheathe and engaged the left coronary artery. A selective left coronary angiogram was performed to visualize the RCA via retrograde flow.

Further attempts to cross the RCA with a Astato 20, Confianza Pro 12 were unsuccessful (Fig. 3d). A decision was made to convert to open surgery for SVG-RCA graft placement. The patient was stable and admitted to the cardiac surgical intensive care unit for continued management following the operation.

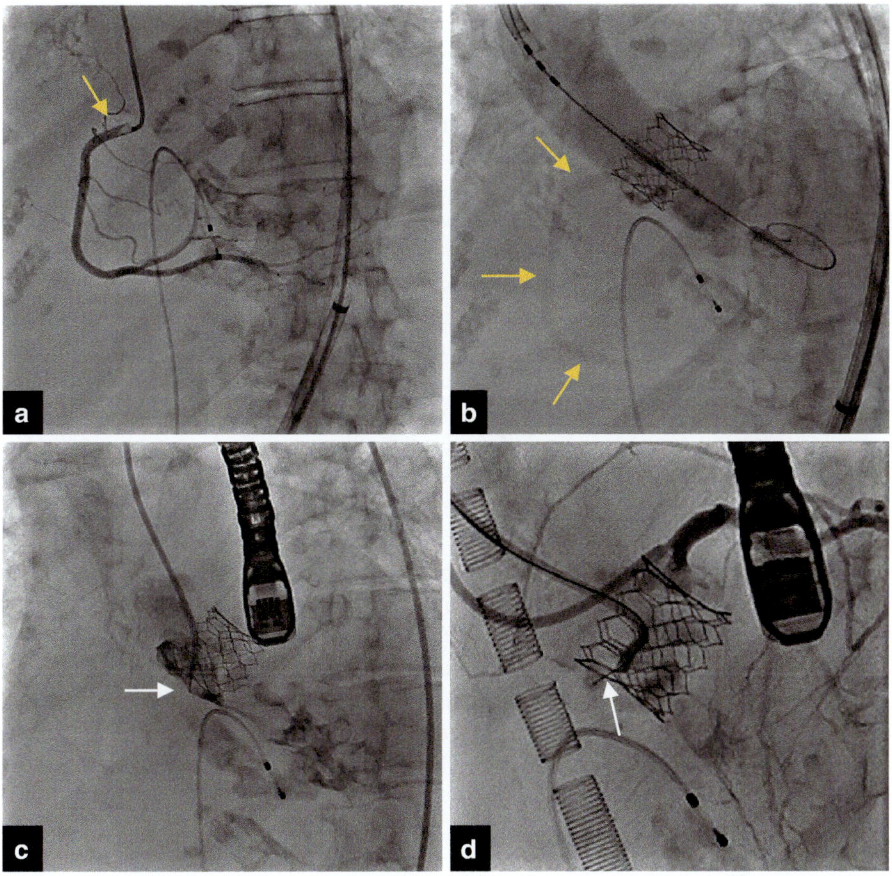

Fig. 3 Fluoroscopic images of the TAVR procedure. (**a**) Right coronary angiogram (yellow arrow) before the TAVR procedure. (**b**) Right coronary flow (yellow arrow) after deploying a balloon-expandable Sapien-3 valve. (**c**) Multiple attempts to engage guide wire (white arrow) to the right coronary artery. (**d**) Blocked right coronary artery ostium (white arrow)

On a 30-day follow-up, the patient remained fatigued with poor appetite since TAVR and CABG procedure. However, her breathing and dizziness have improved. She complains of drainage from her incision sites managed by home health. Since the procedure, she denies chest pain, shortness of breath, dizziness, syncope, pre-syncope, orthopnea, paroxysmal nocturnal dyspnea, fevers, chills, and gastrointestinal bleed. TTE 30 days following the operation demonstrated decreased aortic valve stenosis, with a mean gradient of 14 mmHg. It also demonstrated a decreased transvalvular velocity, as well as mild mitral valve regurgitation (Fig. 1e, f, Video 8). Cardiac CT post-TAVR with volume-rendered images also showed closure of the pseudoaneurysm (Fig. 2f).

5 Discussion

Acquired pseudoaneurysms of the Sinus of Valsalva (SOV) are infrequent cardiac anomalies that result from a tear within the intimal layer of the aorta, causing blood to collect within a false lumen. This is usually as a result of traumatic surgical or interventional procedures, as well as complications of infective endocarditis and paravalvular abscess [1–4]. These pseudoaneurysms can be diagnosed on computed tomography and affect the right coronary sinus in 80% of cases, noncoronary sinus in 16% of cases, and left coronary sinus in 4% of cases [3–5]. Complications of pseudoaneurysms include valvular compromise, dissection and rupture, aorto-cavitary fistula formation with an adjacent cardiac chamber resulting in shunting, and thrombus formation resulting in embolization or occlusion of the coronary artery [1, 3–5]. Surgical repair of aortic root may be performed; however, transcatheter closure using Amplatzer occluders has been reported [1, 6]. Successful TAVR implantation using a self-expandable Medtronic CoreValve under rapid pacing has been described in an aortic stenosis patient with an SOV aneurysm of the right coronary sinus [7].

Our patient developed an acute coronary artery occlusion (COA) following TAVR, a rare but serious complication with a 30-day mortality rate of 35–40% and peri-procedural mortality of 10.4% [8–10]. COA can occur immediately after valve deployment or in a delayed fashion duc to tissuc ingrowth and thrombosis [11, 12]. Risk factors include low coronary ostial height, shallow sinus of Valsalvas, balloon-expandable valves, previous surgical aortic prosthesis, female sex, and older age [8, 9, 11]. Coronary occlusion more commonly affects the left ostia due to closer proximity to the aortic valve. However, RCA ostia occlusion has been demonstrated in 17% of occlusion cases [8, 9]. COA may result in marked hypotension and hemodynamic instability, requiring immediate cannulation of the coronary ostium to restore blood flow [13]. However, the wire cage in TAVR can make coronary ostium access difficult. Therefore, mechanical support should be considered via extracorporeal membrane oxygenation (ECMO) or surgical revascularization by cardiopulmonary bypass grafting (CABG) if the coronary flow is not immediately reestablished [8, 13]. In a review paper describing 96 patients who developed coronary occlusion after TAVR, percutaneous coronary intervention (PCI) was attempted in 82 patients with a revascularization rate of 89% and mortality of 16.4% for successful PCI patients. Roughly 16% of patients required immediate cardiopulmonary bypass, while 40% of the ten patients that underwent CABG died [8]. Another case of RCA occlusion during TAVR demonstrates the unique creation of a stent tunnel under the native valve leaflets toward the left coronary sinus to maintain RCA blood flow [11].

Coronary prevention techniques are recommended in patients with a high risk of coronary occlusion [11, 14]. Pre-procedural computed tomography can help delineate the anatomical relationship of the coronary ostia to aortic root complex and native leaflets, and can help assess coronary perfusion techniques [8, 15, 16]. Additionally, others have advocated placing a guidewire with an undeployed stent within the coronary artery during deployment of the valve prosthesis to prevent difficult access, as well as treating significant coronary artery disease before valve placement [11, 13, 15, 16].

Key Points

- Acquired pseudoaneurysms of the SOV are infrequent cardiac anomalies but should be acknowledged in the pre-TAVR evaluation.
- Coronary artery occlusion following TAVR is a rare but serious complication with relatively high procedural mortality.
- The main risk factors for coronary occlusion during TAVR are low coronary ostial height, shallow SOV, and previous surgical aortic prosthesis.
- Coronary protection techniques may be used in cases with high risk for occlusion.

References

1. Li S, Sethi P, Kelly SC, Sheikh M, Stys M, Stys A. Recurrent ischemic stroke: a manifestation of a sinus of Valsalva pseudoaneurysm. S D Med. 2018;71(8):346–8.
2. Hilal T. Chronic rupture of the coronary sinus of Valsalva with pseudoaneurysm formation. Oxford Med Case Rep. 2014;2014(7):120–1. https://doi.org/10.1093/omcr/omu047.
3. Park HO, Byun JH, Moon SH, et al. A case report of pseudoaneurysm of left sinus of Valsalva invaded into the left ventricle with severe aortic regurgitation. J Cardiothorac Surg. 2018;13(1):1–4. https://doi.org/10.1186/s13019-018-0754-1.
4. Lee CC, Siegel RJ. Sinus of valsalva pseudoaneurysm as a sequela to infective endocarditis. Tex Heart Inst J. 2016;43(1):46–8. https://doi.org/10.14503/THIJ-14-4841.
5. Iida H, Sudo Y, Sunazawa T, Ukita H. Acquired pseudoaneurysm of the sinus of Valsalva. Tex Heart Inst J. 2008;35(2):186–9.
6. Szkutnik M, Kusa J, Glowacki J, Fiszer R, Bialkowski J. Transcatheter closure of ruptured sinus Valsalva aneurysms with Amplatzer occluder. Rev Esp Cardiol. 2009;62(11):1317–21. https://doi.org/10.1016/s1885-5857(09)73359-6.
7. Hendry C, Della Siega A, Nadra IJ, Robinson SD. Successful transcatheter aortic valve replacement in a patient with a sinus of Valsalva aneurysm. JACC Cardiovasc Interv. 2014;7(4):2013–4. https://doi.org/10.1016/j.jcin.2013.07.021.
8. Akinseye OA, Jha SK, Ibebuogu UN. Clinical outcomes of coronary occlusion following transcatheter aortic valve replacement: a systematic review. Cardiovasc Revasc Med. 2018;19(2):229–36. https://doi.org/10.1016/j.carrev.2017.09.006.
9. Joshi U, Duvvuri P, Barzallo M, Mungee S. Acute ostial right coronary artery occlusion during valve deployment of transcatheter aortic valve replacement leading to acute right ventricular failure: a perfect storm and successful navigation. Cureus. 2020;12(12):2–7. https://doi.org/10.7759/cureus.12373.
10. Ribeiro HB, Webb JG, Makkar RR, et al. Predictive factors, management, and clinical outcomes of coronary obstruction following transcatheter aortic valve implantation: insights from a large multicenter registry. J Am Coll Cardiol. 2013;62(17):1552–62. https://doi.org/10.1016/j.jacc.2013.07.040.
11. Abramowitz Y, Chakravarty T, Jilaihawi H, Kashif M, Kazuno Y, Takahashi N, Maeno Y, Nakamura M, Cheng W, Makkar RR. Clinical impact of coronary protection during transcatheter aortic valve implantation: first reported series of patients. EuroIntervention. 2015;11(5):572–81.

12. Kleiman NS. Delayed coronary obstruction after TAVR: a call for vigilance. J Am Coll Cardiol. 2018;71(14):1525–7. https://doi.org/10.1016/j.jacc.2018.01.067.
13. Manchester A. Managing the risk of coronary occlusion during TAVR. Nurs N Z. 2001;7(6):21.
14. Kanei Y, Qureshi W, Walker J, Kakouros N. Guide extension-assisted stent implantation at ostial right coronary artery creating stent tunnel during transcatheter aortic valve replacement. Cardiovasc Revasc Med. 2020;21(11):50–3. https://doi.org/10.1016/j.carrev.2020.04.022.
15. Perry TE, George SA, Lee B, Wahr J, Randle D, Sigurðsson G. A guide for pre-procedural imaging for transcatheter aortic valve replacement patients. Perioper Med (Lond). 2020;9(1):1–11. https://doi.org/10.1186/s13741-020-00165-1.
16. Zhang G, Luo J, Chen G. Right coronary occlusion following transcatheter aortic valve implantation: two case reports. Front Med. 2016;10(3):351–5. https://doi.org/10.1007/s11684-016-0465-8.

Index

O. Koren et al. (eds.), *Complex Cases in Structural Heart Intervention*,
https://doi.org/10.1007/978-3-031-05965-0

L

M

N

P

R

S

T